My Mother's Hip

Lessons from the World of Eldercare

My Mother's Hip

Lessons from the
World of Eldercare

LUISA MARGOLIES

Foreword *by* WALTER M. BORTZ II, M.D.

TEMPLE UNIVERSITY PRESS
Philadelphia

Temple University Press, Philadelphia 19122
Copyright © 2004 by Luisa Margolies
Published 2004
Printed in the United States of America

⊗ The paper used in this publication meets the requirements of the
American National Standard for Information Sciences—Permanence
of Paper for Printed Library Materials, ANSI Z39.48-1984

Library of Congress Cataloging-in-Publication Data

Margolies, Luise.
   My mother's hip : lessons from the world of eldercare / Luisa Margolies ;
foreword by Walter M. Bortz II.
      p.   cm.
   Includes bibliographical references.
   ISBN 1-59213-237-5 (cl. : alk. paper) — ISBN 1-59213-238-3 (pb. : alk. paper)
      1. Aged—Medical care—United States.   2. Hip joint—Fractures—Patients—
Biography.   3. Osteoporosis in women—Complications.   4. Aging parents—
Care—United States.   5. Caregivers—United States—Psychology.   6. Care-
givers—United States—Family relationships.   7. Parent and adult child—
United States.   I. Title.

RC954.4.M37 2004
362.1'9897'00973–dc21   2003055245

2   4   6   8   9   7   5   3   1

In memory of my mother, June

"Life brings such sweet sorrows,
But death brings no tomorrows."

—June A. Margolies

Contents

Foreword

PLATO OBSERVED, "The unexamined life is not worth living." Examination and self-reflection seem to be rare qualities. If this is true of life as whole, it is particularly true of the last of life. A logical excuse for such lack of insight into the deep nature of the far reaches of life would simply be its relative rarity, until now. When one observes that there are as many people alive in the world today older than sixty-five as in all prior world history put together, you can create at least a semblance of an explanation of why old age has lacked a conceptual framework. Conferences, journals, Nobel Prizes, study courses, and so on elaborately detailed the identifying parameter of what it means to be young, or middle aged. We all have some ideas about the job description of earlier life, but what of later life? What is it really? What can it be?

To these questions the answers are just now being revealed. *My Mother's Hip* is a beautifully conceived and executed true story. It is a vivid, highly personal narrative describing the impact of an accident not only on its victim, but on the family, the social convoy, of the victim. Revealed throughout the progressive narrative written by Dr. Luisa Margolies, loving daughter and deep observer of life, are the unexpected encounters and recognitions that are generated after a fractured hip. As epidemic as this unforeseen event is, it is entirely possible that the events disclosed here will become even more commonplace. In his charming book *The Medusa and the Snail*, Lewis Thomas mused on the future moment when all disease is eradicated. Thomas wrote, "Then what? What on earth will we die of? Are we to go on forever disease-free, with nothing to occupy our minds but the passage of time? What are the biologists doing to us? How can you finish honorably, and die honestly, without disease? Accidents."

Throughout our early history, it is interesting to observe, survival on the Serengeti for millions of threatened years, 200,000 generations of our ancestors, was specifically dependent on movement, and thereby on the structural integrity of our legs. As long as their legs were sound, our ancestors were able to move with their families to follow the game that followed the rain. The energetic equations balanced. But as soon as the legs gave out, movement, and thereby survival, was at risk. Such linkage is apparent throughout nature.

It is perhaps a collective vanity to think that modern man and woman can flout this tight historic relationship between movement and survival. Maybe we can; but maybe we cannot, as this fine history illustrates. Maybe the fractured hip is the talisman that predicts death. But what if it is not? Medical science has elaborately detailed the body's magnificent capacity to heal, even until the moment preceding death. But the body needs help in its curing efforts. Ignorance and neglect of these supportive strategies echo throughout the book.

This book, although highly specific in its clinical detail, is really an allegory for basic life processes that affect us all. The value of the book lies in its unblinking assessment of the general themes struck at life's furthest reach. Aging is clearly one of life's most poignant passages. May Sarton observed that it is that part of life when we have the chance to be more who we really are than at any earlier time. Such precious self-actualization should provide not only rich intellectual and emotional satisfaction; it should also permit life to proceed to its rightful spiritual climax in which reunion with the infinite may truly be achieved with grace. Approach to grace is an option, but one that will be more possible as our species progressively matures.

Old age has been termed "a surprise." If it is, it is only because we have failed the oracle at Delphi's exhortation to "know thyself." Old age is new, but it is gradually becoming familiar. As mythology and ignorance fade before new science, much fear of aging will be erased. Widely proclaimed these days is the "right to die." Inherent in this is the insistence on the inclusion of dignity in the act of dying. There can be no reasonable challenge to these presumptions. Less widely identified, however, is the responsibility to live, which is the immediate corollary to right to die. In my inner view, having been born and having lived in this world create a responsibility to live life in as meaningful a manner as we can construct. The older we become, the more have we lived and accumulated responsibility to sustain vitality. Therefore, old age becomes a tension point between a dignified death and a sustained, meaningful life.

It is just this battlefield that I look forward to as my future decades beckon. It is just this battlefield that Dr. Margolies describes in *My Mother's Hip.*

—WALTER M. BORTZ II, M.D.

Acknowledgments

I AM GRATEFUL to the many individuals who played an indispensable role in bringing *My Mother's Hip* to fruition. Family, friends, neighbors, and colleagues offered different kinds of support that were vital in shaping my vision of the book.

First I thank my husband, Graziano Gasparini, who encouraged me to write this book and has supported me unflinchingly throughout all my professional endeavors, no matter how far away from home they might take me. I appreciate his earthy philosophy, passed down through several generations, regarding the aging process: the problem with old age is that it arrives unannounced and one is never quite ready to receive it. *My Mother's Hip*, because of fortuitous circumstances, also arrived unannounced and I hastily put aside other projects to work on this book while my memories were fresh. Graziano and our son Graziano Andres understood that my caregiving responsibilities as a daughter often competed with my other roles as wife and mother. Later, both Grazianos provided constant feedback during preparation of the book.

I will always be beholden to the Assaels, Epsteins, Fines, Lambergs, and Newmans of the community of Palm-Aire, Florida, who acted as a surrogate family during my mother's long illness and provided much-needed solace. Meris Alcazar and Sandy Doyle, who will recognize themselves in the book, were loyal to the point of abnegation and contributed important details to the story of my mother's care. Drs. Anthony T. Schiuma, William A. Flignor, and Steven G. Sackel showed genuine compassion while treating my mother and were sensitive to the social ramifications of providing medical care to a frail, elderly patient. Helen Assael and Evelyn Newman, close friends of Mother's, read the manuscript and offered heartfelt comments. As a "general" reader during the book's evolution, Evelyn often reminded me that I must speak clearly to different generations.

I am indebted also to anthropologist Lambros Comitas for providing affiliation at The Institute of Man in New York; to author David Nevin, my cousin through marriage, who enlightened me about the ins and outs of the contemporary publishing world and offered crucial feedback throughout; to editor Joan Pollack, who during the early stages of the book's preparation advised me that less is more; and to Anthony Taylor at the New York Academy of Medicine Library, who was always pleasant and helpful during my months of library research. My colleague, the late Jacob J. Climo, "tested" the manuscript in his graduate seminars on aging at Michigan State University, and ethicist Daniel Callahan shared challenging thoughts about the state of our medical system and facilitated my use of library resources at The Hastings Center. The geriatrician Walter M. Bortz II offered critical insights on successful aging, as did orthopedic surgeon Joseph D. Zuckerman, whose seminal writings and research on hip fractures may one day transform the way we care for hip fracture patients. Jeanie Kayser-Jones, Gina B. Aharonoff, and Mary E. Tinetti sent me packets of reprints and research material, much of which would have been difficult to locate under other circumstances.

I am fortunate to have had the input of many persons who read and commented on different drafts of the manuscript from the perspective of their areas of expertise. Walter M. Bortz II, Joseph D. Zuckerman, Shirley Armitano, Penny Collins, Joan Pollack, Audrey Wolf, and my colleagues Barbara Pillsbury, George Ann Potter, and Jacob J. Climo read the entire manuscript, sometimes more than once, and provided critical feedback. I also benefited from the incisive comments of those who kindly agreed to read certain chapters: Mary Ann Bardes, Barbara Bode, Robert Carneiro, Robert J. Catanzaro, Hector Cintron, Victor H. Frankel, Sue Gilman, Joan Halperin, Gary Miller, David Nevin, Jan Pasquerella, Blossom Rosen, and Nick Taylor. Their various voices have enriched the final rendition of the book.

Janet Francendese, editor-in-chief at Temple University Press, brought uncommon professionalism and her rigorous editorial expertise to guiding this book through the numerous stages of publication. I am thankful for her unswerving commitment. Matthew Kull, Ann-Marie Anderson, and Jennifer French at Temple University Press as well as project coordinator Lynne Frost and copy editor Susan Deeks were also essential contributors to the production process.

I am grateful for writer William Zinsser's reminder that the best gift you can give when writing a personal history is the gift of yourself. As long as your story has integrity, your version is validated. This is *my* story of my mother's hip, and to be able to tell it openly I have chosen to protect the privacy of some of the protagonists by using pseudonyms. The names of all physicians and institutions involved in my mother's medical treatment have also been changed.

My Mother's Hip

Lessons from the World of Eldercare

My Mother's Hip

MY MOTHER, JUNE, would have wanted me to tell her story. She was that way. When she had her first child in the late 1930s, she was terrified because nobody would tell her what child-birth was like. She had an uncomfortable breech delivery without anesthesia, and afterward she told everyone the smallest details. They listened. When she underwent a radical mastectomy in her early thirties, she told everyone she had been hospitalized for breast cancer. The subject was taboo, though, and nobody wanted to hear about the big "C." Word quickly got around the neighborhood that Mother's death was imminent. She soon realized that frankness served no useful purpose, so she stopped talking about her illness. She was ahead of her time, and this was one of the few occasions when she decided it would be best to remain silent. Throughout her lifetime, we had many talks. I learned what it was like to be a working woman in the 1950s, when not many women left home; what it took to nurture a happy marriage; what growing up as a first-generation American was like; how to balance a career and family; and much more. It was natural that Mother and I would talk about her hip fractures and that she would tell me about events that cropped up during her protracted treatment. I learned a lot about hip fractures just from being by my mother's side.

Few people suffered from hip fractures years ago because they rarely lived long enough to experience the consequences of severe osteoporosis, a chronic disease characterized by bone fragility and associated with aging. Now we are in the midst of an "elder boom" in which the population older than sixty-five is ten times larger than it was nearly a century ago. John Riley, Jr., and Mathilda White Riley, pioneering researchers on aging, have called the expanding number of old people a "social phenomenon without historical precedent" (1994:16). This trend is unlikely to change soon. The graying of America will be fueled by the coming of old age of some 76 million baby boomers who will celebrate their eighty-fifth birthdays between the years 2030 and 2050.

Two factors have contributed to this demographic revolution. The first is longevity. Average life expectancy, a mere forty-nine years at the beginning of the twentieth century, may well be higher than one hundred by the middle of this new century. The second is the growth rate. The elderly are growing much faster than the rest of the population, and their demographic composition is changing as more and more people survive well into old age. Seventy-five is no longer "old" compared with the growing ranks of octogenarians and nonagenarians who now constitute the fastest-growing segment of the American population.

The traditional population pyramid has already disappeared. Many people are concerned about the "squaring" of the pyramid and what they consider to be a skewed demographic structure. Will the new demographic realities create an enormous dependent aged population incapable of caring for itself? Or will we experience a social epiphany as our aging populace achieves novel and creative ways to confront the challenges of advanced old age? Will our aging baby boomers live longer and better, or will they face the specter of chronic, degenerative conditions as they approach the twilight of their lives?

Optimists believe that as life expectancy expands, morbidity will be "compressed," resulting in added years of healthy living because infirmities will cluster at the end of one's life. The breach between our life expectancy and our natural life span will narrow. Leonard Hayflick, the author of *How and Why We Age* (1994), predicts that by midcentury we will attain our natural life spans in full possession of our physical and mental faculties and die swift deaths as we approach our 115th to 120th birthdays.

Pessimists claim that as life expectancy increases, so will the debilitating chronic conditions associated with old age, putting onerous pressure on a health-care system that is ill equipped to deal with them. Health status *does* decline with increasing age; old people *are* less resilient; and major problems *do* tend to arise among the old as chronic conditions undermine their autonomy and ability to function. Modern medicine has certainly played a cruel trick on the elderly. Saved from sure death from infectious diseases now easily manageable, thanks to medical advances, the elderly await an old age marred by osteoarthritis, osteoporosis, cardiovascular disorders, Alzheimer's, and other degenerative diseases that seriously compromise their quality of life. Undoubtedly we have come to a crossroads in the history of medicine as we face the new longevity revolution.

My mother's hip is every mother's hip. The inescapable reality of our times is the epidemic growth of age-related diseases, like osteoporosis, that demand new kinds of medical approaches. Osteoporosis is both a common and a serious disease that leads to hip fractures. Hip fractures, in turn, are life-threatening and require extensive periods to heal. How many elderly women can survive such a protracted period intact? How many elderly women can navigate the route to a successful recovery on their own? Not many. Complications can be transformed into consistent patterns destined to terminate poorly. Repeated crises can reduce one's chances and tip the prognosis negatively. An elderly woman may achieve a tentative truce with a chronic condition, but a hip fracture and its ensuing complications can upset the delicate balance. Victims of hip fractures die of complications every day, and if they manage to survive, they are often unable to care for themselves.

We hear about "little old ladies" all the time. The patronizing "little" refers to the obvious physical abnormalities of frail elderly women who look shrunken and caved in as a result of the decrease in bone mass—osteoporosis—that leads to collapsed vertebrae and hip fractures. Women with collapsed vertebrae have a pronounced curvature of the spine, called kyphosis. These women walk slowly and unsteadily and may need a cane for support or a companion to guide them. They are a frightening reminder to younger women of what may await them if they live long enough.

When I looked at my mother, I never saw a "little old lady." Inside was an ageless beauty who did not feel or act old until well into her sixties, when she was stricken with polymyositis, a rare muscular disorder. Even then she carried on and tried to maintain control over her life. She was not one to allow a chronic condition hinder her independence. It was not until she fell that I had to admit: This is my mother, June—a frail elderly woman with a double hip fracture.

September 19, 1993. Nearly five months had elapsed since my mother broke her two hips—a week short of five months, precisely, since she had suffered a spontaneous hip fracture and fell to the floor, jarring her other hip and cracking it. The prognosis was guarded. Mother did not expect to survive the double hip surgery, but she breezed through, only to embark on a period of extended rehabilitation whose object was to return her to the way she was before. For five months, Mother was in and out of the hospital, bouncing back and forth among rehabilitation, intensive-care, and nursing facilities. She made it home once, for only nineteen days. As she worked her way through the medical maze, the possibility of recovering her former self became increasingly elusive.

She was determined to walk again, but her good intentions were barely relevant to the broader picture. Instead of regaining her mobility and cherished independence, Mother suffered repeated complications that left her vulnerable to more relapses later on. Finally, she reached her limits. She yanked the oxygen tube from her nose and refused all medication. "I've had enough," she said. "I'm tired of the whole business. I want to quit." That evening, she had trouble breathing and went back to the hospital. Now Mother was in the intensive-care unit at Boca Raton Medical Center fighting for her life.

For five months I hovered over my mother. We discussed many of the ramifications of her hip fractures and their treatment. I participated in her recovery as her caregiver and medical advocate, and I observed the unfolding events not only as a daughter who suffered enormously watching her mother decline but also as a medical anthropologist who could relate this personal experience to the broader issues elders and their families face when a life-threatening medical crisis occurs. At times it was difficult for me to remain calm and collected so I could carry out the tasks of participant-observation, the sine qua non of the anthropological approach. My intense involvement with my mother—my role as a daughter—kept intervening in my effort to analyze events objectively, and I realized that if I had any hope of understanding what I had observed, I would have to force my anthropological sensibilities to reign. Seeing my own mother as a frail, chronically ill woman with limited options, compelled by circumstances to spend the last months of her life in an institutionalized setting, was a powerful and discordant experience, almost like seeing her floundering in a foreign world, hopelessly immersed in an exotic culture. I, too, was sucked into this maelstrom. I had no notion of what awaited her in her medical travails or of what the outcome would be.

My mother's hip fractures sent me on my own philosophical odyssey and medical inquiry. I wanted to cut through the intellectual tangles and arguments about the meaning of chronic illness—her illness, in particular. I spoke extensively with her doctors. I interviewed the supporting cast; many of the medical professionals who were involved in her treatment served as key informants. Later, I read her journals and notes. I visited nursing homes and rehabilitation facilities. I attended gerontology meetings and conducted research in medical libraries. I also searched for clues in her extensive medical records. They were of crucial importance in piecing together a consistent story of Mother's hip fractures and helped me delineate the patterns of medical care. I lived with these documents for many months and treated them almost like living informants—they allowed me to verify and corroborate the events I observed directly and those described to me. They served as a series of checks and balances to buttress the validity of the medical details discussed here.

Thanks to these approaches, I realized that there are valuable lessons to be learned from my mother's experience that can aid others. Her story in itself is important, because hip fractures are occurring in epidemic proportions. But her story would be incomplete without relating it to relevant issues about aging and chronic disease, housing arrangements, ethical dilemmas, caring for elderly parents, and how our health system treats the elderly. Even if you do not have a mother who breaks a hip, similar issues will crop up in the course of caregiving, because chronic illness is becoming a more intrusive element in the lives of Americans as the age barrier is pushed to its limits. These issues should be aired. Those who have not yet confronted them as patients are likely to do so as caregivers, because a drawn-out medical event such as a hip fracture involves the entire family.

Issues or lessons? I use the term "lesson" in the following sense: "a useful or salutary piece of practical wisdom imparted or learned" (*New Century Dictionary of the English Language*, 1946:943)—as in, my mother's experience taught me valuable lessons. The lessons are organized as separate sections and arranged to build directly on the chapters that precede them. Feel free to read the lessons in sequence or to skip around. If you want to learn about the issues that cropped up during my mother's treatment, then read the lessons as they appear. If you prefer to follow the story without interruption, then save the lessons for last.

CHAPTER ONE

Coral Bay Memorial Hospital

"I broke my hips."

APRIL 28–MAY 18, 1993: 20 DAYS • The emergency calls came around dinnertime in Caracas, but I was not home to receive them. I was taking advantage of my husband's business trip to work late at the office and catch up with my field notes. Our housekeeper, Carlota, was at the door when I walked in at 9:00 P.M. I did not like her grim look.

"Marisa called," she said, referring to my mother's helper, "and your sister-in-law called twice. Your mother had a bad fall early this morning and was taken to the emergency room of Coral Bay."

"Did she break anything?" I asked.

"I don't know, but Marisa sounded very worried."

"Well, hold dinner," I said. "I'm going to try the hospital number Marisa left."

I knew this would be a chore. My stomach was churning at the thought of Mother's fall, and I expected difficulty with the Venezuelan phone lines. It was after 10:00 P.M. when I finally got through to Coral Bay Memorial Hospital in Fort Lauderdale, Florida. The operator refused to connect me with Mother's room because it was so late and told me to call back in the morning. Next I called Marisa, who explained that she and my father had been at the hospital all day. He was exhausted and now asleep.

Mother had called for help in the early hours of the morning. Marisa found her sprawled on the rug in the bedroom hallway. She was in severe pain and could not move. She was also fully conscious and refused to complain. Marisa brought Mother the cordless phone, and she called 911 herself. Within five minutes, an emergency team arrived with a special stretcher and administered a painkiller. Mother asked to be taken not to the nearest hospital, as is customary in an emergency, but to Coral Bay Memorial Hospital, where she could be met by her family internist. After bringing in an orthopedic surgeon to handle her case, the emergency-room team took an electrocardiogram, X-rayed her hips, and performed various preoperative diagnostic tests. They swathed her hips in special pressure bandages to hold them in place. Marisa was with her when she was moved to the orthopedics floor later that day. Mother was calm but complained that her legs felt "dead" and that the hip bandages were too tight. She instructed Marisa to call her two children and inform them about the impending operation.

My last call that evening was to my older brother, Noel, a gynecologist–obstetrician who lives in the Chicago suburb of Oak Park. The news was not good. He informed me that Mother had broken *both* hips and had to have immediate surgery. Nevertheless, she had spoken to Noel and told him to remain calm.

"Noel, are you sure?" I asked, panic-stricken. "I've never heard of anyone breaking both hips at the same time."

"Yes, I'm sure. I spoke with her internist, and she has to have emergency surgery. She's resting comfortably, and she's scheduled for tomorrow afternoon."

"Noel, there must be a way to avoid surgery. It's too risky. Remember what happened last winter when Mother was going to have a minor outpatient procedure on her finger? She ended up in the hospital because of an extremely high white count, and her cardiologist told me she wasn't a candidate for surgery."

"Unfortunately, there's no choice. The area will become infected. It has to be cleaned out. Without surgery, she'll be in a wheelchair for the rest of her life. What kind of life is that? There's simply no choice."

We were both silent. Finally I said, "Noel, I'm scared, really scared. What can I say? Mother won't come through the surgery. You *must* get on the first plane tomorrow—please! Somebody has to be there with her."

"I can't. I have several births scheduled for tomorrow. I won't be able to get away."

Noel's specialty often forced him to work around-the-clock, and he disliked leaving his patients in the hands of a covering physician. "Okay, I'll make my own arrangements," I replied. "Somebody in the family has to be there."

I ate no dinner that evening. I was so upset I could not sit still and paced back and forth most of the night, wondering how this accident could have occurred. I did not think my seventy-eight-year-old mother would survive the operation. She had fibrosis of the lungs and was not supposed to have general anesthesia. I knew that her chances were poor, yet no other options occurred to me. I prepared my passport and papers and packed a small bag for the trip I would surely have to take the next morning.

On Wednesday morning, severe tropical rains caused a blackout and flooding in Caracas. Although I would have preferred to be with my mother before the operation, it was impossible to leave early enough. At 8:00 A.M., I called my travel agent and told him to prepare a round-trip ticket to depart that afternoon and with an open return. I asked him to deliver the ticket to the house, then sent Carlota to the bank to withdraw several thousand *bolivares* for my taxi and departure fees.

I called Coral Bay again, and even though the operator insisted it was too early, she reluctantly rang Mother's room. "Mother, I'm so glad I finally reached you," I said. "They wouldn't put me through last night. Tell me what happened and how you are."

"Darling, I'm having surgery at one o'clock this afternoon. I broke my hips. I don't know how it happened. I was sleeping on the living-room couch because my back hurt. I was worried about Dad and went to check on him."

"Oh, Mother, how many times have I told you not to get up at night? You need your rest. Why didn't you call Marisa? She left the bell by your side for just this purpose. Why didn't you use it?"

"Frankly, I don't know why. I think I also had to go to the bathroom. When I got to the linen closet, I knew I was going to fall. I could feel it. I didn't lose my balance. I just went down very gently."

"Where was Dad when all this happened?

"Dad was in the bathroom."

"I can't believe this story. You never fall."

"Well, I did. I asked Marisa to bring me the telephone and even managed to call 911 on my own. I haven't slept much lately. I keep worrying about Dad, who's been wandering around at night."

"You don't have to watch over Dad every minute. That's one of the reasons Marisa's with you. That's why she gave you the bell. Why didn't you call her?"

"I really don't know. As for the surgery, I'm not afraid. Whatever will happen will be. I know I may never wake up, but I'm going to enter surgery without fear."

"Mother, I'll be thinking of you every minute. I can't get there before the operation, but I'm flying up this afternoon and will be there when you wake up. Believe me, you're going to come through this because you're a very brave person. I know you'll be fine, and I'll see you later today. And, as we say here in Caracas, *suerte!*"

"Darling, I'm not afraid, believe me. I know what the situation is, and I accept it."

"Mother, have faith. I'm on the way, and I'll see you this evening."

I then called Kathy Summers, my parents' Medicare processor, and asked her to pick me up at Miami International Airport at 6:00 P.M. In addition to handling Medicare paperwork for the elderly, Kathy offered rides to and from the airport. Luckily, she lived near my parents and was always willing to come for me.

Kathy was waiting for me at the international flights exit. The plan was to drive by the house to drop off my bag, then head straight to Coral Bay. But as we were pulling into my parents' home, Dad arrived with Marisa. I jumped out of the car.

"Dad, how did it go? How is Mother? How was the operation?"

Dad turned and looked at me. He appeared confused and startled. "It was terrible," he said. "It's not good."

I was shocked. "What happened? Marisa, tell me quickly. What happened?"

"Señora Luisa, don't worry," she replied. "Señora June is fine. Your father became hysterical when she came up from the recovery room. He kept saying, 'It's Albert; it's Albert.'"

Dad was in a bad way, Marisa told me. (I'll explain later how Marisa became part of the family picture.) After all, they had been at the hospital since shortly after breakfast. The operation took four hours, and Dad was very nervous. After a seemingly endless wait, Mother's surgeon appeared and told Dad that everything had gone smoothly. Her condition was stable.

Mother was half-asleep after she was wheeled in from the recovery room. Dad took her hand. "June, June, wake up, wake up. June, answer me," he implored.

Mother managed to respond, "I'm fine, I'm really fine," but she was too groggy to continue. Dad was reluctant to leave, but he finally agreed to go home before Mother was fully awake.

"Dad, listen to me. Mother came through the operation well and is waking up," I said. "She's fine, and I'm going to visit her now."

Dad barely glanced at me and continued walking upstairs. I said good-bye to Kathy and carried my overnight bag to the second floor. I grabbed the car keys and prepared to leave for Coral Bay right away.

It was 9:00 P.M., after visiting hours, when I arrived. I did not ask anybody's permission to go up. I just walked briskly through the lobby as if I worked there and took the elevator to the fifth floor. I did not even stop at the nurses' station; I went directly to Mother's room. Her eyes were still closed, but she was beginning to come out of her deep sleep. She was flushed, and her face was slightly swollen from the massive dose of prednisone she had been given just before the operation. I wrapped her hand in mine.

"Mother, open your eyes. I'm here, and you've come from the recovery room. Dad is home now and exhausted. It was a long operation, but you're going to be just fine."

Mother slowly opened her eyes. "I can't believe it's over," she said, "and I'm alive. I thought I was still waiting to go in. You mean the operation is really over? I can't believe it."

Mother looked comfortable and was in no pain. I was thrilled that she had come through so well. By no means did I think the path to recovery would be smooth, but she clearly had surmounted the first hurdle. She was happy to see me and smiled contentedly. I did not stay long but promised to return early the next day.

That night I established a pattern that would continue for the next few months. I called my brother and told him the results of the operation. Every evening thereafter, after I had left the hospital and while he drove home from his office, we chatted on the phone. Now I gave him the full report: No complications of any sort had arisen during the long double procedure. Mother had pulled through, and furthermore, she had done surprisingly well.

Was I too optimistic? Mother had a few strikes against her. First was the matter of her fractures. Bilateral hip fractures were rare and usually resulted from a severe skeletal trauma. Joseph Bianchi, her baby-boomer surgeon, had performed only one such operation in his entire career, and that was on a woman much younger than Mother who had fallen from a tree. Few orthopedic surgeons have handled more than one or two cases.

Another strike was Mother's chronic muscle disorder. For fifteen years she had suffered from polymyositis, a one-in-a-million autoimmune disease characterized by progressive muscle degeneration. (The one other case I had heard of was that of Laurence Olivier, who wrote about his illness in *Confessions of an Actor* [1982]. The "sweet prince" died a peaceful death in 1989 after a long bout with the rare condition.)

Mother was on a downhill course characterized by flare-ups, painful spasms, and chronic fatigue, alternating with brief remissions. She frequently mentioned that in the morning her body was down, like a computer; each part was locked into place, making movement awkward and difficult. Mother felt like the Tin Woodman in L. Frank Baum's *The Wonderful Wizard of Oz*, but a few minutes under a hot shower acted as the oil can to loosen her up and prepare her to face another day of constant pain. The disease soon began to manifest itself in other ways. Her hands twisted out of shape, and she developed dry rales, or rattling, at the base of her lungs. Immunosuppressant drugs and maintenance doses of the steroid prednisone barely managed to hold her complicated condition in check.

Mother actually required two operations, or bilateral surgeries. Her X-rays showed an intertrochanteric fracture of the right hip and a displaced subcapital fracture of the left hip. She would need two separate procedures: pinning of the shattered right hip and total replacement of the left hip. On the day of the surgery, Dr. Bianchi decided to perform both operations at the same time. Despite her medical status, Mother sailed through the double procedure. Not only was her internist, Arnold Risden, pleasantly surprised, but even her surgeon was relieved that she had experienced no complications. Dr. Bianchi actually congratulated Mother after the operation. "You are a very strong woman," he said, "very brave. I've never seen a woman as strong as you." They exchanged pleasantries. Dr. Bianchi was from an Italian family. So was her son-in-law, Mother told him.

According to Dr. Bianchi's operative report (using plain language to describe extremely complex procedures), Mother's right hip—the side with the intertrochanteric fracture—was prepped and draped in the usual manner. Dr. Bianchi began the open reduction and internal fixation by making an eight-inch incision from the level of the greater trochanter down the side of the thigh and dividing the subcutaneous tissues and muscles. He drilled a hole into the neck and head of the femur and inserted a "lag" screw to hold the vertically shattered bone together. Next, he screwed a steel plate over the outer length of the femur to "fix" or align the fracture in place. He copiously irrigated the wound with antibiotic solution and found it to be "dry" (thus, no drains were required). Dr. Bianchi closed the wound in layers, using self-absorbing sutures for the muscles and subcutaneous tissues, and large staples on the skin. He applied thick sterile dressings to the site of the incision.

Mother was then transferred from the special fracture table to a regular operating table with a hip-immobilizing device, and turned on her right side, with great care to pad the right axilla. Then her left hip—the one that showed a displaced subcapital fracture, in which the head of the femur had almost been decapitated—was prepped and draped. The fracture table was removed from the operating room, and a new set of instruments was brought in. Dr. Bianchi left to rescrub and regown before beginning the arthroplasty. A representative from the manufacturing company also scrubbed and brought in a variety of titanium and polyethylene components. A laminar airflow system was used to create a highly sterile operating field and prevent bacteria from entering the large wound. Dr. Bianchi made another eight-inch incision, but this time, instead of repairing the fractured bone with screws, he gave Mother a completely new hip. Specialized tools like chisels, reamers, rasps, drills, and mallets were used to fit her with a sophisticated ball-and-socket prosthesis that allows universal range of motion. Dr. Bianchi cut the fractured femur to the proper angle and removed the femoral head. After testing various trial sizes, he tapped the definitive artificial head into place and bonded it with cement. He irrigated the wound, inserted drains, and closed the incision in layers. An abduction splint was placed between Mother's legs to keep them parallel and prevent the dislocation of her new hip. She was carefully moved from the operating table to a bed and rolled to the recovery room. Dr. Bianchi noted that "the patient tolerated both procedures well under general anesthesia and left the operating room in stable condition."

Dr. Bianchi had performed the two types of surgery that currently exist for treating femoral-neck fractures—a hip arthroplasty, or total hip joint replacement, in which the head of the femur is replaced with an artificial ball and socket, and an internal fixation in which the fractured bone is held together with screws. Some orthopedic surgeons believe that the decision to use one method or the other depends more on the art than the science of medicine. Total hip replacements result in fewer postoperative complications but often need to be redone after ten to fifteen years of wear and tear. Internal fixation is permanent and allows better movement. However, internal fixation fails more often, resulting in a re-operation rate of some 20–36 percent. Overall mortality at the end of a one-year period is similar for the two procedures.

We were fairly confident that Mother would gradually regain her strength after the operation and go on to complete a program of physical and occupational rehabilitation. I had nagging doubts, but I kept them to myself. There were too many unknowns to consider. Still, Mother was a fighter and would do her best. Noel was emphatic over the phone that Mother should get out of bed the next day, cough frequently and vigorously to clear her lungs, and exercise with the spirometer, a plastic breathing device that helps surgical patients maintain optimal lung capacity.

Mother had a Foley catheter in her urethra so that the urine ran directly into a plastic bag, which prevented the dressings from getting wet while she was bedridden. Noel also stressed that it was important to remove the catheter as soon as possible because it could cause an infection. But the attempt to remove it after a few days failed. Mother could not wait for the nurse's aide to respond to her call for a bedpan, so the catheter was reinserted. Mother developed a urinary infection, which was treated with an antibiotic. The Foley catheter was a source of constant embarrassment and concern. When Mother started therapy, she had to drape the bag over the wheelchair's armrest, making sure that the plastic tube was not twisted. The bag followed her from the bed to the wheelchair, from the wheelchair to the bed, back and forth like an albatross. Eventually, the doctors decided to leave the catheter in, even though it meant risking another infection.

But I am getting ahead of myself. For the first few days, Mother did not move from her bed and was attached to a pole holding an intravenous infusion of painkillers that included morphine. She administered this patient-controlled analgesia by pushing a button at the end of a cable, although the maximum dosage was regulated by computer. Mother was comfortable in the first few postoperative days and did not experience any throbbing until pills replaced this ingenious device.

Both doctors, Bianchi and Risden, were pleased with Mother's progress and planned to discharge her to a rehab center within two weeks. Dr. Bianchi estimated that she would be in the hospital a week longer than usual because of the double fracture. Therapy began almost immediately, with exercises carried out in a prone position. Two days after surgery, a student therapist started Mother on a series of leg lifts and rotation exercises. It immediately became clear that her left side—the one with the complete hip replacement—was more flexible and less painful than her right side. For all practical purposes, this became the "good" side and the one Mother was rolled onto. One is not supposed to turn onto a newly operated hip, but Mother had no choice.

On the third day, Mother sat up but was too dizzy to leave the bed. Her doctors were adamant about getting her moving. The longer a hip-fracture patient is immobile, the greater are his or her chances of developing a blood clot or lung complication. Mother wore special stockings to prevent an embolus and was instructed to "wave" her feet every so often, but nothing is as effective as getting out of bed. The therapist persevered and brought a wooden board to the bed, sliding it under Mother's legs and enabling her to move them with less effort. Twice daily, with the therapist's help, Mother exercised to strengthen her hip muscles. Within a few days, she could easily do ankle pumps, gluteal sets, and quad sets on her own. But she could not do the exercises that involved lifting her legs off the bed. The quad roll, for example, was a real killer: It required Mother to bend both knees while her heels remained on the bed. Then she had to straighten each knee and try to kick toward the ceiling. Mother's therapist helped her, lifting each leg up and counting out the seconds. On day four, the nurses transferred Mother to a wheelchair, and from this point on she did one of her two daily sessions in the small therapy room down the hall.

Mother had to follow a few precautions in the strictest sense. Otherwise, she could easily dislocate her recently implanted prosthesis. She could not point her toes inward (although outward was part of the exercise program) or bring her legs together. Nor could she flex her hips more than 90 degrees. She could sit up in bed but could not lean forward, and she could sit in the wheelchair but not bring her legs up.

How Mother broke her hip was a mystery. None of us could understand it, despite her severe osteoporosis. For a few days, this was the main topic of conversation. Obviously, the question should have been not "How did Mother fracture her hips?" but "Why did she fall?" She did not have balance problems and rarely fell. Now we were holding daily postmortems on the cause of her fall. At first, she blamed Dad, who had a tendency to wander. Sometimes he would forget to come back to bed, and she would get up to look for him. Dad's wakefulness was getting to be a problem between them, yet Mother could not bear to sleep in separate rooms. To recapitulate, on the night of the fall, she was sleeping on the living-room couch because of her bad back. She heard Dad get up and went to investigate. She saw the quilt bunched up in the walk-in closet opposite the hallway where she fell. Dad had disappeared—or, at least, she did not see him. Was he lying under the quilt, smothered, as she surmised? Actually, he was back in bed, but Mother had already fallen.

In another version, Mother said that she got up to go the bathroom and decided to check on Dad. She did not trip. She did not lose her balance. She felt weak and knew she was about to fall. "My body went down gently," she said. "There was no time to avoid it. I yelled for help. I couldn't possibly get up."

Mother fell on a Wednesday; she had been complaining about throbbing in her right hip since the previous Saturday. By Sunday, she could not walk and spent the entire day on the couch. On Monday, after a painful day on the couch, she called her rheumatologist, Dr. Kroeber. He told her to take the analgesic

Darvocet and wait until Friday morning, when she had a scheduled appointment. Mother now felt that Dr. Kroeber had given her the wrong advice: He should have told her to go directly to the nearest emergency room instead of prescribing the analgesic, which left her feeling woozy. Darvocet is a narcotic that can cause lightheadedness and affect balance, yet it is not much more effective than plain aspirin.

We kept going over this point. "Mother, did you tell Dr. Kroeber *emphatically* that you could not walk? Did you tell him about your sudden pain? Were you clear enough about this?"

"Yes, of course, and I'm really angry," she answered. "I don't even want to talk to him over the phone."

"Well, he is your rheumatologist and should know what has happened. Maybe he can give you advice about your medication."

"O.K., I'll call him, but not right now. Not yet."

I called Dr. Kroeber myself and told him what had happened. I felt he should know, especially when Mother did not show up for her appointment. I had always liked Dr. Kroeber, who received patients in a relaxed, smiling manner and never treated them as if they were too old to get better.

"How could this happen?" I asked, "particularly after eighteen months of salmon calcitonin injections to strengthen her bones?"

"I don't know. These things just happen. You know, your Mother is no spring chicken."

I chuckled. I was not offended. Dr. Kroeber always teased Mother, "You know, you're no spring chicken." In truth, she was remarkably resilient and plodded along despite the constant ups and downs. But shortly after Dr. Kroeber assured Mother that everything was about the same, she experienced the disastrous event the elderly are warned about—*don't fall!* Mother was not a faller, yet she blamed herself, which I thought was ridiculous. Just a month earlier, she had clipped an article from *Arthritis Today* on improving one's balance and preventing falls. Did she have a premonition she would fall?

Elaine Simmons, the visiting nurse who came to the house to administer Mother's weekly salmon calcitonin injections, thought that she had sustained a spontaneous fracture. This view is consistent with the intense pain she began to feel a few days before falling. Perhaps if Mother had gone to the emergency room right away, the hairline fracture would have healed on its own with bed rest. Now she had a monumental disaster. Elaine's explanation made sense: Mother had suffered a spontaneous break, went down gently, and the other side—the side that received the brunt of the fall—also broke. Elaine said that this was not unusual; indeed it was becoming increasingly common as the population grayed. I liked this theory. It explained why Mother simply went down, without tripping or losing her balance.

I told Mother about this. "Now let's forget it," I said. "There's no point in going over and over the reasons for your fall. It's already done. Now we have to concentrate on getting you walking, so you can come home quickly."

But Mother continued to hold a grudge against Dr. Kroeber. Later, when I began researching osteoporosis, I developed considerable animosity of my own. At best, he had shown poor judgment in telling Mother to take a narcotic painkiller that could dull her mind and make her shaky. At worst, he had made a serious mistake whose repercussions would soon play themselves out. I found the "take-a-pill-and-rest" approach dictated over the phone particularly offensive. Mother was a disaster in the making, yet the best her rheumatologist could come up with was, "take some Darvocet and get some rest." Certainly, he had been warned a year earlier when Mother suffered repeated compression fractures of the vertebrae, which are usually a harbinger of hip fractures.

Dr. Kroeber was well aware of the association between corticosteroid therapy and bone fractures and knew that prolonged steroid therapy causes severe osteoporosis, leading to collapsed vertebrae and fractures of the proximal femur. Standard textbooks on bone diseases in the elderly point out that the sudden onset of severe pain in the pelvic region of osteoporotic patients probably indicates a fractured femur. The doctor of a patient with steroid-induced osteoporosis should send her to the nearest emergency room immediately. Mother's anger began to subside as she became preoccupied with more pressing matters, such as her impending therapy. Now I was the angry one.

• • •

Mother was comfortably ensconced at Coral Bay. Although she was a Medicare patient, the hospital was not fully occupied, so she was given a large private room with a sofa and comfortable armchairs. This made life easier for visitors, as well. After the initial hellos, I settled Dad on the sofa, where he napped before leaving. Fresh flowers or potted flowering plants from well-wishers stood on the end table, and we placed Mother's many get-well cards on a large bulletin board facing her bed.

We settled into a routine of sorts. I normally went to the hospital at noon and stayed with Mother through lunch. Then I made the twenty-minute drive home and picked up Dad and Marisa. We all went to the hospital and kept Mother company until dinnertime. At 6:00 P.M., I took Dad home so Marisa could drive to her English-language classes. The objective was to maintain a semblance of normality within a context of tremendous abnormality.

Mother was fully engaged with her surroundings. She had a good appetite—she had no special dietary restrictions—and seemed to be in stable health, despite the trauma. Her mind was on matters at home and everything she had left pending. Her folders were still sitting open by the living-room couch; I went through them and brought the bills up-to-date. Each day, I took paperwork to Coral Bay, and we discussed the routine running of the household. For the past year, she had managed the bills by herself because Dad was beginning to show signs of forgetfulness.

Although Mother was attentive to her personal affairs and made a point of being well informed, she constantly upbraided herself for falling. Her greatest fear was that she would fall while being transferred from the bed to a wheelchair. Then, she reasoned, the operation would be undone, and she would have to start all over again.

I had planned to stay for about two weeks, enough time to see Mother settle into the rehab unit at Sacred Heart Hospital of Fort Lauderdale. I brought work with me, and while Mother and Dad napped, I corrected my husband's book proofs. Graziano, a preservation architect and photographer, had recently published a book on Venezuelan houses; it had proven to be a best-seller and was now due to appear in English. We had co-authored several books on Venezuelan popular architecture, so I was asked to review the text.

"Mother," I griped, "this is turning out to be an enormous job. It's time-consuming and boring. I should be paid for my time."

"Don't be ridiculous. You're doing this for your husband."

"I'm only kidding. But I'm having trouble concentrating. You know, instead of sitting here and working on this, maybe I should be taking notes on what's happening to you."

She smiled. "Well, I've always told you you'll learn a lot more about aging firsthand from us—after all, we're in it—than from all those gerontology conferences you attend."

The truth, though, is that I felt too anxious to take notes. I was always taking notes for my anthropological research and rarely left the house without a notebook. But now I found it hard to be detached from my mother's illness. Nevertheless, even though I expected this medical event to conclude promptly, I decided to jot down a few observations and keep running notes on the unfolding events.

I forced myself to be pleasant, even cheerful and friendly, with the nursing staff when I certainly was not in the mood. I felt that Mother would be treated better if her daughter appeared unruffled. I wore my most colorful outfit—a hot-pink bodysuit and flowing Indian skirt in tones of pink, turquoise, and yellow. Everybody, including Mother, admired this inexpensive ensemble I had acquired at the Himalayan Arts Center in New York. My ethnic dress lifted my mother's spirits, and I did not have to think about what to wear. I just threw on the same outfit every day. My high-heeled shoes with leather soles were an indispensable accessory: From the time I reached the nurses' station, several yards from Mother's room, she could hear me clacking my way down the hallway.

"Mother," I said on one of the few occasions we were alone, "I want you to have something that will accompany you when Dad and I are not here." I took a laminated, wallet-size image of Dr. José Gregorio Hernández out of my shoulder bag and stuck it in the flap of her executive planner.

"Just hold it in your hands and pray to him. Put his image under your pillow or in your drawer. Whatever you do, remember: He's always with you."

"I know," she replied. "Don't worry. I'll take good care of him."

Mother had read, and even edited, most of my articles on José Gregorio Hernández, the Venezuelan physician and folk saint who, in the early twentieth century, had shown an inexplicable gift for curing even the strangest, most intractable illnesses. Dr. Hernández was a deeply religious man, a "saint" who never turned away even the poorest patient. When he died in 1919, struck down by one of the few motorcars that circulated in Caracas, people immediately began assembling at his graveside, imploring him to perform posthumous miracles. Dr. Hernández gained fame for his curative powers and is currently undergoing the Roman Catholic church's arduous canonization procedure. He has become known as simply "José Gregorio Hernández."

While working with many of his devotees, I came to understand that hope and faith in a higher being are indispensable components of the curing process. Why not give Mother something symbolic to believe in, I thought—especially such a powerful conduit to God as a saint in the making? Mother was not religious in the formal sense, but she was deeply devoted to God and needed spiritual support. I myself was not a devotee of José Gregorio Hernández, but I had witnessed several inexplicable cures in the course of my research and respected what he stood for. Amidst the highly technological world of Coral Bay Memorial Hospital, the nurses looked at me skeptically when I told them about his miraculous cures. But it did not matter to me what Mother's nurses thought. I felt that praying to a curative saint would help her to have hope.

Right from the beginning I was conscious about the impact of Mother's accident on Dad's health. My parents were devoted to each other, and except for the birth of their two children and Mother's one visit to me while I was studying anthropology in Mexico City, they had not been separated in over sixty years. As teenagers in the Bronx, when it was common for young people to roam the neighborhood as a "gang," they enjoyed a few years of "group" courtship. When they finally became betrothed, they had no money and had the bad luck of starting off their marriage at the height of the Depression.

Dad, like many other young men at the time, had trouble finding a decent job. He was a math whiz who had completed a year at City College before dropping out "temporarily" to earn a living. Necessity led him to the beauty business by sheer chance, and he spent thirty years as a stylist at Best & Co., a small, elegant department store on Fifth Avenue. What started out as a temporary position to tide my parents over the Depression ended up being Dad's accidental career.

Mother was one of the few working mothers of her generation. Despite her impressive résumé, she always claimed that she had to work to supplement Dad's income and was therefore not a true career woman. Later I realized this was not the whole story. Entering the work force as a young mother was her way of reaffirming that she was in good health and that it was time to put her bout with breast cancer behind her. She was an accomplished stenographer and worked her way up from the secretarial pool to executive assistant of the CEO of several advertising firms.

When Best & Co. unexpectedly closed in the early 1970s, Dad at age sixty found himself the victim of ageism despite being too young to retire. After he received several job rejections, Mother decided to intervene. By then, she had spent several years as the assistant to the Controller of a major car rental company. She dropped five years from Dad's age and approached the head of personnel, asking that her husband be considered for an entry-level position. Dad joined the pension department and finally found the kind of career that had eluded him for over forty years. Relying on his math skills and sharp attention to detail, he set up a nationwide tracking system in the days before the personal computer and soon became an indispensable component of his department.

My parents were the oldest members on the staff and served as their coworkers' surrogate parents. They repeatedly put off retirement because they enjoyed their jobs and relished the routine. When the firm relocated its headquarters to the Midwest in 1980, Dad had every intention of going with them, but ultimately he and Mother decided against the move. After the company offered Dad part-time work at any of its locations in the continental United States, he and Mother reluctantly decided to "retire" to South Florida.

Even though Mother had a well-paid career, she identified herself as a homemaker, wife, and mother in deference to Dad. "My husband's comfort and wellbeing are the most important to me," she wrote in her journal. "If these two requisites are filled, it helps add up to happiness. I cook the things he likes to eat, keep the house clean and neat, and to top it off, I have a job outside the home, which is an important part of our income. Everything is shared without pointedness." Dad was not as articulate as Mother, but he walked the dog, did the marketing, and was always kind and considerate. On their 35th anniversary, Mother reminded Dad that mutual dedication had been the secret to their long marriage.

I worried about my eighty-three-year-old father. I tried to ensure that his routine was as normal as possible, but this, of course, was merely an illusion. How could life be normal when we spent most of the day every day at the hospital? He liked to have dinner at exactly 6:00 P.M.; now I prepared dinner whenever we returned from the hospital. Further, Dad was still recovering from cataract surgery, and his chronic heart condition required careful monitoring. We talked about what he would do when I returned to Venezuela. Marisa wanted to continue her nightly English classes, and I encouraged her to do so, even though it was an enormous inconvenience. Noel was adamant about not leaving Dad alone in the house for even a few hours. Dad, however, did not want outsiders around.

Dad's reluctance to have outsiders in the house had been a constant topic of discussion over the past few years. He had balked at the notion of having anything come between him and his precious freedom. My parents had worked out an effective system for managing the household, with each compensating for the other's deficiencies. Dad tired easily, but he could still drive and had full use of his hands. Mother orchestrated their days and covered for Dad's occasional forgetfulness. Each was the other's caregiver in their shared determination to run their own household without help.

As Mother's polymyositis worsened, I knew there would be occasions when I could not be there. I offered to bring a helper from Caracas, but Dad repeatedly refused. After Mother had a flare-up, I was convinced that the time had come for full-time help and begged Dad to give it a try. "Carlota's sister Marisa is still available and is dying to come to the States," I told him.

"No, I don't think so. We like to be on our own."

"Dad, you and Mother need help, and this is a person I can trust."

"I'd like to think about it."

"What is there to think about? Give Marisa a three-month trial. If either side is dissatisfied, you each go your own way."

It took a few more phone calls to persuade Dad (Mother was too sick to argue), and within ten days Marisa and I were in Florida. I liked her the moment we met. Her sister Carlota had been with me since my son Graz was a toddler, and I felt that this would work. Marisa, the youngest of six, had never left Barranquilla, Colombia, and jumped at the opportunity to see the United States. Although she was thirty-three, Marisa looked more like a college student than a grandmother's helper. She had studied physical therapy for a semester and was pleased to be working with an older couple. Marisa and my parents agreed to try the arrangement for three months. Marisa's job was to help my parents with sundry tasks; they paid her a small stipend and covered her basic expenses. Eighteen months later, she was an integral part of the household.

Now Dad and I mulled over his staying alone in the evening. "Dad, I'm concerned about your being alone in the house when Marisa's at school. Suppose you don't feel well. Suppose you have chest pains. What would you do?"

"Well," he started to laugh and replied, "I'll just lie down on the floor and hope for the best."

"Dad, I'm afraid you've given the wrong answer. I really don't think you should be alone in the evening. If you didn't have a heart condition and were still driving, maybe yes, but not the way things stand now. I'm upset about returning to Caracas and leaving you alone. Just please me. Let's get a person in while Marisa's at school."

"I don't want anyone else in my house. She'll probably just sleep the time away."

"Dad, maybe you're right. But do it anyway, just to give us peace of mind. It's only for a few weeks, while Mother's at Sacred Heart."

"Well, I'll think about it."

"Please do," I said. "I have to make the arrangements soon."

"I don't need anybody. It's a waste of money."

"Dad, I don't want Mother to worry about you when I go home. It's just a temporary arrangement. Or maybe you'd rather stay at the hospital with Mother while Marisa's at school, and then she can pick you up on her way home."

"No, I'd rather be at home in the evening."

"Well, let's talk about it again tomorrow."

I was already upset about something that had happened the previous Sunday, Marisa's day off. I had decided to do the marketing while Dad stayed with Mother at the hospital, and I told them it would take me about two hours. I returned to the hospital two-and-a-half hours later. Dad was upset, and Mother seemed practically unhinged. "What's the matter with you, Dad? You look like you've forgotten that I went to the supermarket."

"What took you so long? I was about to call the police," he said.

"Dad, you know it's impossible to get the groceries in less than two hours. I even went home and put away the perishables. Why are you so upset?"

"He's been driving me crazy," Mother said. "Maybe you should take Dad home."

"Well, I know one thing for sure. I'm not going to leave the two of you alone anymore."

Mother continued, "He called Noel and told him to call you at home."

"Why didn't you just call me yourself?" I asked.

"Dad couldn't remember the phone number."

"But, Mother, you know your own phone number. It certainly wasn't necessary to call Noel in Chicago."

Mother looked sheepish. "Dad got me very upset, I forgot my own number but had Noel's written down in my planner."

• • •

Mother looked ethereal. She was usually propped up on several thick pillows, with her favorite cardigan draped loosely around her shoulders. Her fine chestnut hair had grown, and I arranged it in a soft ponytail. Then I wrapped the ponytail on top of her head with vibrantly colored ribbons. The two natural streaks of white on each side fell softly away from her center part, making her look like the Gibson Girls of bygone days. Mother had always been strikingly beautiful, and even now, in the throes of a major medical crisis, she was lovely to look at.

Mother charmed the student nurses, and they came around every day to chat. She picked up a variety of tips from her student informants that she expected me to act on instantly. Mother's doctors were also fond of her. She was a good patient, alert and uncomplaining. When Dr. Risden asked how she felt, she inevitably replied, "Not too bad; coming along." Dr. Risden peppered his medical reports with such phrases as "very pleasant," "nice," and "very nice lady." Mother was thoroughly likable but eager to get out of the hospital and start the rehab program at Sacred Heart.

I, on the other hand, was anxious and could scarcely pull myself away from Mother's hospital room to do anything for myself—as if my mere presence would keep Mother safe. Mother's forceful demeanor could hardly compensate for fifteen years of chronic illness and an impaired immune system. So many things could go wrong. The most frequent complications of hip surgery are sepsis, anemia, thromboembolic disease, respiratory difficulties, pneumonia, urinary-tract infections, and pressure sores. Not only can these complications upset the rehabilitation process; they can lead to death. Mortality rates range from 1.3 to 16 percent in the immediate postoperative period. Pulmonary embolism, the most frequent cause of death, starts out as a blood clot in the veins that, if not treated promptly, can break off, move to the lungs, and become life-threatening. I tried to block all this from my mind.

Everything went smoothly for the first few days. Mother's Day was a disaster, though. I had taken Dad shopping to pick out something for Mother. The minute we walked into the department store, he started acting like a zombie. I held his arm and had to walk him from one place to another.

"Let's get out of here," he said. "I don't have anything to buy."

"Dad, remember: We're here for Mother's gift. It will only take a few minutes."

Dad was restless. I left him on a stool in the cosmetics department and told him to wait for me there. I picked out a brightly striped canvas carryall and matching cosmetic case for Mother, something she could use when she left the hospital. I had it gift wrapped and looked forward to taking the cheerful package to the hospital. Luckily, Dad had not moved when I got back.

Early Sunday morning, the phone rang. It was Mother. She was sobbing and barely intelligible. I sat up in bed. It was only 7:30.

"Mother, please, take a deep breath and tell me what happened."

"Dr. Bianchi was in to see me this morning, and he said I may need another operation. Enough is enough already!"

"Wait a minute, Mother. I don't understand. Everything's coming along so well. Tell me exactly what happened."

"He said that if the incisions continue to drain, he'll have to open them up and clean them out."

The incisions had started to drain two days earlier, and Dr. Bianchi was treating Mother with intravenous antibiotics. He had also called in an infectious-disease specialist and was waiting for the results of the culture. If the infection turned out to be deep-seated, Dr. Bianchi would have to operate again. I was upset that he had been so blunt. He could have waited until after he had received the test results—or, at least, until after Mother's Day.

The tension of the previous few days broke loose. Mother lost her composure, and I felt rotten.

"Mother, please, let's wait and see. They just started the antibiotics, but I'm sure—I feel it in my gut—that the infection will clear up."

"I can't bear the thought of another operation," she said. "It's enough. How much *mutchering* [torturing] can a person take? I'll never make it. I won't go through it again."

"You're right, Mother. I agree with you. You've done extremely well, and now no more operations. We'll come over at noontime. Please calm down. This is bad for you. I just know it will be all right."

The panic in her voice subsided. "I'll see you in a little while."

"And Mother, I can't tell you how happy I am to be with you on Mother's Day. We'll be over as soon as they let us in."

I called Dr. Bianchi. The hell with Mother's Day. He repeated what Mother had told me. Fortunately, when the results of the culture did come in, they showed a superficial infection caused by *Escherichia coli*, a bacterium normally found in the intestinal tract. Possibly, once the Foley catheter was removed, Mother's damp diapers provided the perfect milieu for transmitting the *E. coli* to the site of her incisions. Now the incisions were heavily dressed, and the amount of drainage slowly began to diminish.

A week later, the wounds were still festering. Mother originally had been scheduled to leave the hospital on May 12, but her transfer to Sacred Heart's rehab division would have to be postponed until the following week. Mother was in a vile mood and reacted poorly to her older sister Gussie's visit. "Another last hurrah," she said. On May 11, she wrote in her diary: "Bad night, so am not in good humor. So sorry to have caused so much trouble. Anyway so tired of all this pain and inconvenience. Poor, poor Daddy. Still draining and infection is still present. Know full well it could happen at any time."

Mother did not express her fears to me. I knew she was worried about the rehab program and being able to walk again. If she did not have a disease that rendered her hands useless, if she had broken only one hip—ifs and more ifs—the situation might have been tolerable. Now there were so many unknowns. So long as no further complications presented themselves, Mother was slated to leave the hospital on May 18.

Noel's mind raced ahead during our daily phone conversations. He was thinking about the future while I focused on the present. Mother's accident brought out stresses between us over what should be done. It was hard to anticipate what Mother's future needs would be, and this uncertainty aggravated the tension. He was concerned about the stairs to their second-floor condominium apartment and doubted that Mother would ever progress beyond a walker. I felt there were too many considerations to be worrying about the stairs and wanted to think ahead one step at a time. Mother had such an indomitable will to succeed that I convinced myself of her ability to eventually walk again—period—without a walker. Maybe it would take twice as long, but she would do it. They could move to a first-floor apartment if necessary or even to a villa, where they would have more room for live-in help.

"They should both really be in a nursing home," Noel said.

"Don't be absurd. Dad doesn't need a nursing home. I don't even want to talk about nursing homes. Mom and Dad want to stay in their own home, and that's what we should respect."

"You know, Dad needs a babysitter," Noel contended. "He cannot be alone. He has to be watched constantly."

"How would you know that? Babysitters are for babies, and Dad is not a baby. Why do you have to denigrate him? I know what you're trying to say, but you can say it another way."

"Well, call an agency and get Dad a companion. He can't be alone while Marisa's at school."

"That's fine," I said. "Dad needs company in case he feels ill. And another thing, Noel: Stop referring to Mother as 'that lady.' Why do you do that?"

He was silent for a few seconds and then responded, "I guess I'm trying to be objective by referring to our mother in the third person. I won't do it anymore."

"Good! Because it really drives me crazy."

We agreed that Mother seemed to have cleared the first hurdles. The incisions were nearly dry; the staples would be removed shortly; and Mother would soon be ready to leave for the rehab hospital. I told Noel that I was satisfied with her progress. I planned to go home before Mother left Coral Bay and return to Florida before she had completed rehab.

Hip Fracture, the Silent Killer
The New Hip-Fracture Epidemic

HIP FRACTURES constitute a global public-health crisis of catastrophic proportions. Thanks to the longevity revolution, the number of hip fractures is on the rise worldwide. The budding epidemic will be felt acutely in the developing nations of Asia, the Middle East, Africa, and Latin America because of the unprecedented graying of their populations. In 1990 alone, some 1.7 million hip fractures occurred worldwide, and the number could rise to 6.3 million by 2050 (Melton 1993:S1). The cost of caring for the enormous hip-fracture population will also increase fivefold as the aging population triples in size.

The incidence of hip fractures varies greatly not only from one population to another, but also from country to country and region to region. Nigeria has the lowest incidence of hip fractures (0.8 per 100,000 persons) and Germany the highest (100 per 100,000). The precise roles that ethnic difference and environmental factors play in explaining this variation have yet to be identified. Some epidemiologists hypothesize that, compared with "white" populations, Africans are protected by greater bone mass and Asians by hip architecture (Frassetto et al. 2000:M590). The occurrence of hip fractures varies more than sevenfold from one European country to another, with the highest numbers in Scandinavia and the lowest in Yugoslavia. This variation has been explained in terms of differing amounts of sunlight, climatic changes, the proportion of animal protein in the diet, and historical events that have intervened in the general environmental picture. In the United States, overall fracture rates are highest in the South and lowest in the Middle Atlantic states. This disparity seems to correlate with demographic patterns, but some researchers note that severe nutritional deficiencies in the early twentieth century (that is, poor nutritional habits in the formative years) led to a high number of fractures decades later (Hinton et al. 1995; Jacobsen et al. 1990).

John Rowe and Robert Kahn (1987) characterize hip fractures as a problem of "staggering" importance for the aging population, reducing the possibility of aging successfully. Women are prone to hip fractures because they have less bone mass than men do and because they undergo rapid bone loss right after menopause. The orthopedic surgeon is likely to have a fairly accurate notion of what awaits him in the emergency room—a "little old lady" with severe osteoporosis who has fallen and cracked her hip. Although hip fractures are a health issue primarily for women (some 75 percent of the estimated 120 fractures per 100,000 U.S. population occur in women older than sixty), their incidence for both genders rises sharply with age. Not only are octogenarians and nonagenarians more prone to falls, but an age-related reduction in bone strength also occurs, making this population shockingly vulnerable to fractures. Bone density of the femoral neck declines by an estimated 58 percent in women and 39 percent in men. The lifetime risk for a hip fracture is three times greater in women than in men, but the gap narrows significantly as men and women age. Then the risk of fracture increases "exponentially" for both sexes, because bone-mineral content and bone strength diminish markedly. By their early eighties, one-third of women and one-sixth of men will have suffered a hip fracture.

It does not take much for an elderly person to break a hip. In fact, nine in ten old people suffer little or no trauma before fracturing a hip. All it takes is a fall from a bed or a chair or a standing position. The cause is not the fall itself, which is secondary to the fracture, but reduced bone strength. Of course, if one falls directly on a hip that is not well padded and bears the brunt of the impact, the fall itself is a contributing factor. But a spontaneous fracture is not unusual in bone that has been weakened by osteoporosis. Some 15 percent of patients complain of pain in the hip area before falling. This pain means that a fracture is actually occurring; the person then falls and has a colossal emergency. Sometimes a person has persistent but moderate pain for a few weeks; suddenly, the symptoms become severe, and the person cannot bear to put weight on the leg. According to some opinions, this acute pain represents the actual displacement of the broken hip.

Hip fractures must be viewed as an affliction with predictable rates and patterns of mortality. All too frequently, a hip fracture is a death sentence: 27 percent of the hip-fracture population will be dead at the end of one year, compared with 9 percent of the general older population. Mortality rates rise precipitously for those who survive the immediate postoperative period and leave the acute-care hospital. The first four months following a broken hip are the most complicated; the next four months after that are almost as complicated. At best, the victims will be consigned to weeks of dependence and possible institutionalization during their attempt to regain mobility. The danger begins to subside only toward the end of the first year. Patients who survive for one year can be regarded as "recovered" because their mortality rates fall back to the level of the general population.

Why do so many hip-fracture victims die? Three significant factors increase the risk of dying: *age* and *health status* at the time of injury and *gender*. These factors not only influence mortality; they also affect the outcome of rehabilitation. The risk of dying from a hip fracture intensifies with advanced age. The older one is, the more likely one is to suffer complications. Old people are less resilient than young people and need more time to recover from traumatic injuries. Fewer than one-third of all octogenarians, and only 6 percent of nonagenarians, are alive and walking one year after fracturing a hip, compared with 80 percent of the younger elderly. The magnitude of the increase in both mortality rates and the inability to walk is not so surprising when one remembers that older patients are likely to be in poor health before the fracture. Those with chronic, degenerative diseases such as osteoarthritis and Parkinson's, which impede mobility and affect the ability to function independently before the fracture, face the gravest risk. Their immune systems are already impaired, and the fracture is the logical consequence of a general decline in overall functioning. Finally, men tend to be older and frailer than women when they break a hip and have a higher mortality rate.

An important caveat: Health status includes not only one's physical but also one's mental condition. Impaired cognitive functioning before a hip fracture impedes recovery and increases the risk of dying. Although confusion and dementia are important pre-existing risk factors, depression *following* hip-fracture surgery also diminishes the chances of a successful recovery. A recent study of the role of social supports in hip-fracture recovery notes that patients are often severely depressed right after surgery, because a hip fracture is "a pivotal event contributing to a restructuring of their lives" (Mutran et al. 1995:S360). The fracture signifies a social death and engenders feelings of despair that can seriously jeopardize progress.

Background indicators emerge as the most powerful predictors of recovery and the ability to walk six months after the hip fracture. Three indicators alone give a 90 percent prediction of being able to live independently again: prior state of health, ability to walk within two weeks of surgery, and living with another person. Patients who meet any two of these conditions have an 80 percent chance of returning home; those who meet only one have a 50 percent chance; and those who meet none have only a 12 percent chance. (According to these criteria, my mother, with two strikes against her, fell within the high-risk group and had less than a 50 percent chance of regaining independence once she left the hospital. She was a poor candidate for successful rehabilitation from the beginning.)

Martyn Parker and Christopher Palmer (1995) have worked out a formula to identify the predictors of successful rehabilitation by grading a patient's pre-fracture condition. The patients who were healthiest before falling receive the highest grade and are most likely to survive, whereas those who had a symptomatic illness causing severe restrictions prior to their injury are given a low grade and are thus at high risk right from the start. Parker and Palmer conclude that the pre-fracture mobility of the patient is the most significant variable that affects the outcome of rehabilitation.

Researchers have come up with different statistics but concur that the prognosis for the hip-fracture population is generally poor. Roughly 25 percent of hip-fracture patients return to the level of independence they enjoyed before the fall; an equal proportion die; and the rest are permanently incapacitated to varying degrees and require long-term care. Strangely, these figures contrast sharply with those from Scandinavia, where some 76 percent of hip-fracture victims go home and are doing well a year after their injury. Why the outcome is so unpredictable from country to country is a problem that has intrigued me since I first stumbled on it. Perhaps differences in the quality of treatment and standards of care during the recuperation period lead to the startling success rate in northern Europe.

Why are so few elderly patients alive and walking one year after surgery? The classic approach of American surgeons is to repair the damage by setting the bones in a functional position. The emphasis is on the acute stage that immediately follows surgery rather than on the prolonged stages of physical therapy and recuperation that bring other specialists into the picture. Surgery, which patients and their families often see as the most difficult hurdle, is actually quite safe. The surgical arsenal for repairing hip fractures has become increasingly sophisticated and failure-proof at the same time that victims are older and more frail than ever. This puts the onus for successful recuperation on how well the treatment is *managed* over an extended period. Rehabilitation brings into focus a whole new set of issues.

Rather than concentrating on repairing the damage surgically and monitoring the all too brief hospital stay in acute care, as is the case under the present system, it is more important to return hip-fracture victims quickly to an ambulatory status (Miller 1978). The key to success seems to rest in the careful coordination of available resources to get the patient walking again. Data from Sweden, where a comprehensive early-discharge and home-health-care program has been developed and tested, show that when highly organized community services are brought into the home, the patient receives care tailored to his or her particular needs and has a better chance of returning to pre-injury status. Getting patients up, bearing weight on the repaired hip, and walking early, then sending them home before they start thinking of themselves as disabled people who have been isolated from normal society, seem to be the most effective ingredients in a successful recovery.

A comprehensive team approach is far more effective than a single-focus treatment plan. A study done a few years ago by the Orthopedic Institute of the Hospital for Joint Diseases in New

York found that the 367 patients cared for by a team showed fewer postoperative complications, fewer discharges to skilled nursing facilities, and shorter stays than those in the non-program group. The results of this innovative integrated approach were unequivocal: Almost 62 percent of the program's patients were free of significant postoperative complications, compared with 15.5 percent of the non-program group, and more than half of the patients eventually were able to move around independently, compared with only 19 percent of the non-program group. The team consisted of the attending orthopedic surgeon, an anesthesiologist, an internist, a nutritionist, an ophthalmologist, a psychiatrist, a social worker, and a post-discharge case manager who coordinated the interdisciplinary activities through weekly patient-care conferences.

The Hospital for Joint Diseases was one of the first institutions to determine that hip-fracture patients need to be treated in a special unit comparable to that created for patients recovering from cardiac surgery. Joseph Zuckerman, director of the hospital's geriatric hip-fracture program, notes that "hip fractures in the geriatric population pose a significant challenge to the health care professionals involved in their care. . . . Unfortunately, many hospitals that care for geriatric hip fracture patients approach them as they would elective orthopedic surgical patients. This does not provide an optimal environment for the recovery and rehabilitation of the patients" (1989:9). Patients are more likely to be discharged to home and returned to their pre-fracture condition if their treatment includes plans for the post-hospital rehabilitation period (Aharonoff et al. 1998; Zuckerman et al. 1993). Since 1987, the hospital's geriatric hip-fracture research center has followed more than 1,000 patients in its registry and assembled a unique body of data that substantiates the benefits of a comprehensive interdisciplinary approach to hip-fracture management.

No doubt, many of the factors that affect outcome are susceptible to change, but such steps, according to Dr. Bianchi, my mother's orthopedic surgeon, would require time and money. "The ways things are going in our medical system," he observed, "there are no good answers." A care plan whereby doctors and other specialists would work in unison to achieve a shared goal by following hip-fracture patients through each phase of recovery would yield better results than the traditional piecemeal approach in which each expert does his own thing and has only a partial view of the patient's progress. Physicians, no matter how fine their individual intentions, are just as hampered by the system as are the patients. Medicare is presently structured to move the elderly patient through the acute-care phase as quickly as is safely possible. Such policy goals are often antithetical to the long-term needs of the recovering hip-fracture patient. Yes, it would take time and money, involving concerted pressure to change the culture of our medical system vis-à-vis eldercare, but it would be more cost-efficient in the long run and might also reverse the unfortunate outcome that awaits so many victims of hip fractures in the United States.

Osteoporosis is responsible for some 1.4 million fractures annually in the United States: nearly 400,000 hip fractures, 700,000 vertebral fractures, and 300,000 wrist fractures. More than 10 million people in the United States have osteoporosis, and 4 million more are likely to develop the disease within the next fifteen years (*America's Bone Health* 2002). Osteoporosis is a systemic disease characterized by low bone mass and micro-architectural changes in bone tissue. The bone becomes porous, with a Swiss-cheese-like appearance in a standard radiograph. People with low bone mass have fragile bones and are at high risk for assorted fractures. As an analogy, a normal skeleton can withstand the weight of an elephant; an osteoporotic skeleton can barely bear the weight of a mouse (Harper 1997). Low bone mass is the crucial factor in increasing the risk of age-related fractures. By age sixty-five, one-third of women will have suffered compression or crush fractures of the vertebrae, leading to diminished height and the appearance of the characteristic "dowager's hump." Vertebral fractures are an important harbinger of more serious fractures to come unless immediate measures are taken to stop the bone loss.

Menopause and aging are the primary determinants for osteoporosis, but other etiologies also intervene: genetic makeup, ethnic background, gender, body size, environmental factors, steroid-drug therapy, prolonged use of other medications such as anticonvulsants, and lifestyle indicators such as diet, level of physical activity, and the use of alcohol, cigarettes, and caffeine. Many of the so-called normal aspects of aging, such as reduced bone density, can be partly and even largely reversed through a prudent preventive and therapeutic program in which the modifiable factors are put to work to benefit rather than harm an aging body. Now that osteoporosis is becoming such an important topic, the public is bombarded with advice whose fundamentals are more anecdotal than scientific. For example, people are warned to take no more than 2,000 micrograms of vitamin A daily, because high doses will double the risk of hip fracture. Or people are advised to drink at least two cups daily of flavonoid-rich tea over a ten-year period to increase their bone density. Scientific research has not confirmed the efficacy of these folk remedies.

Women build bone mass in their youth and attain a maximum density by their early thirties. From then until premenopause, little bone is lost—some 3 percent per decade, and only in the proximal femur. The picture changes abruptly in the first five years after menopause, when bone loss occurs at various sites, accelerating rapidly because of a sharp decline in estrogen and androgen concentrations. Bone is steadily lost thereafter, slowing only during the seventh decade. Overall, a woman's bone density declines by about 30 percent between age fifty and eighty.

By the time a fracture occurs, severe bone demineralization and structural changes are usually far advanced. More than 20 percent of the bone-mineral content has already been lost before the thinning becomes apparent on a standard X-ray. The disease is silent and largely asymptomatic until a fracture occurs, at which point it may be too late to reverse the process of bone loss. Bones are living tissues in a constant state of regeneration. The old notion that bones are inert structures probably derives from the fact that earlier generations were taught little about their skeletons when they were in school. Sandra Raymond, former executive director of the National Osteoporosis Foundation, once commented that people are shocked when they suffer a fracture because they never realized they had osteoporosis. They pay attention only when a prominent person falls and breaks a hip: When England's Queen Mother broke her left hip, for instance, everyone marveled at the spirited ninety-seven-year-old's resilience. Pope John Paul II was only sixty-five when he lost his balance while stepping from the bathtub, fell, and fractured his hip. He never regained the agility and vigor of his middle years and has aged before his time, thanks to the unfortunate slip. Ronald Reagan cracked his hip on the eve of his tenth decade, and although he survived, he never recovered the ability to walk. These dramatic examples are known to all and remind us of how unexpectedly and violently osteoporosis can claim its victims.

Every ten years, we get a completely new set of bones as the result of the cycle of bone reformation by which 10 percent of our bone mass is "turned over" annually. Old bone is "resorbed" through the activity of osteoclast cells, and new bone is replaced or rebuilt through the activity of osteoblasts. Any disturbance in this dynamic process of bone resorption–formation will upset the delicate equilibrium and lead to a greater rate of resorption, resulting in bone loss. Under normal physiological conditions, the rate of bone formation equals or outpaces that of resorption, but under the influence of factors known to intervene negatively, bone loss occurs because resorption outpaces bone formation.

We have two types of bone—trabecular and cortical—whose proportions vary from one part of the skeleton to another. The light, spongy trabecular bone makes up some 90 percent of the bone in the axial skeleton and is located in protected inner areas such as the marrow cavities near the ends of long bones, the vertebrae, and the pelvis. This bone is composed of horizontal and vertical plates that form a sort of open latticework whose strength depends on the density of its components. If the reformation process is disturbed, trabecular bone is the first to be affected because it is more metabolically active than cortical bone. As the horizontal plates lose their density, the vertical struts buckle, and the strength of the entire latticework is imperiled. The trabecular struts are then prone to collapse, because they are vulnerable to pressure from different directions. Once the struts are weakened, trabecular bone is lost more rapidly than cortical bone. William Stini notes, "The risk of failure under stress is greatest at sites where trabecular bone plays a major role in weight-bearing activities" (1995:403). Compression or crush fractures of the vertebrae (about 40 percent trabecular bone) are usually the first sign that osteoporosis is in the making.

Cortical bone, which is denser than trabecular bone, makes up the appendicular skeleton forming the limbs and ribs and constitutes some 80 percent of the body's total bone mass. Whereas trabecular bone diminishes slowly in quantity, the compact cortical tissue that makes up the hard, outer shell of the bone is continually being remodeled. When the process of bone reformation is disturbed, an excessive amount of cortical bone is lost, compromising the strength of the bone and ultimately leading to osteoporosis.

As we age, other factors intervene. Bones are the principal depositories of calcium, which is released into the blood to meet the needs of muscles and other organs to keep our bodies functioning at optimal levels. Aging bodies are less efficient than younger ones in mobilizing calcium, and calcium is leached from the bones to fulfill the demand. Over time, this process leads to osteoporosis. Aging also weakens the structures that support the bones. The hip joint is basically a ball (femoral head) and socket (acetabulum) supported by the muscles of the thighs, abdomen, groin, and buttocks. The joint is also supported by ligaments and tendons and cushioned by cartilage and fluid-filled sacs called bursae. A protective layer of fat serves as natural padding for the entire area. This supporting structure of the hip joint weakens with aging. Walking and shifting from one position to another exert differing forces on the femoral head, which, without the requisite support, becomes more susceptible to injury.

Sadly, few reliable scientific studies exist on the relationship between cortisone therapy and "secondary" osteoporosis, the type of osteoporosis induced by drug therapy (as opposed to "primary" osteoporosis, which results from menopause or aging). Further, little information is available about the true incidence of osteoporosis in patients receiving corticosteroids, and even fewer longitudinal studies have been done to determine how rapidly and when bone loss occurs. Oral corticosteroids, hailed as miracle drugs when they were introduced in the 1940s, can be extremely toxic with prolonged use. After ten years of continued maintenance-level dosage, the clinical condition of patients who have taken corticosteroids is considerably worse than that of patients who have never taken them. The latest word on the long-term use of steroids, based on recent studies, is that they do more harm than good.

We do know that corticosteroids have a deleterious effect on bone architecture. They significantly decrease the length, weight, and density of the femur and tibia and may cause osteonecrosis of the femur head. This is a serious complication that results in microscopic cracks and fatigue fractures because the blood supply to the femoral head has "died." Corticosteroids induce bone loss by inhibiting the formation of new bone and stimulating the loss of old bone, upsetting the continual process of bone remodeling. Corticosteroid-induced bone loss is distinctive. In regular osteoporosis, the horizontal plates are lost faster than the vertical struts; in steroid-induced osteoporosis, however, the vertical and horizontal trabeculae are equally thin, producing a peculiar translucent appearance to the bone. Corticosteroids also inhibit the absorption of calcium from the intestines to the bones and retard the production of vitamin D, an important aid in intestinal calcium absorption. The pronounced thinning of the skin in patients on steroid therapy makes them particularly vulnerable to a fall-induced fracture when the force of the impact is directly over the hip.

Barbara Lukert and Lawrence Raisz note that about half of all patients on steroid therapy will lose bone and sustain a fracture. The bone loss seems to be most pronounced in the early weeks of therapy and most rapid in the areas of the skeleton containing the greatest proportion of trabecular bone: the spine, ribs, pelvis, and hips. Although smaller doses have less dramatic effects on premenopausal women, postmenopausal women lose bone even on low-dose therapy. Patients on doses of more than 7.5 milligrams daily will suffer the most significant bone loss and are at grave risk for a spontaneous hip fracture (1990:354–357).

My mother did not escape the consequences of prolonged steroid therapy. After a few years of a maintenance-level regime, her back began to curve inward, and it was apparent—at least, to me—that she was getting shorter. Mother finally went for a bone-density test and took the news of 50 percent bone loss in the hip area calmly. "To the supermarket with osteoporosis!" she wrote in her journal. She was more concerned with her throbbing back and put it down to chronic arthritis rather than to bone loss in the lumbar region: "Most difficult to stand straight and for any length of time. Very, very disturbing." Mother soon suffered several compression fractures of the vertebrae and spent most of 1992 on the living-room couch. When she was finally able to hobble around, I had her fitted with a dorsolumbar corset made of molded plastic and metal stays to support her spine. This odd-looking contraption joined a copious collection of hand splints that, when worn together, gave her a distinctly robotic semblance. By Mother's last visit to her rheumatologist a month before she fell, her torso had collapsed, and her posture had changed markedly. "Patient is hunched over with accentuated kyphosis [curvature]," he noted. A second scan indicated that, despite an aggressive course of salmon calcitonin injections, Mother's bones continued to thin.

An alarming trend over the past twenty-five years is the inexplicable rise in falls and fall-induced injuries and deaths. Finnish researchers note that fall-induced injuries have increased by nearly 300 percent, and deaths resulting from falls have increased by 80 percent (Brody 1999). These falls cannot be explained entirely by global aging, but U.S. researchers have shown that age does constitute a risk factor for falling. About 40 percent of the population older than eighty fall each year, and 5 percent of these falls result in fractures (Tinetti 1988:1701).

Old people are at greater risk for falls for a variety of reasons. Sometimes the cause is easily identified, such as Parkinson's and other neurological diseases that lead to disturbances in balance and gait. But more often, increasing frailty pushes one into the at-risk group. Declining vision and hearing; cardiovascular and arthritic conditions; the use of multiple medications or certain drugs, such as antidepressants and antihypertensives; and an episode of acute illness set the stage for a fall-induced injury. These medical factors are not easily changed. Other causes are situational. Poorly lit homes, slippery stairs, dangling cords, and loose area rugs are obvious traps, which rarely are altered in time to prevent a fall. Bathroom and kitchen hazards, clutter, and obstacles create a dangerous physical environment to be navigated. Some people are so fearful of falling, observes the geriatrician Muriel Gillick, that they are afraid not only of going outside but also of moving out of a chair (2001:9). Ironically, the home setting is far more treacherous than the outside environment, but the aging occupant is so accustomed to living with household dangers that she or he does not recognize the threat they pose to safety. Most falls occur at home, and nearly 30 percent of the elderly who live at home fall each year.

One of the best pieces of advice that a doctor can give elderly patients is: "Don't fall." In terms of accidents, says the geriatrician Walter Bortz, falls are to the elderly what car collisions are to the young. A fall and a subsequent hip fracture can be lethal because "mobility and life are tightly linked. . . . As long as we can move, vitality endures. Subtract movement from us, and survival is threatened" (1991:66). Then the "disuse syndrome" kicks in. Immobility leads to all sorts of pathological consequences, such as musculoskeletal fragility and cardiovascular deconditioning that in the long run can only be prejudicial to one's physical well-being (Bortz 1993:1007).

A study published recently in the British medical journal *The Lancet* suggests that four fall-related factors play an important role in determining who is likely to break a hip. They are slow gait, difficulty in doing a heel-to-toe walk, small calf circumference, and poor vision. People with this set of factors are twice as likely to suffer a hip fracture as those without them, and people who have low bone density in conjunction with the four fall-related factors are six times as vulnerable (Dargent-Molina et al. 1996).

The age-related loss in skeletal muscle mass, known as sarcopenia, increases dramatically after age seventy and leads to reduced muscle strength, which in turn leads to falls. Sarcopenia is readily reversible, despite its prevalence. A regular program of resistance training can compensate for the age-related decline in muscle strength that affects balance and gait (Tseng et al. 1995). Even in the tenth decade of life, frail men and women show gains similar to those of young people. As for the hazards that make the home environment a dangerous place, the elderly can be shown how to remove potential obstacles and negotiate the stairs, bathroom, and other danger spots. Potential fallers can be identified, assessed, and taught how to improve their physical condition and safeguard their environment.

Today a simple but effective device is available to prevent hip fractures among chronic fallers: the hip protector, an elastic undergarment with padded pockets that cover the hip joints on both sides. The purpose of the padding is to divert the force of the impact from the bone to the surrounding soft tissue. A recent large-scale study carried out in Finland reports that, among persons who were wearing a hip protector when they fell, hip fractures were reduced by some 80 percent (Kannus et al. 2000). Hip protectors are widely used in Scandinavia and are just beginning to gain popularity in the United States. The American public is still largely unaware of their existence, and the medical community should campaign for their use among people with a history of falling.

Any attempt to manage the growing incidence of hip fractures must begin with prevention, a concept that has yet to receive the focus it deserves in our health-care practices. The problem begins not with the fall, which is merely the direct cause of the fracture; it begins with preventing the loss in bone density that accompanies normal aging. If only a minute proportion of the funds expended each year on hospitalizations for hip fractures (some $8–15 billion, according to estimates) were earmarked for prevention, the deadly consequences of osteoporosis could be confined. If we also take into account the indirect costs of caring for hip-fracture patients during the long recovery period, then prevention is certainly the most effective long-term strategy.

Until recently, estrogen-replacement therapy was the only approved pharmacological treatment for preventing osteoporosis. Estrogen therapy halts the rapid decline in bone density that begins soon after menopause; estrogen slows the rate of bone loss from 2 percent to about 0.5 percent annually during the first five years after menopause. The Farmington Heart Study, which has followed nearly 3,000 women throughout their lives since 1948, shows that estrogen therapy has a protective effect for women younger than seventy-five. Not only does estrogen increase bone density by some 11 percent in women who have taken it for seven years; it also reduces the risk of hip fracture by more than 60 percent.

Nevertheless, a Catch-22 situation exists. Women rarely have hip fractures in their fifties and sixties, and if they take estrogen for a few years to stem menopausal bone loss, they will not protect themselves from age-related bone loss later on. The picture is not entirely clear. It appears that short-term estrogen therapy (one to five years) will slow menopause-induced bone loss but cannot protect women against osteoporotic hip fractures twenty-five years down the road (Ettinger and Grady 1993).

Once a woman stops hormone therapy, she is basically on par with women who never took estrogen, because the estrogen's protective effect wanes rapidly with age. Two clear factors affect bone density. One is related to estrogen; the other is related to age. The age factor kicks in for those approaching their eighties. Most authors argue that even five to ten years of postmenopausal estrogen will have a "trivial" effect on bone-mineral density at age seventy-five. Bone density is only 3.2 percent higher among seventy-five-year-olds who took estrogen during menopause and then stopped than among woman who never took it at all. In fact, women who underwent hormone-replacement therapy simply to relieve the symptoms of menopause may be worse off than women who never started it in the first place, because estrogen withdrawal is followed by accelerated bone loss equivalent to that occurring right after menopause. It may prove necessary to start estrogen therapy at menopause and never stop, thus providing continuous protection against age-related bone loss and reducing the risk of hip fractures among women in their eighties. Treatment can be targeted even to women with osteoporosis years after menopause. Estrogen will not only slow their bone loss; it will also increase their bone density by 3–10 percent, thus reducing the risk of hip fractures by a third. Today, estrogen is commonly prescribed in combination with progestin as hormone-replacement therapy (HRT) to lower the risk of endometrial cancer in women with uteruses.

Hundreds of medical articles attest to the beneficial effects of hormone-replacement therapy on bone health and discuss its protective effects for other diseases such as osteoarthritis, colon cancer, Parkinson's, and Alzheimer's. However, in light of the compelling findings of the Women's Health Initiative, due to end in 2005 but partly terminated in mid-2002, women should undertake long-term hormone-replacement therapy gingerly. In the double-blind clinical trial, one group received Prempro, a combined estrogen and progesterone pill, and the other received a placebo. The study has demonstrated unequivocally that women who have continued hormone-replacement therapy for more than a year are at somewhat greater risk than are non-users for breast cancer, heart attacks, strokes, and blood clots. Each additional year of use increases the risks.

Despite its proven benefits in preventing bone loss, estrogen is a known carcinogen. Before the findings appeared, many orthopedic surgeons recommended hormone-replacement therapy unconditionally because the benefits clearly outweighed the disadvantages. Some continue to recommend hormones despite their known risks, while others skirt the issue and tell women to discuss the matter with their gynecologists. Without doubt, the trial's results raised more questions than answers and have left women thoroughly confused. The controversy rages in numerous medical journals, because not all experts are willing to accept the new findings as the last word, and others are wary of extended hormone-replacement therapy. A few physicians have bravely taken a firm stance, advising only short-term therapy to treat hot flashes and other symptoms of menopause while cautioning women still on long-term therapy to stop because the potential for harm outweighs the known benefits (Grady 2003; Grodstein et al. 2003; Solomon and Dluhy 2003). Each possible user must become her own advocate and carefully weigh the pros and the cons before embarking on an extended course of hormone-replacement therapy.

Women have more choices than ever, thanks to advances in diagnostic techniques and new treatments. There is no reason for osteoporosis to be a silent epidemic once women get the message that they can protect themselves against this potentially mortal disease. Early screening to detect the onset of osteoporosis is becoming as common as mammography, and breakthrough medications to maintain or restore bone density are multiplying. Sensitive biochemical markers also exist to measure the rate of bone turnover and can be used with bone-density tests to make a highly accurate assessment of the condition of one's bones.

Although the steps to good bone health are not difficult, they do require a concerted, multi-strategy approach. Women should have a bone-mineral-density test at menopause and periodically afterward to monitor their bone condition. The most common technique, dual energy X-ray absorptiometry (DXA), is a simple test that measures bone density at the spine and hip. This non-invasive X-ray, which takes about five minutes, uses a scanner that passes over the lower body as one lies fully clothed on a table. Bone density is measured in T-scores, or standard deviations (SD) from the average peak bone density of a young adult. People with T-scores between −1.0 and −2.5 SD have low bone mass, or osteopenia. Those with T-scores lower than −2.5 SD have full-blown osteoporosis. Hip-fracture risk increases threefold for every SD decline from the average (Cummings et al. 1993). The bone-density test is an accurate measure of bone health and should be used as a guide in deciding which strategies to pursue.

The first steps in preventing hip fractures are weight-bearing exercise, calcium supplementation, and short-term hormone-replacement therapy around the time of menopause. A proper exercise regime and a prudent diet may even halt the continued decline in bone mass if started early enough. A balanced exercise program should include weight-bearing exercises such as walking, which puts stress on the lower body's bones, and strength training, which works muscle groups against some degree of resistance. (People with balance problems can do strength-training exercises in a pool. Not only does the water provide resistance, but it also reduces the forces exerted on the hip when moving.) The purpose of the dual exercise regime is to slow the pace of bone loss and strengthen the supporting structure of the hip socket. People who have a tendency to fall should also include tai chi chuan or yoga to improve their balance. Calcium supplementation should be undertaken together with vitamin D, which helps regulate the deposition of calcium in the bone. Exercise and calcium supplementation work synergistically with hormone-replacement therapy to prevent the rapid loss of bone-mineral density that occurs right after menopause.

For women who are concerned about the possible long-term effects of hormone-replacement therapy, alternatives are available that maintain optimal bone health. The U.S. Food and Drug Administration (FDA) has approved four medications other than hormone-replacement therapy for the prevention or treatment of osteoporosis. They are classified as antiresorptive medications because they slow the rate of bone resorption during the remodeling cycle.

Alendronate, introduced by Merck in 1994 as a revolutionary therapy to reverse bone loss, blocks the osteoclast cells from attacking and breaking down bone. Alendronate is one of a new class of drugs called "aminobisphosphonates," which take up residence in the osteoclasts, where bone resorption takes place. Fosamax, as alendronate is known by brand name, does not actually stop bone resorption; it decreases it to normal levels. It is not only a selective inhibitor of bone resorption, but it also builds normal bone quality by reversing bone loss. In a three-year study of 1,000 women in thirty medical centers worldwide, a dose of 10 milligrams daily of Fosamax was shown to increase the participants' bone mass in the hip area by nearly 8 percent. The drug must be taken first thing in the morning with a full glass of plain water and at least a half-hour before eating or drinking anything else. The patient must remain upright to prevent absorption problems and to ensure that the drug is delivered directly to the osteoclasts. In 2000, a 70-milligram tablet to be taken once a week was introduced, thus reducing the frequent side effects of heartburn and nausea. Alendronate has also been approved for prevention in the form of a 35-milligram weekly tablet.

Risedronate, which is marketed as Actonel, is the other bisphosphonate that works to prevent and treat osteoporosis. Tests have shown that Actonel increases bone density by 3–4 percent in the hip region and reduces the incidence of hip fractures by nearly 50 percent. Actonel, like Fosamax, can be taken daily or weekly. To recapitulate, the bisphosphonates Fosamax and Actonel are used to prevent and treat osteoporosis. By increasing bone density in the spine and hip, they lower the risk of vertebral and hip fractures. They are also the medication of choice for treating osteoporosis derived from steroid and other types of drug therapy.

Raloxifene, approved in 1997, derives from a class of drugs known as selective estrogen receptor modulators. Raloxifene hydrochloride, or Evista, acts on the bone much as estrogen does. Although Evista is not as effective as estrogen in stopping bone loss, clinical studies have shown that, during the first three years of therapy, the drug produces positive changes in blood lipids that may protect against heart disease and possibly lower the risk of breast cancer. Evista's long-term effects on fractures are not yet known, but preliminary results are promising. Evista should be approached cautiously, because it can have undesirable side effects, including hot flashes, joint pain and swelling, and blood clots.

Salmon calcitonin is available as a nasal spray or subcutaneous injection. Calcitonin, whose brand names are Calcimar and Miacalcin, is a naturally occurring hormone that increases vertebral bone density. It is known to relieve the pain associated with bone fractures, but its effect on hip fractures has yet to be demonstrated. Fortunately, the search for promising treatments is continuing, and several new drugs are on the horizon. These include anabolic medications, synthetic steroids available elsewhere but awaiting U.S. approval, and injectable bisphosphonates that reduce bone loss and stimulate new bone growth. In terms of therapy, the available choices are developing at a pace that will allow women to protect their bone health without endangering their general health.

How many baby boomers were taught about the dynamic regeneration of their skeletons every few years? How many received the message about the vital role of prevention as a "health" investment for their later years? Not many. Only when menopause escaped from the closet did baby boomers become aware of the damaging effects of osteoporosis. The problem is not simply a matter of menopause but a public-health crisis with serious consequences for the elderly.

Young women must be encouraged from adolescence to take care of their bones and pursue a maintenance regime before they enter their thirties. The message to "size up your bones," touted in *Prevention* magazine's monthly section on women's health, calls for early detection and action and is becoming as commonplace as the call for breast cancer screening was a few years ago. Slowly but surely, the educational message from the medical community, the media, and the Internet is reaching the public: Osteoporosis can be both prevented and treated. It is up to women, not their doctors, to ensure that longer lives will reap longer years free of the threat of hip fractures and permanent disability.

CHAPTER TWO

Sacred Heart Hospital

"She's not in her room.
She's in therapy right now."

MAY 18–JUNE 18, 1993: 31 DAYS • On the twentieth day following surgery, Mother transferred to the Physical Medicine and Rehabilitation Department at Sacred Heart, almost a hospital within itself. Patients there are considered well and strong enough for an intensive period of physical and occupational therapy. They are told to bring a week's change of clothing—no more hospital gowns for these patients—and are expected to eat together in a small dining room as part of their total treatment. The goals of the holistic hip-rehabilitation program are admirable. These include mastering an exercise regime to increase muscle strength and endurance and learning the guidelines that will enable patients to perform home activities. The idea is to encourage them to achieve the goals in a homelike setting within a specific period of time.

Mother sounded fine when we spoke on the phone, but there were problems from the start. The staff was pushing her too hard, she said, and she was constantly exhausted. After a two-hour therapy session in the morning, Mother lunched in her room. Then she took a short nap, fully clothed, on top of the bed. The afternoon was completely occupied. She was scheduled for an hour of occupational therapy at 2:00 P.M., followed by another two-hour physical-therapy session that ended before an early dinner. Some aspects of the program were easy for Mother. She could do any exercise that involved lying flat on her back. The ankle pumps, quad and gluteal sets, hip flexions and abductions, knee extensions, and quad rolls were a more concentrated version of what Mother had already practiced at Coral Bay.

Standing up was another matter altogether. These exercises were based on the premise that one had one healthy leg and two functional hands. One had to hold on to a countertop or heavy chair and exercise the operated leg. Mother ran into trouble right away. For example, in the hip-extension exercise, she had to lift the operated leg straight back without bending forward; the foot also had to clear the floor. Mother's hands could barely support her weight, and she tended to treat her left leg, the one with the total hip replacement, as the "healthy" leg because it was more flexible and gave her less pain. Mother was game. She did well at walking the length of the room between the exercise bars, but she tired easily and needed to rest on the padded mat.

Mother was actually miserable but confided this only to her diary. "So worried about making it," she noted on arrival. On May 19, she wrote: "First full day here in Sacred Heart—Disaster!" On May 20: "Second day—a little day. Horrors of horrors of horrors of horrors—tooth falls out!" On May 21, she noted: "Fourth day here—imprisoned—not much better. Mamma gone 35 years today. Spoke to her last night—when will her memory fade in my mind—when I go to sleep forever? So, so weary—23rd day since operation." And on May 22: "Fifth day here. Will it ever end? Tough day. Male attendant, not happy with it."

I was not with Mother during her stay at Sacred Heart's rehabilitation unit and could not reconcile the dark thoughts she expressed on paper with our frequent conversations, in which she professed a deep determination to walk out of there. I called her every day, but Mother seemed constantly to be away from her room. "She's in therapy," the floor nurse said, or, "She's in the dining room." "Call back later" was the stock answer every time I got through. She complained to me about her fear of never being able to walk again. Her roommate, the food, and the nursing attendants were all unsatisfactory. She was unhappy, as well, with her attending physiatrist, Dr. Alice Hicks, who had few social graces and had put in but a single appearance, coinciding with Mother's admittance to the rehabilitation unit.

"Mother, think of this merely as a means to an end," I said. "You're only going to be there for a short time, and then you're going home. Talk to Dr. Borosky [the department head]. Tell him you can't tolerate the occupational therapy and need to rest after lunch. Ask to be moved to another room. Come on, now—do you want me to call him?"

"No, don't! You'll only stir things up, and they'll kick me out of the program. The whole notion in that occupational-therapy room is absurd. It's ridiculous to sit there after lunch, throwing rings onto a spool. I don't see the point to it, and frankly I'm just too tired. It looks like I'm not going to be here much longer anyway. I understand they're going to do an evaluation next week."

The occupational-therapy program was meant to get the patient beyond the stage of shuffling up and down a practice room with a walker. Guidelines had been drawn up for activities that healthy people routinely take for granted, such as getting in and out of a car, sitting down, standing up, going up and down stairs, going to the bathroom, bathing, dressing, and cooking. But no guidelines existed for people with double hip fractures.

This was not a custom-designed program for those who deviated from the norm. Mother was given a set of ten "commandments" loosely known as "Body Mechanics." They were barely relevant to her needs. For example, commandment number nine proclaimed: "When lifting objects from below your waist, keep your back straight, bend your knees and use a reacher as needed. If you have had hip surgery, you may reach under a counter by sliding your operated leg back behind you and bending your non-operated knee; hold on to a stable surface and follow your TOTAL HIP PRECAUTIONS, if indicated." True, physical therapy provides the opportunity to participate actively in your own recovery, but what did these complex body mechanics accomplish for a patient with arthritic hands who had trouble maneuvering a walker? What were you supposed to do when you had no unoperated leg to compensate for the injured one?

Mother complained angrily that "they" had taken away the special walker that had been customized by the Coral Bay therapists and paid for by Medicare. Her walker had wheels and extra padded armrests for her elbows. I made many phone calls from Caracas about that walker. Finally, getting nowhere fast, I told Marisa to head over to Coral Bay Memorial Hospital, go to Mother's old room, and unobtrusively walk her walker out of the closet. Because Medicare had paid for it, the walker was hers to keep. The therapists told her so. Marisa did exactly what I instructed her to do, and when I called the next day, Mother had her old walker back and was happier during the therapy sessions.

"Seventh day here," Mother observed on May 24. "When can I think of ever walking? Will be evaluated on Thursday." She explained that, if the evaluation went as expected, she would be discharged at the end of the week.

"They're going to dismiss me," Mother said, her voice trembling. "I've gone just about as far as I can."

"Mother, what do you mean by 'dismiss' you? Do you mean they're going to discharge you? Are you walking?"

"I can shuffle back and forth with the walker, but that's about it. I can't get out of bed by myself. I can't go to the bathroom. I can't even get out of the wheelchair."

"But how can they dismiss you if you can't really walk?" I asked. "Who decides? You or them? Let's wait for the evaluation and see what they have to say. I'll ask Noel to speak to Dr. Borosky, and we'll take it from there. I'll fly up beforehand, and we'll work out what's best for you."

"I'm almost sure I'm being dismissed. I've failed the program. There's nothing more they can do for me."

I was puzzled. How could Mother be discharged if she could not walk? Wasn't the whole point of therapy to train people to carry out the activities of daily living? Could anyone seriously believe that ten days of rehab would prepare people to function in the real world? Wasn't this awfully premature?

I called Noel. "Mom's absolutely correct," he said. "I've spoken to Dr. Borosky, and they plan to discharge her on Friday. But she's obviously not ready to go home yet. It will be very complicated. She'll need a hospital bed, a wheelchair, and nursing care. I've discussed it with Mom, and she's decided to go to a nursing home—Pine Manor, across the street from Sacred Heart."

Mother had reached a "plateau," according to the evaluation, and therefore was no longer eligible to receive Medicare benefits. If she chose to stay at Sacred Heart, she would have to do so as a private patient and pay for her bed and therapeutic sessions. I did not like the idea of Mother going to a nursing home, particularly one that neither of us had seen. Just the term "nursing home" scared me. Noel explained that Pine Manor received a lot of patients from Sacred Heart's rehabilitation unit and that he expected to check it out when he visited Mother over the Memorial Day weekend.

I spoke with Mother on Friday morning, the day she was scheduled to transfer to Pine Manor. Yes, they were planning to move her, but she was not sure when. She was very tired and could not complete the physical-therapy session the afternoon before. She had gone to the session, which involved doing exercises on the mattress pad, but had to return to her room to rest. I was upset by Mother's voice. She seemed to be gasping for air at the end of each sentence.

"Mother, what's the matter? How are you feeling? Why are you short of breath?"

"I'm just very tired. I didn't even realize I'm short of breath."

"How long has this been going on? You didn't have this on Wednesday. You must tell the nurse immediately that you're having difficulty breathing. Mother, do you promise?"

"Yes. I'll call her now."

"Fine. I'll get off the phone right away, but I'll call you back first thing tomorrow morning."

I called Mother at least a half-dozen times early Saturday, but the operator kept insisting that she was out of the room. Finally, I demanded to be put through to the nurses' station and was told that Mother was in therapy. When I called back later, the nurse claimed she was in the dining room. I knew that Mother, with her shortness of breath, could not be in the dining room. (Noel was getting the same runaround.) I called the operator again, and she repeated that Mother was simply out of her room. In fact, Mother was not simply "out of her room." She had been rushed to telemetry, an intermediate-care unit, where she was hooked to a non-invasive heart monitor and placed on oxygen.

When I called the telemetry unit on Sunday morning, I was told, "No, I can't put you through until noon."

"Why not?" I asked. "I've been trying to get through for two days, and for two days the operators and floor nurses have insisted that my mother is out of her room. They seem to have been

unaware of her transfer to your unit. Now her condition has worsened, and I must speak to her. I'm calling from overseas, and it's
not that easy to get through."

"Well, I'll put you through this one time."

At last Mother's voice came on the line. She was feeling better, she said, but she was going to be moved again. In fact, the
nurse was with her that very minute and could explain it better
than she could. The nurse took over and explained that Mother
had congestive heart failure and was being transferred from
telemetry to the intensive-care unit (ICU), where she would be
more closely monitored. She was stable and coming along well.
(So why did she need to be moved to the ICU?) She put Mother
back on the line.

"Look, Mother, hang in there. I may not be able to speak to you
directly once you're in the ICU, but I'll be in touch with your
nurse and with Noel. I'll come up as soon as I can pull the arrangements together."

Congestive heart failure was just an educated guess. Dr.
Borosky dictated on May 28: "Today, while transferring herself
from a wheelchair to the platform, she became severely short of
breath and tachycardic [excessively rapid heartbeat]. The patient
denies any chest pressure or discomfort whatsoever. She just
states she felt short of breath and had some palpitations. Of note,
the patient is very frail. It's very difficult for her to move because
of severe deformities of rheumatoid arthritis as well as osteoarthritis and osteoporosis." The doctor also noted slightly decreased
breath sounds at the base of Mother's lungs. He ordered an ECG
(electrocardiogram), which was normal and showed no changes
from the one done when she had arrived in the rehab unit. Dr.
Borosky did not discard the possibility of a pulmonary embolism,
pulmonary edema, pneumonia, a myocardial infarction, or angina.
In other words, he discarded nothing and seemed to be unaware
of Mother's medical history. Most likely, he surmised, she had
had an acute episode of shortness of breath. He recommended a
chest X-ray and an examination of blood gases, as well as bed rest
and nasal oxygen. Mother's chest X-ray was not good. It showed
"bilateral pleural effusions," or fluid in the lungs, a finding that
suggests congestive heart failure under average circumstances.

This was undoubtedly the reason for her immediate transfer to critical care.

The doctor drew pleural fluid from Mother's lungs to make her more comfortable and to collect a specimen for analysis. The light-yellow fluid indicated a chronic active inflammation, but the significance of this result would not become evident to me until many months later.

• • •

I took a late-afternoon flight. Kathy was waiting for me at the airport and drove me directly to the house. Dad and Marisa had just come from the hospital and were in good spirits. "Mother was responding well," he said in a relaxed fashion. I was pleased with Dad. He looked and acted like his old self. His color was good, and there were no signs of forgetfulness as he recounted Mother's progress and her efforts to make it through therapy.

It was too late for me to go to the hospital, so I called Noel, who had already spoken with Dr. Risden. Mother's congestive heart failure was under control, and Dr. Risden was optimistic that she would be able to return to rehab soon—if not at Sacred Heart, then somewhere else where the program was less taxing. I was reassured and decided not to call the critical-care unit. I would get a good night's rest and arrive on time for the 9:00 A.M. visiting period.

I do not know why I called the ICU early the next morning. I expected to go there shortly. But the nursing staff had thoughtfully told Noel and me to call whenever we felt like it. The nurses' station put me through to Mother's nurse, Emma.

"There was a problem last night," Emma said hesitantly. "I'm sorry I have to tell you this. Your mother had a heart block around nine o'clock, and it was necessary to act at once."

"What do you mean by a 'heart block'?"

"Her heart stopped, and we had to work on her. We had to do CPR."

"You mean resuscitate her?"

"Yes. It was necessary to intubate her. We nearly lost her last night," Emma said.

"What do you mean by 'intubate'?"

"We had to put your mother on a mechanical respirator. She was in acute respiratory distress."

"But she was fine all day yesterday. She sat up in a chair and chatted with my father until dinnertime. Why didn't you call us when this happened? Why didn't you call the house? Why didn't you call my brother?"

"We didn't have any of those numbers. We called your cousin. Your cousin was informed."

My cousin? My cousin Mark—my only cousin living in South Florida? I did not understand why Mark was involved. I had prepared a yellow-lined sheet with phone and fax numbers for Noel and me and had given it to the head nurse at Coral Bay, with explicit instructions that it be attached to Mother's medical chart and follow her to Sacred Heart. Still, was it not the responsibility of the Sacred Heart staff to make sure they had the necessary phone numbers, including that of Mother's husband?

My stomach was churning, my legs were quivering, and my hands were shaking as I hung up. It was impossible. The unimaginable was about to happen. I had to get to the hospital instantly. I dressed and tried to compose myself before speaking to Dad. He looked so innocent that I could not bear to destroy his equanimity.

"Dad, I'm going to the hospital now. I just spoke to Mother's nurse. There was some sort of problem last night, and I want to see how she is."

"I'll come with you."

"No, Dad, you stay here. I'm ready to leave. I'll come back for you later, and we'll go over together after your lunch."

I do not recall all the details. I stood nervously at the nurses' station in the critical-care unit while Mother's nurse informed me that her condition had stabilized. She pointed me in the direction of Mother's room, just a few paces away, but I could not see in because the glass wall was curtained off.

Nothing prepared me for the sight of my mother. She was absolutely still, but the hissing and beeping of the monitors and life-support systems sent intermittent sounds through the silent air. She was raised up high in the bed and lightly covered with a sheet. Her hands were loosely tied to the rim of the bedrails. The ventilator to her left, beyond her range of vision, regulated the number of breaths per minute, assisting her on every fifth breath. The whooshes were accompanied by a staccato beat synchronized with her heaving chest. A rigid tube ran from the ventilator into Mother's mouth and down her throat to her lungs; it was held in place with opaque tape that ran above her mouth and around under her chin. A device, called a facutron, was attached to the wall behind her head to suction the secretions from Mother's lungs. Wires ran from Mother's left side, converging in a thick lump under her chest wall, where a temporary pacemaker had been inserted. Tangled cords ran out of her right side and were attached to a Swans-Ganz catheter whose monitor was bolted to the wall. This invasive device had been plunged into Mother's heart chambers through her veins. The monitor looked like a computer screen and showed assorted information concerning her heart function in vivid colors. A pulse oximeter was attached to her right thumb and glowed like an incandescent lamp. This seemingly innocuous instrument was of vital importance in measuring the amount of oxygen in Mother's blood. Numerous clear, thin plastic tubes ran from a Heplock tube in Mother's vein to a jumble of infusion pumps hanging like miniature coats from a metal rack. Each plastic sack contained a crucial liquid that would prevent her organs from shutting down. A Foley catheter, the only object I was familiar with from Mother's Coral Bay stay, was hanging from the foot of the bed, completing this dreadful scene.

Mother's hands and arms were swollen with fluid. I wondered, since she was so thin, whether the edema was apparent to the nurses. Mother's head was pushed grotesquely back by the position of the ventilator tube, and her mouth hung slack. Her face was frightfully angular, with hollow cheekbones jutting up like unexpected knolls in a flat field. Her color was pasty.

How could this have happened in the space of two weeks? On May 15, I had left my spirited mother in full recuperation. Now she was attached to complex life-support systems.

"Mother, Mother, can you hear me?" No response. She appeared to be in a deep coma. I stayed for a few minutes, then searched for Emma. I wanted the details.

But Emma was not on duty, and my cousin Mark ended up describing what had happened. He and his wife, Judy, had dropped in for an unexpected visit, and by chance they witnessed Mother's profound crisis. While quietly conversing, Mother suddenly slumped down and cried out, "My God!" Then she was fine, and apparently nonplussed she continued the conversation. All at once, Mother jerked up with a shocked expression and cried for help. But before Mark or Judy could move, she recovered and insisted she was fine. A few minutes went by, and after crying out for help, Mother slumped over for the third time. Mark ran for the nurse. Mayhem followed. "Code red, code red, code red" reverberated through the loudspeaker. Within seconds, nurses and aides rushed into the room; the double doors slammed to and fro as people hurried in and out with equipment. Mark and Judy were hustled out and told to wait in the critical-care waiting room.

My mother was clinically dead. In a matter of seconds, a nurse was pounding on Mother's chest. Finally, her heart began to beat, and she was intubated. Mark told me that he was in the waiting room for nearly two hours while the staff stabilized Mother. If these extraordinary measures had not been taken, Mother would not have been alive when I arrived from Venezuela. What was less clear was why this had happened. How could a so-called episode of breathlessness conclude in sudden clinical death? I also wondered how much time had elapsed before she was resuscitated. Would she have brain damage if she came out of this? The nurse assured me that Mother was not in a coma but was heavily sedated so the respirator could do its work.

Mother was now in the midst of a pitiful situation she had repeatedly warned me about—one that she never wanted to be in under any circumstances. Five years earlier, following Dad's myocardial infarction and near brush with death, my parents had signed living wills. They used standard forms but had added the following: no cardiopulmonary resuscitation (CPR), no artificial ventilation, and no feeding tubes. I felt ambivalent about Mother's present situation. It seemed to me that her wishes about extraordinary measures had been violated. But despite this violation, I was grateful to find my mother alive, no matter how grim the prognosis. I was relieved to hear that even more invasive procedures, such as electric paddles, electrodes, and emergency surgery, had not been used to resuscitate her heart.

"Did you know that my mother has a living will?" I asked the nurse. "She would have hated the idea of being put on a respirator. I'm so thankful she pulled through, but it's a real conflict."

"Believe me, the only thing we thought about was saving your Mother's life. We didn't know she had a living will. Now that we're aware of it, we'll consult with you while you're here. And bring a copy of it when you come back this afternoon."

"Well, now that it's done, I'd like to read her living will again first. I also want to discuss my mother's condition with her physician."

I knew they would mark Mother's chart with the code "DNR," for "do not resuscitate," if I brought in the living will. I did not want this to happen, because I did not believe that Mother was terminally ill. She was in no position to speak for herself, so I would have to be her advocate.

I dashed down the long corridor to call my brother. Noel had postponed his Memorial Day visit and was scheduled to arrive on the evening of June 3. Jane, his assistant of twenty years, put me through at once when she heard the urgency in my voice.

"Noel, I'm at the hospital, and the news is not good. Mother had a crisis last night. She had what they call a heart block, and her heart actually stopped. She's on life-support systems and seems to be unconscious. See if you can get an afternoon flight and come right away."

"I don't think I can do that. I have appointments all afternoon and no one to cover for me. I have a complicated delivery later tonight. I'll see what I can do about changing my flight, and I'll get back to you tonight."

"Noel, you need to come as soon as possible. This is an emergency. It's nothing like Coral Bay, as awful as that seemed at the time. Mother looks ghastly. She could easily have died last night. You need to fly down today."

I had to go home and collect Dad and Marisa. I told Dad that Mother had had a respiratory crisis and was being helped to breathe by a machine. I did not use the term "heart block" or mention the cardiac resuscitation. We carried a chair into Mother's room and pulled Dad as close to her side as we could. I admonished Dad not to touch any of the tubes. We lowered Mother's bed so he could reach her hand, and there he sat, stroking her edemic fingers and talking to her softly.

"June, open your eyes now. Come on, you've been doing so well." Dad looked at me and asked, "How did this happen so quickly?" Surprisingly, Mother did open her eyes and stared knowingly at Dad. Then she glanced my way. She was still heavily sedated, but I knew she was happy to see us and not at all surprised that I was there.

Dr. Jack Hafner, Dad's cardiologist, had been called into the case. Apparently, Mother had experienced arrhythmias, or irregular and erratic heartbeats, throughout the two days before her heart arrested. Dr. Hafner explained many weeks later that it is not uncommon for patients with lung problems to experience heart arrhythmias. But when Mother was transferred to the ICU, the doctors were still looking for heart problems and incorrectly surmised that her trouble stemmed from congestive heart failure.

I detested the words "congestive heart failure," which are not as ominous as they sound. The term simply means that the heart's pumping action is impaired and the body's oxygen requirements are not being met. Fluid is forced into the lung tissue and collects in the pleural space between the lungs and the chest wall, producing the characteristic symptom of breathlessness. As the condition worsens, the shortness of breath occurs even while the person is resting. A stethoscope positioned at the base of the lungs indicates the presence of rales, or moist, crackling sounds. At the "heart" of heart failure is the impairment of ventricular contractile force. Since she had entered the ICU, Mother had received digoxin, the generic version of digitalis—the drug of choice for improving cardiac output and relieving the symptoms of atrial or ventricular arrhythmias. Mother was given an average dose of 0.125 milligrams but immediately had a toxic reaction, leading to heart block. Her advanced age, petite size, and frail condition all contributed to a rapid buildup of the drug in her bloodstream. This was not unusual. According to the American Heart Association, "toxic manifestations of digitalis include such rhythm disturbances as ventricular premature beats, *heart block*, and atrial tachycardia with a conduction block" (1980:195; emphasis added). Heart block interferes with the normal conduction of electrical impulses, preventing them from traveling through the heart's muscles.

It seemed to me that the digoxin should have been prescribed more cautiously. The elderly are sensitive to medications such as digitalis because their kidneys do not eliminate wastes as efficiently as do younger people's, making them vulnerable to adverse reactions. They should be started off on low doses to prevent serum digoxin levels from building up in the blood. This could have been accomplished easily with the 0.125-milligram tablet, which is designed to be broken into halves.

Dr. Hafner was convinced that Mother had a strong heart and would pull through, but it would take a few days. The only way to counteract the toxic levels of digitalis was to infuse the body with fluids and flush the drug out through the kidneys. It was a matter of waiting patiently.

By late Wednesday, it was clear that Mother's heart was normalizing. Her heart rate was regular; her elevated blood pressure had dropped considerably; her pulse rate was steady; and the oximeter showed that her blood-oxygen saturation level was consistently higher than 90 percent. Mother's nurse mentioned that I might think about introducing a feeding tube. I had initially rejected this suggestion because it was the only procedure stipulated in Mother's advance directive that had not yet been instituted against her wishes. Noel (over the phone) and Dr. Risden also prevailed on me later in the day, insisting that without adequate nutrition Mother would be unable to ride out the crisis. Now I was the bad guy. If anything happened to Mother, I would be responsible for having failed to authorize a lifesaving procedure. If Dr. Hafner was correct, Mother had had a life-threatening crisis but was not terminally ill. Therefore, every effort should be made to pull her through. That was how I thought at the time, and I knowingly went against Mother's living will. I wanted Mother to live. This was probably the sickest moment of her entire life. I went along, although saving Mother would not be easy.

I was drained—tired from the flight the day before, tired from the excruciating tension, and tired of trying to be strong for my ailing father. I was tired of shuttling back and forth throughout the day for the four thirty-minute-maximum visiting periods. To boot, I was not convinced that Dr. Hafner was correct. I understood the business about the heart block but was still confused about what had brought on Mother's problem.

Noel called late. This time, I gave the report. I had half expected to see him that evening, but now it was too late. Obviously, he had not managed to rearrange his schedule. He had moved his flight up, though, and planned to arrive early the next morning and meet me at the hospital.

"By the way," he said, "if I were you, I would take everything out of Mom and Dad's accounts, their CDs, their money markets, and put it all in your name."

I was stunned by this suggestion, although he undoubtedly intended it to make things easier. "What do you mean by that?" I said. "There's no need. It isn't right. Everything that involves Mom and Dad—absolutely everything—I discuss with them. I would never do a thing like that."

"Well, maybe you ought to think about it."

"Look, I'm completely exhausted. The only thing I can think about right now is Mother lying there on life supports. I'll see you tomorrow."

Even if Mother's heart continued to stabilize, the considerable problem of the pleural effusions—the fluids that had collected in the pleural space between the chest wall and the lungs—remained. I expected to speak to Mother's pulmonary-disease specialist in the morning. Dr. Roberto Castronuovo, an Argentinean who had lived in the United States for more than thirty years, was a stickler about making early rounds and comparing each day's test results with those of the previous day. He was not as sanguine as Mother's cardiologist about her prognosis. I recalled that the portable sitting X-ray taken of Mother's chest the day before she arrested showed that she had large bilateral pleural effusions as well as pulmonary infiltrates "compatible with pulmonary edema from congestive heart failure" (as the radiology report read). Another X-ray, taken the day after she was intubated, showed that the "congestive heart failure" had worsened. Dr. Castronuovo was treating Mother with prophylactic doses of the antibiotic clindamycin and intravenous infusions of the diuretic Lasix.

Twice he had drained the thick fluid from Mother's lungs with a special needle. He said we would have to be patient; that we had to be hopeful. He expected Mother's lungs to start clearing and wanted to know the etiology of her lung fibrosis, a condition characterized by an abnormal increase of connective tissue. Had Mother had pneumonia or a similar illness? I explained that the tissue scarring evident in her chest X-ray was probably a consequence of her rheumatoid condition, but had never caused her trouble.

I left the hospital briefly. When I returned, Noel was standing at the foot of Mother's bed. Mother was still in a deep sleep, and Noel was staring at her with a shocked expression that mirrored mine of a day earlier. I knew that he was as shaken as I was. The ICU staff may be used to working with critically ill patients and life-threatening situations—some people, I understand, even relish the challenge and excitement—but for those of us forced to confront this for the first time because of a parent's illness, it is frightful.

Richard Selzer (1993) was right when he observed that even the conscious patient exists in a state of reverie in the ICU. The patient is immobilized not only by his or her delicate condition, but also by the physical attachment to the tubes and machines. The continuous harsh noises of the respirator, and the beeps and alarms of the remaining equipment, compound the dreamfulness already achieved by heavily sedating the patient.

The patient's family exists in a nerve-racking state of anticipation. Will the patient get better or get worse? What is there to talk or think about except the patient's condition? We are on hold and our lives are momentarily suspended; nothing exists except the patient. We maintain a constant vigil.

I trembled when the ICU's pneumatic double doors swung closed behind me, isolating me from the rest of the hospital. In this world of whispering and muted tones, the ubiquitous machines seemed to dominate. The normal bustling sounds of routine patient care were far away and disconnected from this solitary confinement. I wondered why ICUs were located in the bowels of hospitals or at their periphery. To reach the Sacred Heart ICU, we had to walk down a long hallway, far from the main entrance;

take a little-used elevator to the third floor; turn down another endless hallway; and walk past the telemetry unit, with its own separate nurses' station.

We stepped out of Mother's room, and Noel intercepted the day nurse. She had not been on duty the night of the heart block but was sufficiently informed to bring him up-to-date. I could tell she was somewhat in awe of him—nothing like having a medical doctor in the family to gain the attention and respect of the nursing staff, I thought. At the same time, I got along well with anybody who spoke Spanish, which usually put me at the level of the licensed practical nurses and orderlies. I depended on my rapport with the medical community's Hispanic members to stay abreast of Mother's condition. It certainly cut through a lot of red tape. Noel had complained that he had a hard time understanding Dr. Hafner's cardiological jargon, and now I felt the same way. While Noel continued his questions, I took a brisk stroll around the ICU. Some twenty beds in glass enclosures were arranged along the sides of a large rectangular space. A small rectangular nurses' station in the center dominated the unit; from there, the staff could not only peer into each room but could also monitor patients from the screens looming overhead. Some beds were empty; some held patients who seemed indistinguishable from those in regular rooms; and others had patients attached to machines of various sorts. Everyone except Mother was conscious. It saddened me to think that she was probably the most critically ill patient in Sacred Heart that day.

I returned to catch a discussion of blood-oxygen levels. After only a day, I knew that the nurses paid a lot of attention to the pulse oximeter and blood gases. Sherwin Nuland notes that the chief task of the ICU is "to maintain a dependable supply of oxygen to the beleaguered cells of the body" (1994:119). As long as plenty of oxygen circulates in one's blood, death is not imminent. The degree of oxygenation of the body's cells spells the difference between one who is momentarily dead and one who is definitively dead—between clinical death and biological death. In the first four to six minutes after a person has stopped breathing and has no detectable pulse, it is still possible to bring him or her back from clinical death without causing permanent damage.

After that brief window, the cells are starved for oxygen, and the possibility of successful resuscitation dims rapidly (Nuland 1994:121). I, the amateur, however, was obsessed not with the blood gases but with the overhead monitors clearly visible from the ICU's entryway. My eye was invariably drawn to Mother's screen when I entered the unit; I searched for her pulse rate before I went into her room and felt relieved to know that her vital signs were still intact.

Mother awakened that afternoon to the presence of her two children. She was drowsy but seemed to understand what we said. I did not mention the heart block but explained that she had suffered a toxic reaction to the medication. Meanwhile, it was necessary for her to breathe with a mechanical ventilator. I knew she was disoriented about time and place, and I told her what day it was and went through the chronology of how many days she had spent in telemetry and then in critical care. I told her that a feeding tube would shortly be inserted through her nose because she had to have adequate nutrition while recovering from this toxic shock.

At this point, Dr. Hafner walked in. "Well, June, you've given us all a fright, but let me tell you, you're going to be fine. You've had a bad reaction to the digitalis, but your body will eliminate the excess amount. In the meantime, I want you to remember that you have a strong heart, a very strong heart, and you're going to be fine. But you do have to be patient for a few days. All right?"

I liked Jack Hafner immensely. He was unfailingly kindly with his elderly patients and ran an orderly office in which he never left a patient waiting unless he had an emergency. Moreover, none of his patients had to handle the dreaded Medicare paperwork, thanks to his efficient administrative setup. I liked his optimistic approach, which was exactly what we all needed. Maybe Mother really was invincible, as Dr. Hafner seemed to imply.

Noel called me again on Thursday evening. He was staying at a friend's apartment in Fort Lauderdale because his wife, Cynthia, was arriving that evening. Marisa was installed in our study, and it would have been difficult to accommodate them comfortably at home.

"You know," Noel continued to harp, "I think you should sell Dad's stocks and put everything into a money-market account.

Anything might happen with Mother in the hospital. Who's handling the bills? Who's controlling the checks coming in?"

"I would never touch Dad's stocks," I replied. (It had taken Dad more than twenty years to amass his modest portfolio.) "It would kill him. What's the matter with you? It's not even a smart business move, because his dividends provide him with more income than any money-market account could. I told you last night, I always consult with Dad first."

I explained to Noel that Mother had handled the bills over the past year, and now I was doing them. Kathy processed our parents' medical claims and helped Mother balance their checkbook. She had been coming to the house once a week for the past year, so it was natural for her to continue the pattern during Mother's hospitalization.

"Who is this Kathy? How do you know Mother can trust her? Who's there to control which checks go into the bank and which ones don't?"

Noel had a point—not about Kathy, but about the checks. Dividend checks from Mother and Dad's stocks and bonds arrived in the mail nearly every day. It was not inconceivable for one of them to end up accidentally in the garbage.

"Noel, I trust Kathy. Mother trusts Kathy. I've told you a number of times about Kathy and her help with the Medicare forms. Thank God, they have Kathy. She's a wonderful person. Anyway, I go over all the paperwork when I'm in town, and everything's always in order. You're really aggravating me tonight. Let it go. I'm just too tired."

"Didn't you tell me that Kathy threw away the paid phone bills?"

"Yes, but that was once, just an oversight. I spoke with her about it, and she saves everything for me to file."

In fact, Kathy threw away all the paperwork once the medical claim had been processed because she put all the information on a spreadsheet of her own design. Mother adored this system; it eliminated excess paper and let her feel that the matter was accomplished. I, by contrast, was not happy with this method and asked Kathy to throw the paperwork into a "done" portfolio. Then I neatly filed the papers when I came to town, properly matching up and stapling together the Explanation of Your Medicare Part B Benefits (EMOB) with its corresponding Explanation of Payment of Benefits from Prudential, my parents' supplementary AARP insurance carrier. This way I had a chronological record of their medical histories in case I ever needed it.

The year before, I had spent three weeks at my parents' house straightening out Medicare forms. After years of handling matters like a professional accountant, Dad had suddenly started throwing the EMOBs into the garbage. This meant that he neglected to apply to his supplementary carrier for reimbursement. My parents were paying nearly $4,000 annually for supplementary insurance but had failed to collect even the smallest sum they were due. I called the Medicare and AARP hot lines and asked for duplicate statements for the past few months. "Medicare sends enough paperwork to wallpaper an entire hospital," one customer representative said. "It can be overwhelming to the elderly." I spent a lot of time processing the forms and saved my parents a few thousand dollars.

In fairness to Noel, he had offered to take care of the backlogged forms in his office, because he had an employee who handled insurance claims exclusively. But I knew the paperwork had to be dealt with regularly, and I had to come up with a better solution. When I met Kathy, after responding to her flyer for airport rides and learning that she also handled medical claims, I asked her to meet with my mother. Mother was delighted with Kathy and accepted the arrangement with enormous relief. Mother detested the Medicare paperwork. Now, in exchange for a modest fee, she was free of this horrendous chore.

On Friday, I drove to the hospital at 8:00 A.M. to catch Dr. Castronuovo while he made his rounds. Mother's most recent X-ray showed some improvement. It was slow, very slow, but if she continued to progress, he would try to wean her off the respirator over the weekend. Although the level of digoxin in her blood was still high, her heart rhythm had normalized. This was a good sign. Nevertheless, I felt vaguely dissatisfied with the explanations. If Mother had such a strong heart, why did this happen in the first place? It was senseless—it was like missing an important piece of a jigsaw puzzle. I went to the nurses' station and asked to see Mother's chart.

"Impossible," the nurse answered. "You'll have to speak with her doctors first. The only information I can give you is to tell you what medication your mother is taking."

"Tell me: Why does everybody in this unit have access to my mother's medical records except her own daughter?" I asked. "With all your access, none of you seems to be aware that she recently had a double hip fracture."

I would figure it out myself without the chart. Mother looked much better today. The sedatives had practically been eliminated so that her lungs would start working on their own, and her face had lost its pallor. Mother was now linked to a nutrition pump and was receiving a can of Pulmocare, a high-calorie balanced supplement commonly used for respiratory patients, through a tube in her right nostril. The Pulmocare was mixed with green food coloring to show that the substance was entering rather than leaving the body. I could not bear to look at the nasogastric tube, but I knew that without it her chances were slim.

We all met at the house for lunch. Noel and Cynthia had already visited Mother and then gone shopping, carrying in a large bag of bagels and a few pounds of lox and fruit. The thought of eating nauseated me, and I had not eaten in several days. But they ate voraciously, and I wondered whether this was merely another way to handle the stress. I had been completely put off by a phone conversation they had had the previous day, after Noel had seen Mother. "What kind of restaurant do you want to go to tomorrow—Thai or Chinese?" Noel asked. "Maybe a fish place?" Cynthia answered. My stomach was queasy after overhearing this exchange.

We were sitting around the kitchen table when Noel started to question me about Dad's home-health-care bills. Several weeks earlier, Noel had insisted that Dad could not be left alone while Marisa attended English classes. Before returning to Caracas, I called the agency I knew best and hired an aide for a four-hour shift in the evening. The agency asked to be paid up front, a week's fee in advance. This was unusual. The customary practice was for the agency to postpone billing until it had been partly reimbursed by the patient's supplementary insurance carrier. Although Marisa had monitored her hours, the aide claimed to have worked overtime and demanded compensation above and beyond what the agency paid her. It was the aide's word against Marisa's, and I was trying to resolve the mess.

"Why did you pick such an expensive agency?" Noel asked. "Four hundred dollars a week is a lot of money. You chose an agency that charges twelve dollars an hour. I'm sure you can find one for a whole lot less."

"Noel, they all charge about the same—maybe a dollar or two less, at the most. I did the best I could in the available time. I had to take care of a lot of things before leaving. I chose Associated because they're reliable and Mother has used them before." For the past year, Associated Nursing's Medicare division had been sending a visiting nurse to give Mother her Calcimar injections.

"You should have spent more time looking around," Noel said. "I'm not going to spend this kind of money. I pay a lot less for my maid at home."

"What you pay your maid is irrelevant. The aide I hired comes from a licensed home-health-care agency, is bonded, and gives personal care. You're making an incredible fuss about a matter of a few dollars." By now my face had begun to heat up. How dare my brother chew me out in front of everyone, particularly when I was the one doing all the work. I tried to stay calm, but my stomach was churning again.

"Look, Noel, it's not important. I'll pay for Dad's care, and with pleasure. I'm not going to argue about it with you."

At that point, Cynthia fled the kitchen, and my brother and I were alone. The discussion was escalating. "Barbara," he continued, using my childhood name, as he always did, "I'm not paying this expense. And I don't think you should pay it, either. Take it out of their accounts. They've always saved for their old age, and now they're in it. This is what their savings are for."

"No. I don't agree with you. Their savings are not there to be eaten away by medical expenses. Their savings are their security, and their stocks provide them with an income. No one can survive these days on Social Security payments alone. They've always said they wanted to leave their children an inheritance. This has always been very important to both of them."

I had not intended to argue with my brother, but we did argue— bitterly. Even today the details are so painful that I would like to pretend I don't remember. I did not realize at the time that arguments between siblings are not uncommon when a parent's life is at stake. We seemed to be bickering about a small sum of money, but I think we were really talking about commitment. I wanted my brother to be there for my parents—to the same extent I was. That is what the whole disagreement was about.

I was still smarting over our acrimonious exchange when Noel started pontificating about Dad. "We need to have a plan. If it becomes necessary, I'll have to take Dad to Chicago with me and put him in a nursing home."

"There's no need for that. Dad's with Marisa in his own home. He already has his own plan. I resent that you're sitting here talking about Dad—our Dad—as if he's a sack of potatoes. Dad's sitting right in front of you, and it annoys me that you ignore him and talk over his head. If you have any plans concerning Dad, then you ask Dad."

I turned to Dad. "Dad, do you want to go to Chicago now—or at any time in the future?"

"No, of course not," Dad answered. "I don't want to go to Chicago. What about Mother? I wouldn't leave your mother under any circumstances, and we don't want to leave our home."

I turned back to Noel. "Well, so much for Chicago. Now you have your answer. It's enough. You might start by consulting with your parents before making their decisions for them."

Thankfully, Noel chose not to answer back. He just glared. I was breathless and headed for the terrace, leaving Noel and Dad sitting at the dining-room table. Cynthia was on the couch, pretending to read a book, and Marisa was hiding in the den. Dad rushed out to me.

"Please, Barbara, calm down. Don't pay any attention to him. Don't get yourself all worked up. What will we do if something happens to you? I need you; Mother needs you. Calm down. It's not worth it. You can't afford to get sick."

Noel followed me onto the catwalk, as did Dad and Marisa. I had forgotten that they intended to accompany me to the hospital. "Be careful driving," Noel admonished. "You're in no condition to drive. Drive safely."

Cynthia came out. "Do you want to have dinner with us this evening?"

"I can't believe you want to have dinner together," I said angrily. "All you think about is eating. I want to be by myself, and the thought of dinner makes me nauseous."

Mother was now fully alert and indicated with her hands that she wanted her steno pad. I brought it over along with a red marker and propped the notebook up on a pillow. The light and the outside stimuli must have bothered her, because she kept closing her eyes.

"Mother, open your eyes. You're awake now, and I want you to see us. You can't write unless you open your eyes."

"Were you here?" she wrote in a spidery hand. "I am not going to have an operation?" I knew that Mother did not remember my earlier explanation, so I repeated what had happened—what day it was and how long she had been in the ICU. I told her that the doctors expected to wean her off the respirator soon, but they wanted to do it slowly, when they were sure she could breathe on her own. Mother managed to write a few more lines: "They are tormenting me. . . . Please take it off; it's hurting me." I looked at the flashing oximeter clipped to Mother's thumb. Her arthritic finger could not take such pressure for long, and now that the sedatives had worn off, her hands were probably throbbing. I removed the oximeter and untied Mother's hands from the bedrails. The nurses undoubtedly would not like that, I thought, as I made Mother more comfortable.

Later that afternoon, Noel and I thrashed through some issues. I apologized for my strong language; he said he was sorry he had not come for Mother's operation. We both knew it was major surgery and Mother might not survive it. I explained that Dad had kept asking where Noel was, where Cynthia was. He could not understand why no one had come. Dad needed plenty of care, too. He was still recovering from cataract surgery and was not feeling well. Dad wanted his children with him, not some hired aide. I wondered whether my brother would ever see that no hired hand could take the place of an adult child. Each of us was a separate child. Noel had his own, unique relationship with our parents. My presence could not absolve him from being there.

Noel claimed he felt like an outsider because I was always there. I contended that I did not expect him to have the same relationship with our parents that I did, yet he had made himself an outsider. "Maybe you're more sensitive than I am," he said, "because I never realized they needed to have things done. Every time I asked them, when we were here, they said they didn't need any help."

I, however, took them to their doctors, did their banking, cleaned and organized the house, shopped for food, and took care of the other errands they invariably saved for my visits. Dad even saved his surgical procedures and sprang them on me the minute I arrived. And I did this all while living abroad. Now I was beginning to feel the stresses of a long-distance caregiver. I had moved to Caracas twenty years earlier after marrying my Italian-Venezuelan husband. At first it was a lark to visit my parents a few times a year, but now I could barely keep up with their growing needs. Noel either had no idea what had been going on or had refused to see it. For the past year, Mother arose and showered every morning, dressed herself, and read the newspaper, then spent most of the remaining day on the living-room couch. Her hands had become useless (despite several surgeries), and only her strong determination and Dad's help kept her going. Mother never explained any of this to Noel. If he had visited regularly, he would have figured out the situation on his own. I certainly never expected to give him a rundown of all the things I routinely did for our parents.

At the heart of the differences between Noel and me lay gender and professional issues. I had the impression that my brother expected me to respond first to my parents' emergencies. In recent years, he was always busy, whereas I was rarely too busy; his time was invaluable, and mine was dispensable; he was on a tight schedule, and my university hours were flexible; he was a medical doctor, and I was a dilettante with a doctoral degree in anthropology who dabbled in book publishing and took exotic field trips to the Amazon and other out-of-the way places, helped by my husband's financial support, my modest salary, and occasional grants. Did he have this attitude because he had been treated differently while we were growing up? Boys were taught that men had to support a family, and girls were taught that women would probably have a husband to depend on. Later, Mother apologized for foisting these ill-conceived notions on us. She was a victim of her times, she said, and had been entirely wrong.

Noel tended to think like a medical professional rather than a son when it came to our parents' care, and his collegial relationships with their physicians interfered with his role as an effective caregiver. I felt that I needed to question Mother's doctors every step of the way and that they needed to inform me about changes in her treatment. I was not challenging their medical expertise, as my brother charged, but asserting my role as an advocate. I did not act as though I knew more than Mother's doctors, and so far I had not offended anybody.

I sensed that Noel was feeling sorry for himself. How could anyone have such sick parents—parents with so many infirmities? I understood because I had often had the same thoughts. Our mother had a rare combination of chronic, degenerative auto-immune diseases, and our father had suffered three major heart attacks. The third, in 1987, nearly killed him and left him a cardiac cripple. In addition to the heart attacks, he had had major prostate surgery, several skin cancers, two hernia operations, a pacemaker insertion, double cataract surgery, and numerous diagnostic procedures—that is, twelve hospitalizations since 1979. Now, a general systemic decline characterized by short-term memory loss complicated the dreary picture.

"Well, tough luck," I said. "We have no right to feel sorry for ourselves. They're the ones who should feel bad. They're the ones with the terrible luck. Still, they've managed to handle their infirmities with dignity and strength."

"Well, perhaps you're right," Noel said skeptically.

"You know, Noel, maybe you will have to shuttle back and forth twenty times or so in the next few months. You can't think about it when it's an emergency; you just have to put everything aside and go. I think that's the least our parents can expect from us. They were good parents—wonderful parents, in fact. They always put our needs first when we were children. Sure, it would be wonderful if our parents could grow old gracefully. But they still have each other—maybe not in the way they wanted, but between the two of them they've managed to function as a whole individual."

Noel and I reached an accommodation of sorts. I had to admit that it was difficult for us to act in unison, because we lived in different countries and saw each other infrequently. Our entire adult relationship had been mediated through our parents, and now we had to act together on our own and do what was best for our desperately ill mother.

That night, Dad had severe heart flutters. He woke up with a start and complained of chest pains. I slipped a tiny nitroglycerin tablet under his tongue and made him a cup of herbal tea heavily sweetened with honey. I probably should have called for an ambulance but surmised that it was an emotional reaction to my quarrel with Noel. Slowly, Dad's flutters disappeared, but I can't say we got much rest that night.

Saturday brought more of the same. Noel and I managed to visit Mother amicably. She wrote, "I'm not crazy? They make you think you're crazy.... Am I crazy? Where am I? ... I'm a prisoner.... Too much effort.... Is this necessary?" Mother was miserable. Her body ached, and she wanted her position changed more frequently. Her chest throbbed from the pounding she had been given the night of the resuscitation. Her throat was swollen and sore from the tube; her mouth was dry; and she craved an orange. The Foley catheter pinched, and she had several bouts of diarrhea.

"First professional treatment by my son and utterly natural." This comment puzzled Noel. Mother also wrote something about a baby, but I could not decipher all the words. The matter of the baby was a mystery whose significance became clear to me only later. "Don't give any money away," Mother continued. She had been staring at the large cross on the wall since she had opened her eyes, and I assumed she was referring to the clergy. I told Mother I was keeping a running record of all her treatments so she would know exactly what had been done to her and why. Mother nodded and drifted off to sleep.

At this point, a rabbi walked into the room, but I did not invite him to stay. Throughout her ordeals, Mother had never asked for a rabbi. She deeply believed in God, but that was a private matter, and she did not feel the need for spiritual counseling. I wondered what the rabbi would think if I told him that my Jewish mother prayed to a Catholic folk saint. The rabbi glanced at Mother with pity. "Hey," I wanted to shout at him, "it's not what you think. My mother will come out of this; she's not dying. Don't look at her like that." But, of course, I did not say anything. I just smiled at the rabbi, and he apologized for intruding.

As I put away Mother's steno pad, a small piece of paper slipped out of her diary. It was torn from the menu for the day Mother had felt the acute breathlessness. She must have known that something was brewing. She scribbled: "Beloved family, darling too, of course Mrs. B. [for Barbara]. . . . I rely on Noel to feel as a brother, to remain your brother, to be someone to turn to . . . so sorry not able to take care of . . . so tired of the pain—Don't forget grandchildren."

Dr. Castronuovo planned to take Mother off the respirator on Sunday afternoon. He was being cautious because he wanted this to go well. The respiratory therapist had tried briefly on Friday, but Mother still needed help every few breaths. When I arrived on Sunday morning, Mother was breathing on her own and was receiving only oxygen from the machine.

Noel and Cynthia came for their final visit. I did not understand how they could leave while Mother was still attached to the respirator. "We'll just have to see how you do," Noel told Mother. "We just have to wait and watch. I'll call Barbara tonight when we arrive in Chicago."

Mother was apprehensive about the respirator. I told her to relax, because if she started hyperventilating, the job would be much tougher. She was already breathing on her own, I reminded her. The matter now was removing the endotracheal tube. Mother wanted her steno pad.

"I've begun to think everyone else is lying to me, and I'm insane," she wrote.

"No, no," Noel interjected, "that's not so."

"No, please, Mother," I added, "you know I would never lie to you, and certainly not about something as important as this. You're going to be drinking a glass of water within a few hours. You're going to be fine. Dad and I will be here with you."

Noel said good-bye, and Cynthia embraced me. I was close to tears and pulled back stiffly. I wanted to respond, to be able to depend on them, but I could barely forgive them for the anguish I had felt the day before. They must have been nervous and upset, as well, but I was still too angry to see it.

"Orange," Mother continued to write. "I want a piece of orange. It's been so frightening. I must be having hallucinations."

"As soon as they take out the tube," I said, "you can wet your mouth. I know it must be very dry. But right now I want you to forget about the machine. You've been breathing on your own all morning. Let me tell you a story."

I told Mother a funny story about a Canary Island woman who flew to Venezuela in search of her long-lost husband and discovered that he had committed bigamy. Finally, the nurse came into the room and asked us to leave while the endotracheal tube was removed. We could come back in about an hour. I took Dad to the coffee shop, praying silently that all would go well. Mother could not afford to backslide. In my naiveté, I expected my old mother back within the hour. I had no idea what being weaned from a respirator actually involved.

When we returned, Mother was sitting up comfortably on newly fluffed pillows. The machine was gone, and her hands were free. But within a few seconds, before she could even speak, a horrible retching began as Mother coughed up accumulated phlegm. She heaved all afternoon in the attempt to rid herself of greenish globs of thick, sticky mucus. I kept passing her wads of soft tissue and encouraged her to bring up as much as possible. Why, I wondered, didn't the nursing staff prepare us for this? Dad looked faint and I felt woozy myself from Mother's continued retching. I was disappointed she could not speak; she made a valiant effort, but had no voice. It was back to the steno pad, where Mother expressed her need for liquid to quench the dryness. Her lips were chapped and split from the tube, and her nose was crusted with scabs from the friction of the feeding tube. Her mouth also bothered her. She had developed thrush, a fungus infection, and needed to be treated with the antifungal drug nystatin. By late afternoon, the heaving had quieted, and I felt confident that Mother would survive the weaning. Her vital signs were normal, but she would have to stay on the feeding tube for a few more days.

I wanted to believe that Mother would bounce back with verve, but the experience had taken a terrible toll. Mother's body was wasted and she was so weak she could not even pull herself into a sitting position. Everything she had accomplished during the ten days of intensive rehabilitation had been annihilated by her seventeen days in the ICU.

Mother was as mad as hell when I returned the next morning. Her helplessness infuriated her. Still unable even to whisper, she wrote, "Because I could not drink the juice as my mouth was too dry, she would not give me anything. . . . I won't look at her again." Mother was furious with the nurse who had either slighted her or had not taken the time to understand what she wanted. She needed plenty of liquids and wanted to know whether she was allowed to drink as much as she could. I watched the two nurses pick up my mother under the arms and drag her to the armchair. I could see she was in pain and started to flinch.

"Please," I said. "Be careful. My mother is recovering from double hip surgery. You're liable to dislocate her hips if you continue to move her that way."

"That's why we ask the visitors to leave when we're working on a patient," one of the nurses snapped at me. "We don't need anybody to tell us how to do our job."

"I understand that," I said, trying to maintain my composure, "but I'm not telling you how to do your job. I'm reminding you of my mother's double hip fracture. Now that she's off the ventilator and can be moved from the bed, there's no point in dislocating her hips." I knew they were doing their job, but I did not like how they were handling my mother. Not only did they lack the slightest notion of physical therapy, but they were obviously unfamiliar with Mother's recent medical history. I thought about Mother's charts, which the nurse had refused to let me see; at least I would have read them.

Now it was Mother's turn to do her job. The feeding tube was coming out, and she would have to start eating—whether she had an appetite or not. Her life depended on it. Dr. Risden and his associate, Richard Ronfeldt, walked in and tried to persuade Mother that she was going to be all right. They exhorted her to eat. They almost made her believe that a good bowl of chicken soup would miraculously restore her health. There were no restrictions. Mother could eat anything she wanted—anything at all—

as long as she received some nourishment. They were going to start Mother on a pureed diet because her throat was sore and she felt an obstruction when she swallowed. Meanwhile, the naso-gastric tube would remain in place so Mother's caloric require-ments would continue to be met through liquid supplements.

Poor Mother. I nagged her endlessly about the food. I brought her a chocolate milkshake from McDonald's. I thought the cold drink would soothe her throat, but she took a few sips and turned away. "I'll finish it later," she said. The next day I brought home-made vegetable soup that I had pureed in the blender with half-and-half to make it thick and creamy. After that, I tried my clas-sic vichyssoise, which Mother claimed was delicious. But that, too, ended up in the ICU's refrigerator. Mother did not want to eat. I was reminded of Richard Selzer's experience in the ICU, where he was literally harassed into eating: "Eat! You must eat! Each day and many times each day he is bidden to eat. . . . You must eat in order to live. But to eat without the blessing of hunger cannot be done" (1993:83).

On Mother's fourth day without the respirator, her nurse inter-cepted me as I walked into the unit. "You know," she said, "I've been a critical-care nurse for a long time, and I've seen a good number of patients like your mother. Your mother is not trying. She's not going to make it if she doesn't start eating. Believe me, I know. I've seen it before. She has come to a fork in the road and has given up."

"Well," I retorted, "you don't know my mother. I don't think you're in a position to tell me whether my mother is or is not going to make it. Even her doctors would not presume this." Still, even though I disliked the message, I listened. The nurse was concerned, and deep down, despite my defensiveness, I knew she was right.

I steeled myself as I walked into Mother's room. "Mom, I'm going to speak to you frankly. I know you have no appetite, and the thought of food makes you want to puke. But we're talking about something more important here than your appetite. You have to eat. It's a life-and-death matter. You've come this far, and I've watched you through every single minute of it. Now you have to eat. I mean it. You have no choice. You must eat so they can remove the tube and get you out of this unit. You've already been here nearly two weeks. I don't care about the visiting hours. Either Marisa or I will be here during every single meal, including breakfast, to help you eat." I knew Mother was listening.

Now I did my part. I went downstairs to the kitchen and searched out the dietitian. If Mother was going to start eating, the food would have to be palatable. The hospital's pureed foods were not fresh; they were preprepared frozen patties. It was impossible to tell what was on Mother's tray. The sight, alone, would make anyone want to gag. Gray, congealed food droppings with little flecks of white fat sat side by side on the plate. Truly, I would not feed such slop to my dog. The dietitian agreed to give Mother a regular menu to mark; then her selection would be pureed and sent up to the ICU. I insisted that the meal be sodiumfree. It did not make sense to permit sodium in the diet while Mother was being treated with diuretics.

Noel called me religiously every evening, but there was little to report, because Mother's progress was so slow. Each time he phoned, he picked at a different issue.

"I think you should go over to the bank and remove everything from the safe deposit box. You know, Mother can even die, and you won't be able to get in."

"Where did you get that idea from?"

"I consulted my father-in-law."

"Noel, all you do is call and tell me you've consulted with your father-in-law. Who asked you to consult with your father-in-law? Why don't you consult with me first? You always give unsolicited advice." I paused for effect. "Maybe you should start listening. Don't involve your father-in-law in our parents' affairs. It's none of his business, and what's more, he knows nothing about Florida law."

"Well, if I were you I'd take the proper precautions."

And the next evening: "Look, I don't trust Kathy. There are too many opportunities for something to go wrong."

"Noel, you're irritating me by harping on this. What are we dealing with here, multimillionaires?"

"Well," he continued, "I want to know if she's registered and bonded by the State of Florida."

"Noel, I trust Kathy; Mother trusts Kathy; Dad trusts Kathy. And that's all you need to know."

I decided to bring the matter up directly with Kathy. She was one of the few people I could talk to, and she phoned me regularly to see how things were coming along. Yes, of course she was registered, she said. Noel wanted to see a copy of her registration when I reported back to him.

"Look, I've had enough. Let it go, Noel. If you have a problem with Kathy, here's her phone number. You can call her yourself and ask her anything you want. But I don't want to hear about this anymore. The only thing I'm interested in right now is Mother's progress, and we have to take that one step at a time."

My husband was my salvation. My conversations with Noel were so unsettling that, when I hung up, I immediately called Graziano to commiserate. There was no resolution in my phone conversations with my brother. I understood that he was anxious and wanted to cover all contingencies, but I felt that many of his suggestions were misguided. I was an anti-planner; I saw no point in planning obsessively for one's old age when the first unanticipated illness could instantly demolish carefully constructed plans.

"How come one parent can handle two growing children," I asked Graziano, "but two grown children cannot manage one elderly parent?"

He quoted a proverb from his native province of Friuli, in northern Italy: "When the parents give to their child, the parents laugh and the child laughs, but when the child gives to the parents, the child cries and the parents cry." Graziano had learned the proverb from his maternal grandmother, and I had heard it many times before. Nothing could have been more appropriate at that moment.

Mother's heart no longer required constant monitoring. Dr. Hafner removed the temporary pacemaker and the Swans-Ganz catheter, and the next day Mother was transferred back to telemetry. But her lungs showed no significant improvement. Mother had had twenty-four portable chest X-rays, which suggested worsening congestive heart failure. I continued to have misgivings about the diagnosis. According to one report, the greater amount of fluid on the left side was consistent with a diagnosis of congestive heart failure. When Dr. Hafner was called in to read Mother's echocardiogram, he was surprised to see a normal left ventricle with a more than adequate ejection fracture rate. This was inconsistent with congestive heart failure. He found no evidence of severe left ventricular disease—or, at least, not enough to cause congestive heart failure. This mystery was left dangling. I assumed that Mother's lungs would slowly clear. It never occurred to me that anything bad could happen once she came home.

• • •

While Mother was still in the critical-care unit, I went to the rehab unit to talk to her physiatrists. Dr. Borosky was on vacation, and Mother's attending physician, Dr. Hicks, had not returned my numerous phone calls. I merely wanted to know whether Mother could return to rehab. I was lucky that day. Dr. Hicks was at the nurses' station and could not avoid me. She was not particularly happy to see me and seemed embarrassed by my presence.

"I'm sorry, but your mother is not a candidate for therapy at this hospital," Dr. Hicks said. "I watched her doing therapy, and she was unable to keep up. She has multiple problems and cannot be rehabilitated here."

"I received a very different impression from the therapists who worked with her," I responded. "They said she was coming along well. It seems to me you have to make some allowances for patients like my mother who have chronic problems. She's probably the first person to enter this rehab unit with a double hip fracture, yet you expected her to complete an accelerated program in the same amount of time as the others. You saw my mother when she was still at Coral Bay. I don't think you should have admitted her to the program under the circumstances you've just described. You should have done an assessment of her medical condition and discussed the requirements with her beforehand. I don't think she would have entered the unit if she had any inkling about the six hours of daily therapy."

"Well, I'm sorry, but I can't do anything for your mother." And with that Dr. Hicks turned her head, making it obvious that she had nothing more to say.

Dr. Hicks's rebuttal stunned me. What a jerk, I thought. I knew she had lied. She had not seen my mother practice in the therapy room—not even once. While Mother was in the ICU, I had spoken with her therapists, and both the therapists and Marisa agreed about this. Dr. Hicks was rude to me, and she had succeeded in making my mother feel incompetent because she had failed to meet the demands of the program.

What really bothered me was Dr. Hicks's attitude. Not once had she called to ask how her former patient was coming along in the ICU. Mother could have fallen off the edge of the earth as far as Dr. Hicks was concerned. I tried not to feel bitter about this, but her indifference bothered me. Every patient, no matter how ill, needs to have some hope, and it is the physician's moral obligation to nurture it. I felt that Mother could learn to walk again under the proper circumstances. It was just a matter of personalizing a program that would give her enough time to compensate for her other health problems. I knew my mother and what she was capable of accomplishing.

But sadly, the system works against patients who are in a category by themselves. Medicare allows only a certain number of days for the rehabilitation of a hip fracture patient. What about a double hip fracture, an occurrence so rare that no guidelines exist? What about a person with a chronic disease who tires easily? What about a person with no upper-body strength or disabled hands? These patients have unique needs. Why does Medicare treat everyone the same? As soon as the patient is "stabilized" or reaches a "threshold," he or she is discharged, regardless of whether he or she can function in the outside world. Who decides, anyway, when a patient is stable? Certainly not the patient. The patient is merely the passive recipient, the invisible partner, in this medical pas de deux.

When it was decided for Mother that she had reached a "plateau," she was no longer eligible for Medicare benefits, even though she could barely walk. She was eligible for only a hurried discharge. Under early Medicare guidelines, patients received therapy in the hospital and went home after a long stay, because hospitals were reimbursed by Medicare for each day of a patient's stay and were motivated to keep him or her there as long as possible. When the rules changed and the average hospital stay was drastically cut, hip-fracture patients began to be discharged not to home but to skilled nursing facilities where they could complete their therapy. The current system harms patients with pre-existing conditions because it practically guarantees that they will be discharged to nursing facilities. Recent studies show that early discharges to nursing homes contribute to the failure rate of hip-fracture patients because they rarely regain their former abilities and end up needing long-term custodial care.

• • •

Mother was in the telemetry unit for three-and-a-half days and continued to improve slowly. I was amazed at the transformation that took place when all the invasive lifesaving gizmos that had kept her tethered to the bed were removed. Graziano could not hide his surprise when he saw Mother. He had arrived from Caracas expecting the worst on the morning of her transfer to telemetry. Instead, he found his mother-in-law reclining on a pile of pillows, looking serene. Mother put on a good show.

"How are you doing, June? You had us plenty worried," Graziano said.

"I could be worse," Mother whispered hoarsely. "I'm feeling fairly well."

"You've had quite an experience."

"I know. Now I can't wait to go home."

Thud, thud! At that moment we heard a crash. I jumped and turned around. Dad had been clinging to the foot of the bed. When he went to sit down, he missed the edge of the chair and sank to the floor. The chair slid over, hitting the floor lamp, which toppled over onto Dad's head.

"Dad, are you all right?" I cried as I ran over to help him. The noise had been so loud that a nurse came hurrying in. Together we collected Dad and determined that nothing was broken. I moved the chair alongside Mother's bed, sat Dad down, and stood on the other side. I was upset. Dad had had a fall with no ill effects just before Mother moved to Sacred Heart. I had better watch him more carefully, I thought. We certainly did not need any more falls.

I looked at Mother's elderly roommate, who was coming out of a diabetic coma and was clearly petrified. She could not express herself clearly and seemed frustrated by this. Her daughter tried to calm and comfort her unsuccessfully.

"No, no, no," she moaned. "I don't want to stay here. I don't want to be ill. I want to leave. Help me, help me!"

"Mammy, please, you're going to be all right. But the doctor says . . ."

And so on, and so on. I felt for this woman and her daughter. I felt sad about the lack of privacy that prevented families from sharing their feelings with one another. I found the moaning disturbing; the poor woman was not handling her hospitalization well. The daughter glanced at Mother and me, and a look of empathy passed between us. Then an aide pulled the curtain around the roommate's bed, supposedly to protect her privacy. But we could still hear her moaning. I glanced at Mother. She had never moaned—not once. Mother had an innate grace. I realized how difficult it was to retain this sense of self when one is so desperately ill.

Mother's bravery reminded me of the story Simone de Beauvoir related about her mother in *A Very Easy Death* (1964). Maman had suffered from arthritis for years, but because her heart was so strong, her daughter rarely fretted. A pedestrian event put an end to that: Maman fell in her bathtub, fractured her femur, and had to be taken away by an emergency service. The femur had not shifted, and the doctor insisted that three months of bed rest would restore Maman to her former condition. A second doctor, however, "doubted whether she would recover in three months. . . . Breaking the neck of the femur was not in itself a serious matter, but a long period of lying still caused bed-sores, and with old people they did not heal. The prone position was tiring for the lungs: patients developed pneumonia and it carried them off" (De Beauvoir 1964:17). In her relatively youthful insouciance, Simone de Beauvoir still was not especially worried. Her seventy-seven-year-old mother was "tough." Then disaster struck. The fall had been caused by a nasty stomach tumor, not a careless move. Now the daughter began thinking not about convalescence but about the death bed. But Maman, in her "desperate eagerness" to get well and please her daughter, was ready to endure anything with enormous courage.

On June 15, two weeks after Mother's heart had stopped, she was moved to the general medicine floor. She was able to speak in a loud whisper, but her new voice had a reedy, imploring quality that seemed to reflect the enormous trauma she had endured. I hoped that Mother's voice would regain its lilt. Mother did not receive much attention on the regular floor. The high point was a compassionate attendant who lavished endearments on her while transferring her to the unit.

"Now sweetheart," he said, "whatever you need, I'm right here. Are you sure you're comfortable?" He gently wrapped a warm blanket about Mother's frail form and took her hand as he wheeled her stretcher down the dimly lit hallway.

I followed right behind. Little did I know that such blandishments scarcely represented the level of care on the general medicine floor. The quality of the nursing care was not comparable to that at Coral Bay—and certainly not to that in Sacred Heart's telemetry unit. I will not go into the awful details except to note that Mother wanted to go home. No doubt about it, Mother wanted out.

On her second day on the new floor, Bruce Zeigler, another associate of Dr. Risden's, informed Mother that her condition had "stabilized" and she was ready to be discharged. I expressed my concerns about going from critical care to home care in less than a week. Mother was still feeble, and I felt that she needed more time to build up her strength. His hands were tied, Dr. Ziegler said. As long as Mother's condition was stable, he had no justification under Medicare's guidelines to keep her in the hospital. According to his reasoning, my mother was an adult with all of her faculties. She was capable of making her own decisions (even though she could not care for herself physically), and she wanted to go home.

I was reluctant to question Dr. Zeigler's word, but should have insisted that Mother stay in the hospital for a few more days to make sure her "stable" condition was truly stable. I could not believe that she was strong enough to go home. She had just come back from the world of the dead. Further, I knew what had happened a few years earlier when Dad's cardiologist rushed him out of Cypress Humana Hospital five days after a mild heart attack. The first day he was home, he had an explosive heart attack that nearly finished him.

The matter of early discharges originated with the introduction of the Prospective Payment System (PPS) and Diagnostic Related Groups (DRGs) in 1983 to stem Medicare abuses. Hospitals receive a fixed rate of payment and are allotted a fixed number of days for each principal diagnosis. Once these limits are exceeded, Medicare reimbursements to the hospital cease, creating an environment in which the hospital is encouraged to discharge patients as quickly as possible. Although some flexibility exists when a patient has complications and needs more time in the hospital, the notion of "stabilized" seems ridiculously vague. The moment the attending physician decides the patient is no longer acutely ill, the patient is booted out, regardless of whether he or she is ready. The system is paternalistic because the patient is merely a passive recipient of externally dictated decisions. Mother was never asked whether she felt well enough to leave the hospital. She was simply informed that the time had come for her to leave. She had to decide whether she wanted to be discharged to a nursing facility or to home.

These days, hospital social workers are actually "discharge planners" who are caught in a "tug of wills between competing phantoms," according to the bioethicists Nancy Dubler and David Nimmons (1992:67–68). Instead of advising patients and their families about their options, the social worker's primary function is to get patients out before they exceed their DRG limits. If the social worker succeeds in discharging a patient before his or her allotted time is up, the unused portion of the fixed reimbursement constitutes a profit for the hospital. This system saves thousands of dollars for hospitals and for Medicare, but it is notoriously detrimental to the patient's best interests. The burden ultimately falls on the family, who must care for the patient at home or find a facility where he or she can complete the convalescence.

Sacred Heart wanted Mother out, and fast. The staff almost seemed to be withholding adequate care deliberately so she would be encouraged to leave. For all the attention she was now receiving, she was better off at home. She could not even turn on her side by herself and was not ready for any sort of therapy. It was like starting over again but with the considerable disadvantage of having survived a near-fatal relapse. By now, Mother had been hospitalized for seven weeks and was going stir-crazy. Psychologically she needed a respite. She yearned to be in her own home, among her own things, within calling distance of those she loved. She needed home cooking; she needed to read the newspaper, peruse her books and papers, and recline on her favorite couch overlooking the beautiful greens. No hospital, no nursing home could possibly compensate for the ordinary things she had lost. It was time for Mother to go home.

I was still a novice at understanding hospital politics. Eventually, I realized that hospitals like to clear patients out before the weekend, and they will probably tell you about it the day before, making it difficult to arrange for home care. I had no realistic idea of what caring for Mother at home would involve, and nobody— from the social-services department to the attending physicians— enlightened me. I wondered whether I would be able to handle it but cast the doubts guiltily aside.

Curiosity prompted me to visit the nursing home Mother would have gone to had she completed her therapy at Sacred Heart. Pine Manor is one of the oldest nursing homes in Fort Lauderdale and is conveniently located across the street from the hospital. I wanted to see the place for myself, just in case. Of course, Mother had already expressed her desire to go home, and I felt she was far too weak to receive the care she needed in any nursing-home setting. The place was run-down, but the nursing director, Susan, was charming and seemed competent. Later I learned that she had a reputation as one of the finest nursing directors in South Florida.

"Don't worry," Susan said. "If you need us, we'll be here, and you can call me at any time. I want you to know that you don't have to move your mother directly into a nursing home from the hospital. She has thirty days from the time she leaves the hospital to the time of entering the nursing home. She will not lose her Medicare benefits if she is admitted before the end of the thirty-day period. Take her home; do what you think is best for her; and when she's feeling a little stronger, you can discuss it with her."

I was relieved by this persuasive argument. It was good to know that the nursing home was there in case Mother needed it. I was also surprised by Susan's familiarity with the Sacred Heart scene. Apparently, it was not unusual for Sacred Heart rehabilitation patients to transfer to Pine Manor. "After all, how many eighty-year-olds can keep up with that type of therapy? The pace is simply too exhausting," she noted.

• • •

Mother was coming home at noon. Sacred Heart's social-services department made the arrangements for a non-emergency van and called a medical-supply company to deliver a hospital bed, an adjustable table, a wheelchair, and a commode early that morning. I expected to set up the equipment in the den so Mother could look out over the golf course, and I hoped to have a few quiet hours to arrange everything before my meeting with Dr. Zeigler to review her medication and discharge plans. But the phone rang at 6:00 A.M. It was Mother, and she was crying.

"Please, Mummy," I said, "try to calm down and tell me what happened. How did you manage to call out so early?" Apparently, an orderly had walked into her room a few minutes before and put through the call. She had been trying to reach the phone for several hours, but it had been placed beyond her reach. Every evening I set up the bedside tray with the phone, tissues, and a glass of water within Mother's reach, and every morning I went through the same routine, because the tray had been moved to the foot of the bed.

"I've had it. I want to die," Mother said. "I won't go on any more like this. It's so humiliating. How dare they come in here and shout at me. How dare they yell at me because I was wet. They treat you worse than an animal."

"Mummy, who shouted at you? What happened exactly?"

"I kept calling for the nurse, ringing the button. Nobody came. Then I yelled for the nurse, and finally someone walked in. [Mother's room was directly in front of the nurses' station.] Something was wrong. The catheter was pinching me. I think it came out, and I was completely wet. The nurse started to scream at me for being wet. I could stay wet all night, for all she cared, and then she slapped my hands. I kept calling for another nurse all night long, and nobody came in until this nice guy walked into the room. How could she slap my hands? I want to die. I want to die right now. I can't go on anymore."

I did not doubt Mother for one second. If she said that something had happened, then it had happened. I was shocked that a nurse—or whoever she was—had verbally terrorized my mother and slapped her hands. It was easy to see that Mother's hands were badly deformed. I was in a rage but tried to control my voice.

"Mother, do you want me to come over right now?"

"Yes. I'm going crazy. I can't take it any longer."

"I'll be over in a few minutes. Remember that you're leaving today. It's not worth getting upset about. You'll never have to deal with those people again. You're coming home. I'll be over right away."

I was determined to have it out with the head nurse, but when I arrived at the hospital, I learned that the guilty party *was* the head nurse—the one on the night shift. The nurses' station was deserted when I left the elevator, and I went directly to Mother's room. She had calmed down but was still sopping wet. Now a practical nurse was seated at the station. I told Mother's story and insisted on seeing the head nurse immediately. The culprit appeared and claimed that my mother had imagined the incident. I said I would talk to her supervisor when she arrived on the floor.

Mother's catheter was checked and reinserted properly; her sheets were changed; and she was dressed in a fresh hospital gown. I helped her with breakfast and collected her few belongings. Dr. Zeigler appeared, and while he was with Mother I searched for the daytime nursing supervisor. I told her that I would send a formal letter of complaint to the hospital. She assured me that nothing like this had ever happened before and that she would speak with the nurse. But I did not believe she would follow through. Once we were out of there, we were old news. I told Mother I had to go home to wait for the hospital equipment and would be back shortly to accompany her in the van.

Advance Directives or Misdirectives?

Interpreting a Parent's Last Wishes

I WAS in a quandary. I had disobeyed every one of Mother's directives. She had given me precise instructions about what she did and did not want to be subjected to if she was incapable of expressing her own wishes. We had gone over her living will many times in the past few years, and I thought I understood. Now I realized that I understood nothing and that her living will was not clear. It was a standardized version distributed by Concern for Dying, the New York organization that created the first living-will registry in the 1960s. The will had two sections: a general philosophical statement concerning the ultimate goals of one's medical treatment, and an optional section for listing specific provisions. When I reread the document in light of the recent events, I realized that the statement of objectives was too vague to be meaningful, particularly when Mother could not speak for herself. It said: "If at such a time the situation should arise in which *there is no reasonable expectation of my recovery* from extreme physical or mental disability, I direct that I be allowed to die and not be kept alive by medications, artificial means or 'heroic measures'" (emphasis added). Mother listed three measures of artificial life support to be refused in the face of impending death: 1) electrical or mechanical resuscitation of the heart when it has stopped beating; 2) mechanical respiration when she was no longer able to sustain her own breathing; and 3) nasogastric tube feeding when she was unable to take nourishment by mouth.

Mother counted on Dad (who was no longer capable) and her children to make the right decisions on her behalf. We each had copies of her living will, but she had never given one to any of her physicians. Mother's failure to inform her physicians is not uncommon. Few patients are motivated to discuss the matter of advance medical directives with their doctors. Recent estimates suggest that only 8–15 percent of adults in the United States have prepared living wills to indicate their preferences for the kinds of medical intervention to be carried out under emergency conditions. The problem may rest not with the patients but with the physicians. Death and dying are not within the realm of ordinary discourse for most physicians. Only 20 percent routinely discuss such matters with their patients, and the vast majority never mention the topic of cardiopulmonary resuscitation (Advance Directives 1994:9).

Contrary to the specifications of the Patient Self-Determination Act of 1990, which requires all hospitals and nursing facilities to inform their patients and residents about advance directives, Sacred Heart failed to do so. Mother's heart stopped beating, and she was resuscitated using extraordinary measures. The ICU team acted quickly and spontaneously to save her life. I doubt they even thought about searching for a living will at the crucial moment. But if the staff had known about Mother's living will, they would not have revived her, even though she was not terminally ill. They told me this, and the idea terrified me.

Had I violated my mother's ethical principles about the goals of medical treatment, or had I simply pulled her back from the brink of death by passively allowing the ICU staff to go about their business? Certainly, I was in no position to act when the critical occasion arose, because I was 1,500 miles away in Venezuela. I realized that, even if the hospital had had a copy of Mother's living will, no staff member in the midst of an emergency would take the time to interpret it. Mother had prepared her living will long before, with plenty of thought. It was easy to do when she was in no immediate danger. Now, after the harsh reality of the ICU, the document seemed inadequate and misleading. I was not sure I understood the ramifications of the different types of "heroic" measures.

Had we prolonged Mother's life through heroic measures so she could gain a few more good years, or had we prolonged it to her detriment, to face a deteriorating situation a little way down the road? I had no idea. Some think that the question we should ask— whether physician or patient—is: "What is the best outcome we can hope to achieve, and how should it be determined?" One should set forth all of the factors and balance the "benefits" against the "burdens." The question of "Should we or shouldn't we?" become more manageable when put into concise perspective.

Some physicians believe that cardiopulmonary resuscitation (CPR) is successful if the patient survives to be discharged from the hospital. Others believe that there are no good candidates for the procedure and the entire matter of CPR should be re-evaluated. CPR was developed in the early 1960s to treat patients who had suffered unexpected cardiopulmonary arrest during an accident or illness. Now it is routinely used to treat dying patients who are often untreatable. The general conclusion seems to be that chronically ill, elderly patients are poor candidates for CPR because of their limited reserves.

No physician, scientist, and ethicist who has written about advance directives has a good answer to the controversy over CPR. Physicians tend to err in the direction of overdoing it. That is their job. In his book *Death and Dignity* (1993), Timothy Quill points out that no matter how good the physician's intentions, the potential always exists to do harm. There are limitations to what physicians can do, and they must examine all possible outcomes in the context of the patient's medical history. Only that will give them the greatest chance to make the right decision. Quill has cared for many patients who survived extreme ordeals. For some, the indignity was worth the treatment because they resumed a normal life. For others whose lives were permanently compromised, the situation was more ambiguous.

The dilemma is difficult to resolve because it can be perceived differently depending on one's place in the medical pantheon. For those who confront issues of life and death daily, the idea of "extraordinary measures" may be extremely flexible. But for ordinary people involved in the care of a beloved relative, life-saving procedures are far from routine. The medical ethicist Ezekiel Emanuel argues that these discrepancies exist because our liberal society lacks a consensus on ethical decisions. Physicians tend to treat patients aggressively and prolong life by default, because without clear guidelines it is easier to give than to withhold treatment (1991:91–93).

All agree, however, that the ICU is a place of last resort, the final attempt to overcome or hold back the ravages of disease. Naively, I thought "intensive care" meant just that: around-the-clock, personalized nursing. Today, a stay in the ICU routinely involves an array of invasive high-tech devices that are employed to do battle against death. Patients are fearful of ICUs because the technology comes between them and sustained human contact— that is, technology displaces the familial presence that can comfort a frightened patient. The Brazilian anthropologist Darcy Ribeiro liked to tell his colleagues that if he had spent another minute in the ICU, he would have died. He had battled lung cancer for more than twenty years, but when he found himself in intensive care in 1995, he felt that he was in "the house of death" (as quoted in Báez 1997:5). Only by disconnecting himself from the tubes and escaping out the hospital's back door was he able to reconnect with the world at large and concentrate on regaining his health.

For Quill, ICUs have become "end-of-life shrines" and CPR "the final ceremony" in a religious choreography whose main ethos is to stave off death (1993:49). Sherwin Nuland sees the ICU as a "secluded treasure room of high-tech hope within the citadel where we segregate the sick so that we may better care for them. Those tucked-away sanctums symbolize the purest form of our society's denial of the naturalness, and even the necessity, of death" (1994:254). But for the bioethicists Nancy Dubler and David Nimmons, the ICU has become "the stage on which are played out many of the most heated ethical debates occurring in medicine today." They conclude that the ICU mobilizes the most aggressive efforts available to help the body function again on its own, even though the "perpetual assault" may be detrimental to the patient's ultimate well-being (1992:306).

At some point I realized that the problem was not Mother's living will. It was living wills in general. There will always be uncertainty about hypothetical directives because none of us can predict outcome. A lifesaving procedure may do just that, or it may consign a person to a living death. Bioethicists have spent a lot of time on this issue, which revolves around the idea of medical "futility." Disagreement arises because physicians often are unable to predict who will survive and who will not. Some bioethicists have argued that we must return death to disease, whereas others insist that the concept of medical futility is an illusion because physicians can never be certain whether extraordinary procedures will benefit the patient.

Although written advance directives can provide important guidelines, it would be a terrible mistake to interpret them literally. Living wills, when properly used, can generate enormous respect for the patient's preferences. Patients should never include blanket limitations, because specific interventions may be perfectly acceptable under some circumstances and objectionable under others. For example, a patient who refuses intubation may find temporary intubation justifiable to overcome a reversible occurrence of acute respiratory failure but unacceptable in an end-stage situation. The bioethicist Mark Wicclair has proposed a seemingly simple solution to the limitations of living wills involving a prudent decision-making model now in use at the Genesee Hospital in Rochester, New York. Patients choose the level of care they desire; each level, ranging from comfort care to critical care, implies a more invasive approach to the treatment plan and is tailored to the patient's immediate wishes (1993:44–46). I was comforted when I read Wicclair's book. I knew I had acted properly even though I had gone against Mother's stated objectives. If the technology existed to give her a chance, then it should be used. If Mother had been able to reevaluate her living will in light of the circumstances, I believe she would have concurred.

Wicclair also suggests that physicians actively engage in discussions with their elderly patients to familiarize themselves with those patients' health-care preferences. I believe that physicians are reluctant to talk about death and regard the topic as largely irrelevant. They consider their primary roles to be healers and saviors, and this type of exchange runs contrary to their professional ethics. The anthropologist and physician Melvin Konner notes that doctors are not motivated to have such talks: "These discussions just aren't a high priority for doctors because they aren't reimbursed for them, they aren't trained for them and they are extremely uncomfortable about death" (as quoted in Beck 1994:58). Doctors also become so bogged down in the minutiae of medical treatments that they forget to focus on the whole patient. They are so busy "fire-fighting," notes one commentator, "that they can't see the forest for the trees" (Kaye Abraham 1994:223).

Given the legal, ethical, and clinical implications of health-care decisions, the lack of communication among medical professionals, patients, and patients' families is puzzling. As matters now stand, the patient, not the physician, must initiate the discussion and plan to continue the dialogue so that changes in technology and in sentiments are reflected in the written document. The proper time to discuss these matters is when the patient is in a position to voice an opinion, not when death is looming in an ICU. "Asking a smothering, half-conscious patient whether he wants to be afforded relief is an inappropriate question," writes the cardiologist Lofty Basta in *A Graceful Exit: Life and Death on Your Own Terms* (1996:231). It is demeaning, in Basta's view, to expect a dying patient to choose rationally. Further, by the time a person is dying, the issue of advance directives has become "largely irrelevant" (Hardwig 2000:29). The dying patient is no longer concerned with treatment plans because he faces a spiritual crisis—the end of life.

What is certain is that only someone who is intimately familiar with the patient and knowledgeable about his or her directives should take on the weighty responsibility of having to interpret last wishes. Sometimes the physician, not the adult child, is the best candidate. The registered nurse and anthropologist Jeanie Kayser-Jones tells a story about one case she observed during her nursing-home research. A woman in her eighties died from a treatable infection because her immediate family did not want any "heroic" measures to be taken. But the heroic measure consisted simply of hydrating the patient with antibiotics. The nursing-home staff was confident that no lawsuit would be served, because it was no secret that the son did not especially care for his mother. He had not visited her in at least two years. The doctor simply let matters lag and made no attempt to persuade the son that his mother should be transferred to an acute-care hospital. Kayser-Jones grappled with her own ethical dilemmas: Outside observers are not supposed to intervene, but she did anyway. By the time treatment started, it was too late, and the woman died (Kayser-Jones and Kapp 1989). Fortunately, very few adult children are as uninvolved as that woman's son, but the story illustrates an important point. One must have an ongoing, dynamic dialogue with the patient to understand his or her health goals.

But even those who are suited to taking on the role of medical advocate suffer greatly when the time comes to interpret another person's advance directives. In *Patrimony* (1991), Philip Roth recalls his experience when his father, Herman, was diagnosed with a malignant tumor toward the end of what had been a long, healthy life. The attending physician wanted to take "extraordinary measures" and attach his dying father to a mechanical ventilator, Roth writes. "And I, who had explained to my father the provisions of the living will and got him to sign it, didn't know what to do. How could I say no to the machine if it meant that he needn't continue to endure this agonizing battle to breathe? How could I take it on myself to decide that my father should be finished with life, life which is ours to know just once? Far from invoking the living will, I was nearly on the verge of ignoring it and saying, 'Anything! Anything!'" (1991:232). To complicate matters, Herman Roth had already soundly rejected invasive procedures for a benign brain tumor. He wanted to live peacefully until the very end, but even so, his son, the celebrated author, tormented himself. With or without the respirator there was no hope, and knowing his father's death would be difficult, Roth finally decided to let go.

Another caveat: Having an advance directive does not guarantee that one's final wishes will be followed. Controversy swirls over whether a doctor must consult a patient or his or her health-care surrogate before withholding extraordinary treatments. Should doctors be required to honor a patient's wishes to keep trying when they find themselves facing a medically futile case? The more likely scenario involves the heavy-handed use of such measures in direct contradiction of patients' wishes. A recent study conducted at Georgetown University Medical Center on the health-care needs of seriously ill people determined that the words "do not resuscitate" did not appear on the charts of half the patients who had asked not to be revived using extraordinary measures. Doctors frequently ignored or were unaware of patients' last wishes. Nearly 40 percent of the patients were put on ventilators for at least ten days or were allowed to endure severe pain, all in the interest of prolonging their lives—or prolonging their deaths, depending on which point of view you take. Patients may want care, comfort, and release from pain and discomfort, but they also want care that is appropriate to the severity of the event rather than senseless and costly treatments. For the moment, advance directives in the context of frank discussions with one's physicians are still the best way to insure that one's wishes will be followed sensibly.

The problem of "misdirectives" has become so pronounced that lawsuits are being brought by patients and their families in an attempt to make medical professionals liable for ignoring living wills and other advance directives. Lawyers argue that treatment against a patient's will is a "form of battery, an illegal attack on the patient's body" (Lewin 1996:14). The lawsuits will probably call the medical community to account for forcing unwanted life-extending treatments on patients without regard for the consequences. The trend toward lawsuits for inflicting unwanted treatment, even in states in which no statutory provisions for living wills exist, points to the difficulty of making end-of-life decisions with any degree of certainty.

Equally frightening are the circumstances under which one's advance directives are brought to the attention of a hospital staff. Unless events are extremely fortuitous, the staff probably will not even learn about existing living wills. Patients' written directives rarely accompany them to hospital emergency rooms or to the acute-care settings many patients enter after being hurriedly discharged from a nursing home. Admitting and attending physicians may be unaware of directives—particularly if they are not the patient's physicians. In short, the chances that one will be physically separated from one's directives are ample.

Until some evidence of the existence of advance directives is attached to one's person, the chances of having one's wishes explicitly known are slim. Neither at Coral Bay nor at Sacred Heart was my mother given a list of options in the form of advance directives. I came to the sad conclusion that she could guarantee that her written wishes were known only by wearing a dog tag around her neck.

CHAPTER THREE

Home

"I didn't think I would live to come home."

JUNE 18–JULY 6, 1993: 19 DAYS • Broward Empathy Care, an agency certified by Medicare, was designated to manage Mother's home care for a period not to exceed nine weeks. The hospital equipment that arrived barely an hour before her scheduled discharge had seen better times. The bed was not as sturdy as a real hospital bed and came with a crank rather than a self-operated motorized control. The wheelchair was a no-frills model, and the bed table, which I paid for as an extra item, had an antiquated knob that had to be adjusted constantly to raise and lower the tray to the proper height. The commode was new and arrived wrapped in plastic, but it lacked a back support and sidebars.

I set up Mother's new room, making the bed with her favorite fitted sheets and doubling and tucking a smaller sheet around the middle of the mattress, as they did in the hospital, so I could easily slide Mother up and down. I rotated the bed to look out at the golf course but decided not to have cut flowers. I did not want the converted den to remind her of her hospital room, which frequently overflowed with wilting bouquets.

I called Medical Mart, the private division of Broward Empathy Care, and told the case manager that I would require help the following week and would call back once we had established a routine. Sacred Heart's social-services department had made a big fuss about hiring an ambulance to take Mother home, but I insisted on a non-emergency van. Two drivers could easily carry my eighty-odd-pound mother in a wheelchair to the second floor.

Mother was ecstatic to be home. The men carried her up without touching the stairs, gently lifting her from the wheelchair into the hospital bed.

"I thought I would never see the house again," she said, sighing. "I can't believe I'm really home. I truly didn't think I would live to come home."

"Well, everything's the same Mother, except for a few gadgets we installed to make your life easier. As soon as you're feeling a little stronger, I'll take you around the apartment so you can see for yourself."

"Fine, but right now I don't want to see the hallway where I fell. I don't want to be reminded of the accident."

We propped Mother up with several pillows, and she spent the rest of the afternoon calling her neighbors and letting them know she was home. The visiting nurse and the health aide from Broward's Medicare division stopped by. Mother's vital signs were stable, and the nurse said that, unless a problem arose, she was scheduled to pay three visits a week. The home-health aide would come every day to bathe Mother and change her bedding. Marisa hovered by Mother's side, bringing her whatever she wanted. We didn't mind running back and forth to fix her pillows; raise and lower the bed; bring water; fetch the telephone, address book, and reading glasses; or fulfill any of the myriad requests she had that first day at home.

Mother was exhausted. After the ride home, numerous phone calls, and the home-health visits, she dined on a creamy chicken soup I had prepared from her recipe the night before and fell into a deep sleep that lasted until late the next morning.

Mother's home-health aide immediately warned me not to allow Marisa to take over nursing functions, and I agreed. I asked the aide whether she could come in the morning, but she said that everyone made the same request, and she could not make any promises. I was eager to set up a routine so I could call Medical Mart again. I was still not sure how much care Mother would need, but I soon realized I would have to hire a private aide. It was important not to duplicate services, because if I did bring in a private aide, Mother would be in danger of losing her Medicare benefits. I should do it discreetly, Mother's visiting nurse said, and make sure that visits by the home-health aide and the private aide did not coincide.

Mother required constant attention from the start. I soon realized how much work was involved in organizing her home care. I did not feel in control of the situation and had a lot of trouble planning coherently. When I settled Mother in on that first day,

I had been awake since her 6 A.M. phone call, made two round trips to Sacred Heart, and converted the den into a hospital room. I had already done the marketing, but now I needed to go to the drugstore for waterproof pads to place under her slip sheet, disposable gloves, and dressings for her bedsore. Mother also had been sent home with an extensive pharmacopoeia and detailed follow-up instructions, but without a set of prescribed pills for the evening. I could not keep the medication straight. Some of the pills had to be given four times a day, some with food, some without food, some cut in two. I posted a chart in the kitchen and prepared the day's medication in small plastic vials.

I could not accurately assess where Mother stood. True, she had survived the ICU and lived to come home. But now that her life had been saved, what was her prognosis? Were her chances as good as they were before the ICU, or had they diminished? I vaguely remembered reading in a medical journal that half of the elderly who survived the ICU died within a year. Mother was debilitated. Her muscles had atrophied from inactivity, and she was painfully frail. The smallest movement increased her discomfort. Moreover, the ordeal was still fresh: She had come home from critical care in less than a week and had been a witness to her own clinical death. She was emotionally battered and exuded sadness.

I had no idea whether she really could come out of this; only a shimmer of hope kept me going in anticipation of her slow improvement. I kept reminding myself of Dr. Risden's advice that recuperation in the elderly is one step forward and two back. The course is rarely smooth.

"How did it come to this?" Mother asked me that first weekend. "Will I ever come back to my former self?"

"Mother, you've already come back to some extent. You pulled through a horrible crisis, and now you have to get your stamina back. It may take time, but you'll come back."

I desperately wanted to believe my own words. I had never lied to my mother; nor would I try to fool myself. I racked my brain. Did I know anyone who had bounced back—anyone at all who could serve as a role model for Mother?

"Mother, remember the story of Norman Cousins [which he narrated in *Anatomy of an Illness* (1979)]. He was in intensive care for weeks with a rare virus and was completely paralyzed. He made a complete recovery after a few months. Even under normal circumstances, Dr. Bianchi said that it takes at least three months to recover from hip surgery. I know this period seems endless, but don't try to rush it."

I wish I had known about Richard Selzer then, because I surely would have told Mother about his extraordinary near-death experience. He surprised even himself by surviving a bout of Legionnaire's disease and returning from the "land of the dead." For twenty-three days he was "ventilated, dosed, defibrillated, probed, suctioned, and infused" in intensive care. Despite all that, his heart stopped. He simply expired and failed to respond to any more tendering. While the nurse was writing out the final report, he heaved awake and nearly scared her to death. Recovering was a painful venture, because once he woke up he became aware of the clinical nuances and felt like "little more than a polyp on a stalk" (Selzer 1993:55). His story certainly attests to the persistence of the human spirit.

But my mother had one glaring disadvantage that Cousins and Selzer lacked: her debilitating and incurable polymyositis. She had entered the critical-care unit under the most foreboding circumstances. She was a chronically ill woman who had already endured years of pain. Could she possibly come back from two broken hips and an arrested heart? Even without complications, the period following a hip fracture is delicate. The patient's emotions are brittle, and this complicates the healing process. Mother's mind, though, seemed as crisp as ever. Although she had had some temporal disorientation, she never had the hallucinations common to ICU patients. Mother did not remember that she had been on a respirator because she had been heavily sedated and drifted in and out of consciousness. She had the physical evidence of intubation—a raspy voice, a swollen and irritated throat, and the loss of several teeth—but no recollection of the machine.

Her worst experience was conveniently tucked away in her subconscious, perhaps to be retrieved at a less painful moment. She was not completely convinced she had been in an ICU at all, and certainly not for seventeen days. She remembered having trouble breathing but nothing after that. Once she "died," she entered a diaphanous world, to return to life only when she awoke. Dad's vigil, Noel and Cynthia's visit, and Graziano's visit were all gone. Her memory loss protected her from the gruesome truth, and I wasn't going to tell her she had died and come back.

The most pressing problem as far as I was concerned was what to feed Mother. The pureed hospital food had been unappetizing. I had gone over the menu with the hospital dietitian to determine the correct mix of carbohydrates and proteins to be given at home. Mother was not supposed to have milk products because it was thought they would thicken her bronchial secretions (a hypothesis that was later disproved), but she was encouraged to eat fatty foods such as ice cream to gain weight. She was not supposed to add salt to her food, but sometimes her blood pressure fell and the visiting nurse told me to give her salt. Mother had no appetite and found my home-cooked meals no more enticing than those in the hospital. In the morning I prepared a tray with oatmeal (with milk and butter), a coddled egg, buttered toast, and tea with milk. Mother complained that the oatmeal was lumpy and the toast was cold. If I didn't spoon-feed her, the tray would go untouched by her bedside.

"Mother, please. You have to eat," I badgered her.

"I'm not hungry; the stuff is tasteless."

"If you'd eat it when it's hot, it would taste much better."

"I'm just not hungry," she retorted.

"You don't have a choice. It doesn't matter if you're hungry. You have to eat to get your strength back. If you start eating, maybe your appetite will come back."

For lunch, I prepared a thick cream soup, chicken breasts poached in freshly squeezed orange juice, and steamed organic string beans with mixed herbs and spices. I cut everything into tasty morsels and set a can of Ensure Plus on the tray. I encouraged Mother to eat on her own.

"Mother, why don't you drink the Ensure Plus? That one little can alone will give you the equivalent of a complete, balanced meal."

"No, it's too much. I'm afraid to drink that stuff. It causes diarrhea."

"Mother, you have to give it a try. Maybe the medication, not the Ensure, has upset your stomach. This stuff is a lifesaver. You should drink at least two cans a day."

"I hate Ensure. The vanilla has a peculiar flavor."

"Well, we'll try the chocolate. You have to drink it. Why don't we pour it over ice. That will make it tastier. Or I can blend in some ice cream and you'll have a shake."

Dinner was more of the same. I went heavy on the condiments to tempt Mother's taste buds. I made meatballs in my special tomato sauce (spiked with peppers and carrots), *carne mechada* (Venezuelan shredded beef sautéed in vegetable sauce), bulgur pilaf with chopped onions and mushrooms, breaded chicken cutlets in tarragon sauce, London broil marinated in balsamic vinegar and pressed garlic, grilled polenta with roasted peppers, Kathy's lemon-glazed banana cake, cream-cheese orange-drop cookies from Mother's recipe, chewy chocolate brownies, and much more. The food preparations were exhausting and kept me in the kitchen almost full-time. But nothing succeeded in stimulating Mother's appetite, and she continued to treat the food as though I had laced it with rat poison.

Marisa helped Mother with her meals, which took an exceedingly long time to eat, while I served Dad. He had developed a voracious appetite and the more Mother refused to eat, the hungrier he became. I usually served him first because he claimed he was hungry the minute I walked into the kitchen. Mother was more than willing to wait and was delighted with this arrangement.

One morning, I finally finished washing the breakfast dishes around 11 A.M. and sat down with a cup of coffee. Dad walked into the kitchen and said, "You're neglecting your mother. Mother needs you."

"Dad, I've been with Mother all morning. You don't mind if I have my breakfast now, do you?"

"I guess you have a right to have your breakfast. Is lunch ready yet?"

"Dad, it's not even eleven o'clock," I said after pausing. "I'm not going to serve you lunch before noon. Sit down with me and have a snack."

I cut fresh cantaloupe into chunks for Dad and put off lunch for another hour. Now that Mother was home, he had developed a new awareness and appreciation of food. Food became the center of his universe. The more Mother refused to eat, the more willing Dad was to forgo his once rigid rejection of carbohydrates and sugar.

"Let Dad eat what he wants," Mother said.

What the hell, I thought. Let Dad eat whatever and whenever he wants. It's probably his way to deal with the constant stress. What difference would it make if Dad ate Mother's full-fat cottage cheese while the low-fat cottage cheese sat in the back of the refrigerator? Who cared if he ate Mother's whole-milk Muenster cheese while his low-fat variety grew mold. Look where Mother's low-fat, salt-free diet got her. Dad seemed to be burning the calories off with nervous energy, anyway.

The one issue we stumbled over—the one that caused Mother consternation and was distasteful to discuss—was her incontinence. Mother had had minor problems before she fell, but she kept them largely to herself. She followed the program of Kegel exercises set out in *Staying Dry: A Practical Guide to Bladder Control* (Burgio et al. 1989). The gynecologist A. H. Kegel developed the exercises in 1948 to correct stress incontinence by strengthening the pelvic-floor muscles. Mother's had improved but weakened again in the hospital. The Foley catheter had to be reinserted when constant wetness caused her incision to become infected, and the catheter accompanied her home more than a month later. Now her other bodily function was creating havoc. The rich, high-protein liquid diet seemed to have wrecked Mother's digestive system, bringing on watery diarrhea during her first few days at home. I bought her a special "fracture pan"—a thinner, more compact version of the standard bedpan—but she was too debilitated to lift herself onto it. The visiting nurse insinuated that Mother was capable of getting herself to the commode. This was ridiculous: She could not even roll over, let alone move from the bed to an unsteady commode. I was not going to risk it. The commode's lack of arm rests and a back rest was dangerous for a person with a history of compression fractures. The bed was also a problem. It was too high for Mother to move from safely, and the crankshaft was stuck.

Mother was humiliated by her loss of control. She loathed herself for having accidents and did not want me to be involved in any way.

"Mother," I said, "this is a private problem just between us. You'll get your control back in a few days. I'll help you whenever you need to be helped, but I want you to call me right away. Don't wait."

Still Mother tried to manage on her own and didn't think it was appropriate for a daughter to be involved in such intimate care. She waited until the last minute or neglected to call me at all. Then I had to rush in, change the bedding, and bathe her. Sometimes we went through this routine a few times a night. It was exhausting. I told Marisa I would take charge of this problem and that she should call me as soon as she heard Mother stirring. Marisa insisted on sleeping on a cot near Mother's bed, and between us, we muddled our way through the first long weekend.

Sunday came, and Marisa left for the day. I asked her to return by 11 P.M., at the latest. Mother had to be turned every half-hour to relieve the pressure on her bedsore, and I needed help. But Marisa did not appear. I managed to turn Mother by myself, adjusted her bedding, and went to sleep around 11:30. At 1 A.M., the front door clicked, announcing Marisa's arrival. A few minutes later, Mother rang for a glass of water, and I went to the kitchen. Marisa followed me. "I'll help you with the water," she said.

"No, Marisa, I don't need any help right now. I needed you earlier to help turn Mother. I specifically asked you to be home no later than eleven. I'm really upset that you came home so late."

"Well, Señora Luisa, I was busy. I was very busy, and it was impossible to come home sooner. I'll explain tomorrow."

"Look, Marisa, you really can't do this sort of thing. You have to come home when you say you will. I need to be able to count on you and not worry about where you are."

"*You* look, Señora Luisa," she said, raising her voice. "I was busy."

"Don't raise your voice, Marisa. You'll wake up my mother. You're in no condition to talk about this now. Be quiet, and we'll discuss it in the morning."

"Don't you ever tell me to shut up ever again. Nobody tells me to shut up—not even my own mother!"

"Marisa, I want you to go back to bed immediately. You're inebriated and not making much sense tonight."

I returned to my room to put an end to this silly conversation. She probably didn't even know what "inebriated" meant. But I knew I had been less than elegant with Marisa. There was no courteous way to say "Be quiet" in Spanish. The only expression is *"callate,"* which crudely translates as "shut up."

I was mad. Marisa was tipsy and had created a scene. She was in no condition to discuss anything, let alone care for my mother. I knew that she would feel the effects of her evening on the town the next morning. This was not the first time Marisa had come home in this condition, but it was the first time it had happened while I was there. Mother had complained to me on several occasions that Marisa could not hold a beer.

At dawn I heard a ruckus in the den and went to Mother. Marisa was in a stupor, and Dad was trying to lower the handrails to help Mother out of bed.

"Dad, what are you doing?"

"Mother wants to go to the bathroom, and I'm trying to help her get up."

"Mother," I cried, "why didn't you call me?"

"I don't want you. I want Dad. I need to go to the bathroom."

"I don't believe this—either of you. It's a good thing Dad couldn't lower the rails. Did you both forget that you can't walk?"

I could imagine the disaster that might have occurred if Dad had succeeded in helping Mother out of bed. They both might have ended up on the floor with broken hips. I tried to fall asleep after escorting Dad back to bed, but my mind flitted around, imagining the multiple scenarios that could play out in the next few days.

At 7:00 A.M., Mother was fully awake and I was in the kitchen preparing her juice when I heard a staccato interchange in the den. Mother had asked Marisa for her reading glasses and the telephone, and she seemed to be dialing several numbers without success. I went to the study.

"Mother, who are you trying to call at this hour?"

"I'm trying to dial the hospital. I have to speak to the director."

"About what?"

"I can't tell you right now. Just dial Sacred Heart for me."

"Mother, the director is not in his office yet. It's too early. I don't even know his name. Let's call back during working hours."

"No, now! Marisa, I want you to call Dr. Gregorio."

Mother had attempted to call Sacred Heart before but had waited until I left the house because she knew I disapproved. I tried to convince her that her feelings were actually fragments of a dream—she was remembering the deceased Venezuelan folk saint José Gregorio Hernández. She claimed to have spoken with "Dr. José Gregorio" during her stay at Sacred Heart and needed to find him because she could not remember what he had told her. Mother dialed Sacred Heart herself and asked to be connected with the director's office.

"I need to speak with Dr. José Gregorio," she said.

"There is no such person here."

"That's impossible. I'm Mrs. June Margolies, and he operated on me."

After being told again that no such person existed, Mother asked for the director's name and insisted on speaking with him. The receptionist refused to put her through. Finally, after Mother had made several unproductive attempts to call the hospital and speak to the director or "Dr. José Gregorio," Marisa came into the kitchen. I was in a black mood from my sleepless night and Marisa had a hangover—just the combination we needed for an explosive showdown.

"Marisa, have you seen the cover for the small frying pan?" I asked. "It's always in the holder on the door."

"No, I haven't. Nothing is missing from the door."

"I don't feel like holding a discussion over a frying pan cover. The only thing we have to worry about right now is Mother. I apologize for speaking to you so sharply last night, but let's wait until we can talk about it more calmly. Right now, I have to prepare Mother's breakfast."

Marisa avoided me all day. I suggested that she take a late-afternoon break and go for a bike ride. She put it off until she had finished helping Mother eat dinner. Finally she was ready, but something was odd. Marisa had changed into the blue jeans she wore to go out. I expected her back in a half-hour. Ten o'clock came around, with no sign of Marisa. Finally, at 11:00 P.M., the phone rang. It was Marisa.

"Where in heaven's name are you?" I asked frantically.

"I just called to tell you that I'm not coming back. Ever."

Now I was ripping mad. "What do you mean, you're not coming back? You're acting like a spiteful child. Come home and we'll discuss this like two mature adults." This action was out of character for Marisa, although she had obviously planned it earlier in the day. Her handbag and address book were gone, and the bike was parked in front of the building. Her clothing was still in her closet; she had left without taking a change of clothes.

Noel called a few minutes after I had hung up on Marisa. This was one time I was glad to hear from him.

"Noel," I lamented, "I think I'm losing it. This time I'm really losing it. Marisa disappeared. She went out for a bike ride and hasn't returned. She should have been home hours ago. But she just called and said she's never coming back. This is the last straw. I don't think I can take another setback. I just can't cope anymore."

"What did Mother say?"

"I haven't told her yet. I didn't want to worry her, and now I can't bear to tell her about the phone call. I'll tell her in the morning."

"Well, it's too bad. You probably realize Marisa was the weak link in this setup. You shouldn't have depended so completely on her. We talked about this before, about having a contingency plan. What will you do without Marisa?"

"I know, I know. I didn't expect her to hang around forever. I know she has a life of her own, but we did have an agreement, and she committed herself to the end of the year. This was something I was going to worry about later."

"She never understood what it means to hold a real job, what a job entails, what a responsibility is," Noel said. "She never worked before. She doesn't realize that all jobs have working hours that need to be respected."

"That's for sure," I added. "I know all about it. This is not the first time this has happened."

"Well, I'm really sorry. I thought she was devoted to our parents."

"She is. That's why the whole thing's so crazy."

"You need to hire help immediately," Noel said. "You shouldn't have to handle this yourself. Hire private help now. Call me tomorrow and let me know what happened."

When morning came, I had no choice but to tell Mother. "I can't believe it," Mother said after I explained the circumstances. "I can't believe she would do such a thing. Where could she have gone?"

"She's probably staying with a girlfriend from school, but I don't have any of their numbers."

"No, I'm sure she's staying with a guy. She wouldn't leave just like that."

"I can't believe she would do this, either, Mother. She's really hurting you, not me."

"You're too demanding, too much of a perfectionist, Luisa. You should have let it go. What difference does it make if she comes home late?"

"You're right, Mother. I could kick myself. I have too big a mouth. If I'd had a clue she would do something so insane, I would have kept quiet."

I berated myself for causing my mother such pain. Mother and Marisa had a special, complex understanding that transcended any minor ups and downs. I was so stressed from the hospital grind that I overreacted. I should have let it ride. Not only did I hurt Mother, I hurt Dad as well.

Marisa was wrong and I was right, but did it matter? I should have had around-the-clock help from the moment Mother came home, but it was too late to remedy the situation. Now I called Medical Mart. I wanted a home-health aide every day for two four-hour shifts. By dividing the hours needed into two segments, Mother's AARP recuperation rider would cover about two-thirds of the fee. I chose Lunice, a Haitian woman who had worked in several nursing homes in the area and was employed part-time as a hospice aide in a private hospital. She smiled readily and was patient with Mother. Our household routine recovered a regularity of sorts. Mother was not displeased with Lunice, but Lunice was not Marisa.

Several days went by and Marisa still did not surface. Dad, usually so mild-mannered, was hurt. "I feel like taking every single bit of her clothes from the closet and burning them in a bonfire," he said. Mother calmly proclaimed, "I know she'll show eventually." I was so angry that I never wanted to see her again, but my anger was slowing turning into worry. She had no money and no place to stay, and her friends and family apparently had no news of her. She was my legal responsibility, and I was concerned that some harm had befallen her.

I filed a missing person's report with the police. They opened a file and asked me to keep them informed. The female detective handling the case said, "This type of reaction is not all that unusual. People disappear every day, leaving no trail, and several weeks later they suddenly appear, giving no logical explanation for their actions."

"Well, you can imagine how worried I am. I don't think she's been the victim of foul play, but you never know. I dread the thought of having to tell her mother in Colombia she disappeared. At least I feel I'm doing something productive by calling the police."

"I want you to contact me immediately if there are any changes, and please let us know if she shows up, so we can close the case."

Within a few days it became clear that my attempt to set up a regular schedule with the visiting Medicare specialists would never materialize. Mother took an instant liking to a soft-spoken Peruvian woman named Julia. While we chatted in Spanish and English, Julia sponge bathed Mother, applied cream and powder, and left her looking and feeling like a different woman. Julia was a caring person, and Mother adored her. After a few days, Julia informed us that she was being reassigned. I called Broward Empathy Care right away and insisted that Julia alone would do. The agency agreed to continue sending her, but refused to set a specific schedule—Julia would come for an hour daily, any time during the regular working day. I was fairly certain she would appear in the afternoon, so I asked Lunice to bathe Mother in the morning, ignoring the agency's earlier warning about duplicating services. Neither Lunice nor Julia would tell.

The physical therapist was scheduled to give Mother three half-hour sessions weekly. On Monday, his first day, he phoned to say he would be unable to make it until Wednesday. I called Broward Empathy Care again and followed up with a call to Dr. Risden, insisting that Mother needed daily therapy. Furthermore, I said, the therapist should come at the same time every day so he would not conflict with her aides, and he should not be allowed to break his appointments at the last minute. I had not moved Mother from the bed for the entire weekend because I was afraid of hurting her by supporting her incorrectly. For her part, Mother was afraid that she would fall again and dreaded having to trust a strange therapist. But she had to resume her therapy. Otherwise, she would grow weaker. We all agreed that she did not want to spend her remaining years tethered to a wheelchair. Noel exhorted Mother by phone: She must get up, exercise her cardiovascular system, and start regaining the use of her muscles. He was concerned at how slowly Mother was progressing, yet I saw day-to-day incremental improvements.

It surprised me that Mother had to start over from scratch. Even if she had not fractured her hips, she probably would not have been able to walk after so many days of enforced immobility. Finally, the therapist arrived. He pulled Mother up gently and sat her at the edge of the bed. After being prone for three days, she was too dizzy to stand up. He taught her some arm exercises and helped her practice the leg lifts she had learned at Sacred Heart. He also showed me how to lift Mother by holding her under the arms and swiveling my own hips against the bed to support myself while walking her to the wheelchair. The therapist seemed competent, but his flippant attitude annoyed Mother. He told her that she would be able to throw away her walker within three weeks—*guaranteed!* I did not think this was feasible, even after the nine weeks Medicare allowed for physical therapy. Mother was plainly too weak.

Within a few days, it became obvious that home therapy was not working. I could hire a private therapist, but if I did, I would jeopardize Mother's Medicare therapy by duplicating services. The Medicare therapist canceled appointments and never made them up. When he did come, Mother had trouble completing the half-hour sessions because she was winded and sweated profusely. She was afraid of damaging her heart.

"I have to sit down," Mother insisted. "Remember what happened the last time I was out of breath? I ended up in the ICU. My heart can't take it. I'm afraid to overdo it."

I called Dr. Risden again. "Don't worry," he said, trying to calm me. "This is normal, because your mother's cardiovascular system has not had a good workout during the past few weeks." So I urged Mother on during her sessions, following behind with the wheelchair to give her a sense of security. Mother quickly managed to walk up and down the length of the living room, some thirty feet, but her breathlessness paralyzed her with fear. She insisted on frequent rests and refused to be bullied by the therapist. In fact, she thoroughly disliked him. There was no rapport. He looked at me when he should have been speaking directly to Mother. He was too somber for Mother's tastes, and she claimed that he smelled like a sour fish. He seemed to know his therapy, but I doubted that he grasped the complexities of her condition. When Mother's back began to ache after the first few sessions, the therapist insisted that she had new compression fractures, fueling her escalating fear.

• • •

Mother's honeymoon with home care ended abruptly with Marisa's disappearance. "This doesn't feel like home, *my* home," she said. "This is not my bedroom; I don't have a lamp to read by. This is not my sofa where I can put my feet up and work on the bills. There's no television in here. This is not the home I knew."

Further, the food was cold, tasteless, inedible, or all of the above. I tried to prepare appetizing meals that would appeal to Mother's taste. I substituted toasted wheat for the "lumpy" oatmeal and pastina for rice, I swirled cold fruit soups with dollops of extra-virgin olive oil in the blender, I tried matzoh balls and potato pancakes, I made *tortilla española,* I prepared Venezuelan *arepas* (corn cakes) with fried white cheese. I could have hired out as a personal chef, but no matter how creative I was, I could not accomplish my objective. Mother toyed with the food while Dad binged away.

Mother was irritable and hard to satisfy in other ways. When she called out at night and I went in to check on her, she sent me away, claiming she wanted Dad. I usually went back and forth several times during the night because Mother could not find a comfortable position for sleeping. After sending me away, she invariably called me right back, complaining that I had not come when she needed me.

One morning, Mother asked me to straighten her hair. I pulled it back carefully and tied it with an elastic band. But that felt too tight, so I replaced the elastic with a ribbon. Now it was too loose, so I removed the ribbon and tucked the ends neatly behind her ears. She leaned her head back comfortably on the pillows, and I returned to the kitchen.

A few minutes later, Dad entered in a tizzy. "Your mother is calling you, and you haven't come."

"Dad, I just finished fixing Mother's hair. I didn't hear her calling me."

I returned to the den. "Mother, what's the matter?"

"You didn't fix my hair."

"Mother, I just fixed your hair. Don't you remember?"

"Oh, yes, but I don't like the way you did it."

"I don't really know what other way I can comb it."

"Barbara, you're very angry. You have a bad attitude. I want you to go away now."

"Mother, I'm not at all angry. Let me try to brush your hair and fix it for you again."

Another time, as dawn approached, I ran in when Mother rang.

"Barbara, get away from me. You stink of wine. You're going to hell with yourself. You don't know how to take care of yourself."

"Mummy, please. Did you wake me up in the middle of the night to berate me?" Now it was my turn to feel offended. Mother was right. I was drinking too much white wine, but I thought she did not know. I felt like lecturing Mother about the beneficial effects of moderate amounts of wine (written up shortly before that in the *Wall Street Journal*) but knew I could not afford to vent my frustration on my sick mother.

"I'm under a lot of stress, Mother. Marisa's departure was the last straw. I'm not getting enough sleep, and I'm worried about Dad's excessive wandering."

"This is too much for you," she replied. "This is not for you. I don't want you to do any of these things. I know you have to go home. It's just a matter of time. I don't want to stay here anymore. I want to go into a nursing home as soon as possible."

"Mummy, let's talk about nursing homes in the morning. A nursing home is not going to solve your problems. Right now we need to bring live-in help into the house. I can't take care of both of you and the house, prepare the meals, and do the errands by myself."

"Of course not. It's just too much. That's why I want to leave."

"No. You should go into a nursing home for one reason—to receive the therapy you need—not because Marisa disappeared or because I eventually have to go home. I'll always be here when you need me. You know that."

"I know, darling. But you have your own life to live."

Mother felt that entering a nursing facility for intensive therapy was a tangible step forward in her treatment plan. In fact, once her mind was made up she wanted to leave right away. Further, the Medicare clock was ticking: If Mother did not enter the nursing home within thirty days of her hospital discharge, she would lose her coverage. I implored her to stay at home for the full month. I felt she would receive better care at home than at any nursing facility.

But Mother not only wanted to leave as soon as possible; she wanted to take Dad with her. We had endless "discussions" about this, and for once we could not reach an agreement. Mother wanted Dad with her. That was all. She was worried about his care in her absence and she didn't want to be alone. No matter how incapable Dad was of providing actual services, he was still her true emotional caregiver.

I disagreed with Mother and felt that Dad would cope poorly with the twenty-four-hour presence of her illness. "Mother," I argued, "why disturb Dad's routine. You know he likes to nap in his own bed, sit in his own chair and watch television, and eat the same lunch every day. I'm sure it will be upsetting for him to be in a nursing home. You have a job to do there, and he doesn't."

"No, I want Dad with me. That way I don't have to worry about him. I'll have him at arm's reach."

I turned to Dad. "Dad, what do you prefer, to stay at home and spend a few hours at the nursing home every day or to move in with Mother for a few weeks?"

"Well," Dad said hesitantly, "whatever Mother decides."

Yet when Dad and I were alone, he confided that he did not want to enter a nursing home because he was not sick. "I want my life to be the way it was before. I want to go back to my usual life."

"But Dad," I contended, "this illness hasn't affected just you. Think of Mother; every day she probably wonders if she will ever go back to the way she was before. Look at my life; I haven't been home in months and I haven't been available for Graziano or for Graz. The whole family's affected. If you stay home, you can visit Mother every day. If you go, you'll be with her all the time. But if you stay, I'll have to hire a housekeeper. You can't stay home by yourself."

"Certainly I can. I don't want anyone else in the house."

"Dad, I'm not going to discuss this with you. You must stay with a housekeeper while Mother's in the nursing home."

The decision was made, but when Dad spoke to Mother, he wavered, saying that he wanted to go with her. I knew Mother would eventually prevail, but for the moment I persuaded her to try it with Dad at home. Now I had to look for a live-in house-keeper. If the arrangement did not work out, Dad could always join Mother at The Palms.

I admit to having had occasional bursts of anger at Mother's internists for not telling me how Mother's home care would affect the rest of the family. Although I was the principal caregiver, none of the physicians had bothered to discuss her home treatment with me, except in the most rudimentary way. I had no idea how long Mother's recuperation would take. I had encouraged her to come home and tackled the logistics of her homecoming with verve. I considered her recuperation a personal challenge but did not have the faintest notion of what it would entail. Nor did I think about it in any terms except Mother's. I forgot that a husband, as well as grown children and their families, were involved. I forgot that Dad tended to fall apart when Mother was ill; now that he was older and had his own health problems, would he be able to cope? I had not given Dad's reactions much thought. As for me, I was a constant presence hovering about my sick mother— and taken for granted. Only her most trusted doctors knew that I lived in South America and worried about my own family too. I had an unspoken set of priorities. My own life and my marriage were of secondary importance while Mother was so ill, but I knew that there might come a time when I would have to put my son before his grandmother. I hoped I would never have to make such a choice.

Most medical personnel involved in a patient's care consider only the patient's desires, not those of the family. But every protracted illness involves the patient's family. It would be more realistic to include the family in the decision-making process and consider the impact of decisions on the lives of everyone concerned. If I had been better prepared, I would have made more pragmatic decisions regarding Mother's home care. I would have been sure to arrange for around-the-clock help from the beginning—at least for the first few days, when she required constant attendance. The way I had fallen into the home-care arrangements constituted a no-win situation. I could not care for Mother, care for Dad, and run the household on my own. It was an overwhelming job.

After the first crucial weeks, the emotional support of the patient's spouse is a powerful element in recovery. Oddly, although the spouse's presence can contribute to the patient's physical recovery, it does little to relieve the patient's depression following surgery. Some researchers speculate that the couple's uncertainty about the future is the reason. The husband is usually older and has his own health problems, and the wife's concerns about his well-being complicate an already stressful situation.

Mother did not want to be separated from Dad for an instant. He was her confidante. He held her hand and sat by her bedside, and they chatted comfortably with a camaraderie acquired through years of a highly compatible marriage. These moments were so intimate that I often left the room. Mother constantly called out for Dad, even at night, and when I came she pushed me away.

Dad seemed disconcerted by Mother's return home and resented the disruption of his routine. Now, instead of visiting Mother in the hospital and returning to his predictable environment at the end of the day, he was bombarded with evidence of Mother's delicate condition. The traipsing in and out of the medical personnel upset him; he could hardly relax in his favorite rattan chair when he had a panoramic view of the goings-on. Before, he had spent quiet mornings in his chair; after a nap and a sandwich for lunch, he visited Mother for a few hours. Then he went home for a quiet dinner and a snooze in front of the TV before retiring. Now he was right in the middle of the activity.

Mother wanted a strong husband to support her in her efforts to recover, but Dad was incapable of doing what she demanded. He tried but could no more relieve Mother's depression than he could solve the Latin American debt crisis.

"Mummy," I finally said, "why do you keep asking Dad to do things for you that you know he can't do?"

"I want Dad; I need Dad," she replied.

"But you know Dad can't turn you or help you get up. He tries, but he's a sick man himself. He can hurt you and himself at the same time. It's very frustrating for Dad when he can't help you. Ask him to do small things for you, like bringing the newspaper or a glass of soda."

"Dad can't even remember to do that when I ask him."

"Then leave him alone. Dad's by your side all day. That's enough. I'll fetch the things you need. All you have to do is ring the bell."

"I'm worried about Dad. Dad is like a child. He can't do a thing for himself."

"I don't entirely agree with you. He may not remember things he did earlier in the day, but we've had plenty of talks about your health. Dad has a pretty good grip on what's going on."

"No, he can't even make a simple decision."

"Then don't torture him, Mom. Let him be. Dad's been very brave these past few weeks, it's been terrible for him, too."

"You know I would never do a thing to hurt Dad. He's the best person on earth. I just don't want to be separated from him, that's all."

"I know, Mom. We'll do our best."

• • •

Early one morning, Mother was restless and insisted on calling Sacred Heart again to speak with the director. I could not reason with her; she had an important message for him concerning his babies. For days, Mother had been mentioning the babies, but I listened with only half an ear. She wanted to know if they were all right and seemed to feel that their well-being was connected to her actions. I was mystified. Mother's single-mindedness impressed me, and finally I acceded to her demands to call the director's office. I passed the phone to Mother after getting his secretary on the line and left the room, too pained to listen to the conversation. When I returned, I asked how the call had gone. Mother said that she had explained her reasons for calling, but the assistant had refused to put her through. No doubt, the woman believed that Mother was deranged.

"Mother, I don't want you to call the hospital anymore. You can't expect them to understand what happened to you. I want you to tell me about these babies."

I had tried to ignore the babies. But I realized that I had done almost nothing to ameliorate her anguish except tell her to forget about it. Now I sat on the couch by Mother's bed and gave her my full attention. For the first time, I listened intently. I decided to treat Mother like one of my anthropological informants—objectively. The story came out, over and over again, and the more Mother talked, the calmer she became.

It was predicted that these children would be born. I saw the father in my dream. He was the director of the hospital and an important man; they [the director and his companion] were lovers for years. The parents wanted the babies for years and would get married afterward. It was beautiful. Things were floating around; the babies were floating around. It was a dark and stormy night. Doors were slamming shut and open, shut and open. The children were born in the church.

I was part of it, in it, floating around. I was protecting the babies, floating around with them in water, inside the church, behind the Holy Grail. People in clown costumes were coming in and out, making sure they were in there protected. They were going to be blessed children. The parents were very happy. It was beautiful, just beautiful. It was such an experience, it came on the screen—it will be announced that they have these three beautiful children—triplets. It's all done, the children are protected. They're all happy.

I was there to check the babies. I was wearing lots of gold things. Only the men belonging to the church were there, coming in and out, in and out, to see that it all worked out. They were in clown costumes. They wanted those children; it was like a miracle. I see it now. I keep dreaming it. It was a very lucky person who was protecting the babies. I was protecting them. It was a very happy feeling, such a beautiful experience."

"Then why are you suffering so?" I asked. "You tell it as if it's a horrible nightmare."

I want to get it over with, give it back to them. You have to have some fantasy sometimes. It was a beautiful fantasy. I had this fantasy all night, a dark and stormy night. The parents would do anything for the people who protected those babies. I don't want anything for it. I just want some extra care. I don't need any money. We have everything we need.

The wind was blowing, there were slapping sounds, the doors shutting and opening. The men dressed in clown costumes kept wandering in and out. I went off to sleep, and the babies were born. They were like little fish, and I was swimming around with them, protecting them. It was a beautiful story."

"Then why are you suffering?" I asked again.

Because I was very sick—sick in intensive care. It was such a wonderful experience, a miracle. They would be blessed children, because they were born behind the Holy Grail. It ended, and I went off to sleep. That's why I came back— to tell the director that the babies are very special babies. They're protected and he must take good care of them.

I felt chilled as I listened, and we sat silently for a few minutes after Mother finished. "This is incredible," I finally said. "It's a very unusual dream, isn't it? I think you are actually remembering everything that happened to you the night of the emergency. The slapping sounds you describe are probably the doors of your room opening and slamming shut as the medical staff rushed in and out. You had what they call an 'out-of-body' or 'near-death' experience. I'm sure of it. It wasn't just a dream. Mother, you've had a mandate from God."

"Yes, I know that. I've known it all along," Mother said. "I've had an extraordinary experience, and there's a reason why I came back and am here to tell about it. I'm never going to forget. It was such a happy experience. If it weren't for me, the babies wouldn't be here now. I must call the director and tell him that he must take good care of his babies."

"No, Mom, don't call. Give me some time to find out the director's name and whether he actually has babies. He won't believe you. He won't be able to understand your experience. He'll think you're crazy."

At the time I was not sure what kind of dream Mother had had, but later I realized that it was part of what Melvin Morse (1994) calls "death-related visions," which encompass near-death experiences, after-death visitations, healing visions, dreams, and other premonitions of death. Mother experienced many of the typical events that others have recounted and that have been compiled by the researcher Raymond Moody, Jr. (1975): feelings of peace and quiet, separation from her body, unusual auditory sensations, brilliant light, a sensation of being pulled through a dark space and suspended, and meetings with spiritual beings clad in white.

Morse believes that deathbed visions allow the dying patient to heal the grief associated with the terminal event by providing glimpses of a blissful world beyond. In near-death experiences, the return is "medicine for the soul," because the returnee comes back for a specific purpose (1994:xii). Sherwin Nuland notes that most people who have had such experiences were victims of a "sudden episode," such as cardiac arrest, a burst blood vessel, or electrocution by lightning, and thus the phenomenon may be biochemical (1994:137–139).

I think it is pointless to look for a scientific explanation for near-death experiences. Anthropologists are used to being baffled by phenomena that straddle the line between the religious and the scientific. I have seen how praying with great faith and fervor to a powerful saint can infuse a person with equanimity and lead to a marked and unexpected improvement in health.

After she told me about her dream, Mother was more serene and seemed to lose the urgency that had made her so critical of her experiences at home. I would not demean Mother's feelings by calling her clinically depressed. It was far worse than that. Seventeen days in intensive care and a near-death experience were too much to bear after having had an accident as rare as a double hip fracture. The effort to come back was too hard. It was almost easier to give up than to keep fighting. "You should have let me die," she said on various occasions. This hit me like a stone. What could I say? I felt powerless. I commiserated with Mother, but no matter how hard I tried to imagine her despair, I could not relieve her loneliness. Hers was a solitary experience, yet the simple will to survive, to go on living, was a potent motivator.

Mother claimed that I yelled at her all the time. The truth is, I never raised my voice. I urged her on, imploring her to eat, sit up, get out of bed, open her eyes. My admonishments irritated her, but I wanted her to live. I tortured her to stay alive. Her life could only be diminished from then on, yet I refused to contemplate her eventual death.

Dad was not doing well. I sometimes felt he was teetering on the verge of a major disaster. He was becoming more forgetful and beginning to show unmistakable signs of confusion. He forgot that Mother had suffered a double hip fracture and could not remember how long she had been hospitalized. The comings and goings were driving him crazy, and his only escape was to hide in the bedroom and nap. I tried to get Dad out of the house. We went marketing together, and I accompanied him to the pool every afternoon for his swim.

Dad kept asking, "What did I do to deserve this?" How could a man as healthy as he was have three major heart attacks? How could someone who practiced moderation all his life end up in such poor shape? Dad wanted his old life back; that was his chronic lament.

My mind flitted back to happier times—my parents' visit to Caracas when I was newly married. This was Dad's first trip abroad, and he relished the bustle of Venezuela's capital. I remember one photograph that Graziano took of us on the grounds of the Botanical Gardens. Dad was nicely tanned from the tropical sun and had a healthy glow. With his trim black mustache, he looked more Italian than my Italian husband, more at home among the European immigrants in Caracas than in his own native New York City. Now he sat beside me, sallow-skinned and frail. I could do nothing except sit and listen patiently.

On one occasion, Dad went to fetch a glass of water for Mother, and Lunice intercepted him, trying to take the glass from his hand instead of letting him hand it directly to Mother. I was next door doing the laundry because our machine had broken.

Dad came looking for me. "This is my home," he cried. "How dare those bitches! Who do they think they are, telling me what to do in my own home? I want them all out. Next thing, they're going to try and sell my home."

I sat Dad down in the neighbor's kitchen and held his hands. He was trembling.

"Dad," I replied, "you're absolutely right. But you're going to make yourself sick. Let's just sit here for a while and calm down. I'll talk with Lunice. Don't forget that Mother needs constant help, and we can't do it all by ourselves. And nobody—nobody— can take your home away from you. It's your home, and only you can sell it."

I left Dad at the neighbor's house and went back to speak to Lunice. I told her that under no circumstances, no matter how well intentioned she meant to be, was she to interfere with my parents, particularly when Dad was trying to help his wife. She should relax in the kitchen when they wanted to be together. In short, she should respect my parents' privacy.

Thanks to Lunice, I was again able to get out and run the household errands: the marketing, post office, banking, medical-supply house, and drugstore. The outings gave me a much needed break from household and nursing chores. Every time I bought something for Mother, I bought myself a little treat as well. I could not contain myself, and I accumulated a lot of superfluous items that I vaguely intended to take back to Caracas. Medicated lip balm for Mother, antiseptic spray for Dad's sore throat, and antacid for my nervous stomach; saline moisturizer for Mother's nose and maximum-strength toothpaste for my sensitive teeth; twelve cans of chocolate-flavored Ensure Plus for Mother, various nail products for me; colorful baskets to store Mother's stuff, the latest fashion magazines for me; ponytail holders for Mother, moisturizing shampoo and conditioner for my damaged hair; hydrocortisone cream, aloe vera gel, and therapeutic lotion for Mother's dry, itchy skin, a disposable shaver for Dad, and sun-block for me—Mother's needs, as well as mine, were seemingly insatiable. I spent a small fortune on over-the-counter drugstore products. It was a harmless if costly diversion and, no doubt, a way to relieve the interminable tension.

The one purposeful personal activity that I refused to relinquish was swimming. I was deprived of sleep, but I knew I had to stay in good physical shape to lift Mother and help her transfer between the bed and the wheelchair. I drove to a lap pool five minutes from the house and jumped into the water straight away. No matter how anxious I felt about leaving Mother, I swam for forty-five minutes, practicing a variety of strokes that constituted my daily workout. I did not lounge around the pool when I finished. I just wrapped myself in a towel and drove home, hoping to find everything the way I had left it. I could not leave Dad alone with Mother—not after he had tried to help her off the bed and walk her to the bathroom in the middle of the night—so I had to swim when a third party was present.

• • •

The Medicare social worker recommended an employment agency specializing in full-time home care for the elderly. I did not want to go to another certified home-health-care agency, of which there were hundreds in South Florida, because the simplest form of help, a certified homemaker, would cost at least $125 a day, and more if she drove. I found Helping Hands Private Care, an agency that averaged about $75 daily; its employees were not certified health aides, but they were bonded and insured. Even this rate was more than double what Noel paid for a live-in house-keeper in Chicago and three times higher than Dad's monthly Social Security income. I explained my requirements to Carol Machado, the agency's director: I wanted an unassuming woman to help my quiet father without making him feel overwhelmed. Carol had the "perfect" woman, petite and unassuming, and would send her right up from Miami. The woman who arrived, however, was built like an Amazon, heavily perfumed, and sported long, lacquered fingernails—not exactly what I had expected from an agency that "specializes in the elderly." Dad was clearly intimidated, and after a brief interview I told the woman I would contact the agency later in the day. I called Carol back and, after expressing my dissatisfaction with the first candidate, was told that a woman named Fay would come on Monday. Fay was a mature Jamaican woman whose last job was with an elderly man who died of cancer. Carol read Fay's references to me over the phone, and we agreed to a trial period.

I told Noel that I would return to Caracas as soon as I had trained Fay and arranged for Mother's nursing-home care. I was about to miss a conference at which I was scheduled to chair a session on aging in Latin America but did not plan on canceling a scheduled trip to the Canary Islands to spend a week with Graz, whose school year was about to end, and to complete my long-postponed research. If Mother's therapy proceeded smoothly, I expected to do a few weeks of fieldwork in the interim.

"Tell Graz to come home by himself," Noel said on the phone. "He's a big boy now."

"No, Noel, I haven't seen Graz in more than six months. I have some school matters to resolve, and I have some professional matters pending, as well. I don't tell you what to do with your children."

"Well, this is a different matter."

"Noel, when are you coming? Mother doesn't remember your visit to intensive care. I need you here now. Will you come and help Mother move to the nursing home?"

"I wouldn't even know what clothes to pack for her. I don't know what to do," he said, sounding panicky. "And I certainly can't come at your convenience. I'm busy."

I was seething. *At my convenience?* I was providing around-the-clock nursing and running the household while my only sibling would not be inconvenienced.

"Noel, I'm asking for Mother, not for myself. She can't go into the nursing home alone. I won't allow it."

"Nobody asked you to do all the nursing. I told you that you shouldn't do it."

"Well whom do you expect to do it? Do you think hired help can replace children? I want you to know that I'm drained. I haven't slept through a single night since I've been here. I'm just not functioning the way I should. Are you going to take care of me if I get sick? If I get sick, our parents won't have anybody to take care of them. Let's just forget the whole thing. I'll take charge of the nursing-home move. I'll just have to act like an only child."

Noel ignored my tirade. "Look," he said. "I think Dad should go into the nursing home with Mom. He can't be trusted at home. At least he'll be safe in the nursing home."

"Don't be ridiculous. What makes you think he'll be safer in a nursing home than in his own home? Do you think they're going to watch him twenty-four hours a day? He can fall; he can have an accident at a nursing home just as easily as he can at home."

"There has to be a solution. He should go into the nursing home. And he has to be stopped from wandering at night. They should tie him up."

"I don't believe I'm hearing this. How can you think of tying up your own father? Let's pretend you never said that, and do me a favor: Don't ever repeat it to anybody else."

"I'm going to call The Palms. I want them to send me information on their nursing home."

"Good. Call The Palms. Ask them all the questions you want. It's good for you to be involved," I answered sarcastically. "But, please, Noel, don't mention that business about tying Dad up. They'll think you're insane. We don't tie up our fathers, no matter how safe we want them to be."

Dr. Zeigler's wife, Gail, a patient-care liaison with a Medicare-certified home-health-care agency, suggested that I visit The Palms. Gail had already spoken to Mother on the phone and had mentioned The Palms when she stopped in to see Mother at Sacred Heart. The Palms was part of The World of Palm-Aire, the "leisure-living" community where my parents lived, and was a five-minute drive from their condominium apartment. The Palms was supposedly one of the best nursing facilities in South Florida. Dr. Risden had also recommended The Palms highly. Mother could not go wrong there, he and Gail insisted. I should not bother shopping around.

• • •

Pamela Peterson in the admissions office at The Palms was a good listener. I had a month's tension bottled up, and she gave me the opportunity to unburden myself. I told her about Marisa's disappearance and the effect it had had on my parents' emotional state. She mentioned that my brother had called and that she was preparing a packet of information to send him.

"Is there anything special he asked you?" I said. "He's a physician and is very concerned about the quality of the nursing facility."

"He asked about the possibility of your father coming in. He also brought up the matter of restraining your father at night."

"Yes, he told me that he's worried about our dad and that the only safe place for him would be in a nursing facility. He thinks Dad should be tied in his bed at night. I had hoped he wouldn't bring that up with you. It really upsets me."

"I explained that we don't use restraints at The Palms. It's against the law. This is the state of Florida and in the state of Florida we do not bind people up. It's against their constitutional rights."

"Anyway, my dad needs to get up at night to go to the bathroom—a few times, in fact."

"The most we allow here is putting side rails up on the bed."

"I wouldn't even permit that, because Dad might fall if he tried to get out of bed alone. I know my brother is concerned about protecting Dad from harming himself, but I don't think restraining a person is the way to go about it."

We discussed the possibility of Dad's admittance to The Palms, although I made it clear that for the time being he would stay at home. I had taken Dad with me to The Palms on several occasions while I was completing the paperwork, and he had enjoyed a few chats with Pamela about his old life in New York.

"You know" Pamela said, "your father is a very sweet man, but I would have to classify him as pleasantly confused."

"I understand what you mean, but you must remember he's under a tremendous amount of stress, and this has led to his confusion."

"Let me know what you plan to do with your father. Right now, we'll concentrate on getting your mother settled in."

Pamela handed me a set of papers, including a booklet titled *A Guide to Your Rights and Responsibilities as a Resident* and another one containing cartoons and general information about advance directives.

"By the way," Pamela continued, "does your Mother have a living will? If so, we would like to have a copy on file, and if not, she should think about making one."

"Right now I can't give you anything, because my mother's living will will have to be rewritten. The one she has is vaguely worded and can be easily misinterpreted. I'll have to discuss it with her and bring you the new version."

I wanted to talk with Mother about restructuring her living will, but she would have none of it.

"I don't see the need to discuss this now," she said. "I don't feel like talking about it. After all, it's over. I'm over the crisis."

"Mother, I know it's over, but it's something we need to think about for the future. I went against your express wishes, and it's a good thing, too. If Sacred Heart had had a copy of your living will or had I taken it literally, you wouldn't be here right now. I'm not going to give the present version to anybody. It's too confusing."

I hid the copies of Mother's living will in my bedroom drawer. I was not going to risk the possibility of having this flawed document floating around. It had to mirror Mother's exact wishes. As far as I was concerned, she had verbally rescinded it by asking me to speak for her if she was unable to make her own decisions. But no one could assume that her "loved one" would be hanging around at the right moment to interpret her directives. The thought was sobering. Mother knew what she wanted, but she refused to talk about it. The discussion was best pushed to the future, as far as she was concerned. I respected her feelings and let the matter of a new living will ride. I hid Dad's living will, too. I prayed that nothing would happen to Dad while we worked through the issues. I would not allow Dad to go on life support should an emergency arise. He did not have Mother's iron will; he would never survive.

• • •

I was not thrilled with our new housekeeper. Fay was an intrusive element in our household. Instead of helping me, she created extra work. I was too tired to make polite conversation. I had no desire to train her, to explain things over and over, or to bother showing her the daily routine. Some of her personal habits irritated me: her constant, loud singing; her red nylon undergarments strewn about my bathroom; and her nauseating sweet cologne, which permeated the house. She did seem responsible and spoke softly with Dad, but every time I turned around, I found her sitting on the living-room couch, browsing through magazines, despite dozens of things to be done. I needed her help in the kitchen, but she disappeared the moment I started the dinner preparations. I reminded her that she would be cooking Dad's meals and that she had to learn his likes and dislikes. The refrigerator was over-stocked, yet nothing suited her tastes. She refused to eat the food in the house and handed me a detailed shopping list of what she required, necessitating several trips to the supermarket to stock up on Jamaican specialties.

Fay rarely offered to help with Mother and, in fact, seemed to dislike her instantly. I explained that my mother was very sick and had to be treated with great delicacy. Even though Fay would be caring for Dad, she was supposed to wash Mother's clothing and bring her anything she needed once she was in the nursing home.

I also had doubts about Fay's character. One night, I was awakened by a ruckus. Fay was standing by Mother's bed, hands on her hips, yelling at Dad: "Now Albert, go back to your room. Go back to sleep. You keep waking me up."

I said sharply, "Fay, lower your voice. You're the one who's waking everyone up. I'll take care of my mother, and I would appreciate it if you would leave the study at once."

The next morning, I went directly to the matter: "Fay, you can call me Luisa, but when you speak to my father, you will address him as Mr. Margolies. You woke me up by yelling at my father. Don't you ever raise your voice to my father again. And don't ever tell my father to go back to bed. He's checking on his wife, and that's none of your business. If you can't understand that, you're free to leave today."

Fay said she wanted to stay and that she would take good care of Dad. But she repeated it too often for my comfort. It was an uneasy peace.

Mother was scheduled to move to The Palms after the July 4 weekend. I encouraged her to sit in the wheelchair for longer peri-ods. I wheeled her around the apartment and out to the catwalk. She got up for lunch and again for dinner. We even practiced walk-ing without the therapist. She looked forward to starting the ther-apy program. But on Sunday, July 4, Mother awoke early with a bad backache. I squeezed fresh orange juice and gave her two Bufferins with it. But when I took Mother her tray, she had not touched the juice or taken the Bufferin.

"I want you to know that I'm not going to eat," she said. "And I'm not going to take any of the medications. They're making me sick."

"What do you feel, Mother?" I asked. "What's making you sick?"

"The medication is upsetting my stomach. I have an excruciating pain in my back. I'm not going to eat anymore. And you're constantly yelling at me. I don't want to see you anymore."

At this point, Dad walked in and said, perfectly lucidly: "Now, June, what is this nonsense? You eat your breakfast. You have to eat to have some strength."

"Mother, today is the Fourth of July, but I'm going to try to reach Dr. Risden so you can speak to him yourself. I'm really frustrated. I'm only trying to help you."

"I just want to die! I don't know why they bothered saving me."

I left an urgent message with Dr. Risden's answering service. Within a few minutes, his partner, Dr. Ronfeldt, called back. He explained that Mother was clinically depressed and that her feelings of helplessness were feeding into her physical condition. He asked her to cooperate by eating and taking the medication. "Your daughter is trying to help you get better, June," he said. "You're doing well, and you're ready for therapy. You can't give up now when you've come this far. I want you to help in your own treatment."

Dr. Ronfeldt prescribed something for Mother's queasiness, and that was the only pill she would take that morning. The tension eased somewhat. I called Aunt Gussie and asked her and Uncle Sidney to come for lunch. If anyone could calm Mother, her eldest sister could. I prepared a salad and ran over to the deli for bagels and dessert. I brewed my favorite Venezuelan coffee blend and set the dining-room table with colorful placemats. Mother sat at the head of the table in her wheelchair, looking angelic and calmly conversing with her guests. The crisis was over—at least for the moment.

Who Cares?

Daughters Care for Their Elderly Parents

THE QUESTION of who will care for the elderly is not as simple as it used to be. Fifty years ago, few middle-aged people had frail, elderly parents. Now, nearly 90 percent of baby boomers have parents who survive to advanced ages. Families composed of several generations are not unusual; nor is it uncommon for an elderly child to care for an aged parent. Parents may require different types and degrees of care, depending on their age and health status. Many people older than eighty-five can manage on their own, particularly if they have a spouse to share the tasks, but nearly half need limited to substantial assistance in carrying out their daily activities and can remain at home only with the help of family caregivers or hired aides.

Transformations in family structure have wrought fundamental changes in the nature of caregiving. Thanks to geographical mobility and the decline in fertility, the extended family is almost extinct, and fewer children are around to care for aging parents. Divorce, remarriage, and multiple career paths for men and women have made rendering consistent care increasingly difficult.

The issue of who should care for the elderly has become muddled with moralistic arguments. Some historians contend that economic imperatives were the moral underpinning of the large extended families of the past. In the countryside, adult children toed the line because their parents controlled the means of production and allocated the family's economic resources. One honored one's parents and took care of them in their old age. Ireland's system of impartible inheritance, for instance, obligated children to seek their fortunes elsewhere. The youngest son, however, continued to live with his parents and was committed to caring for them throughout their lives. This child was amply compensated on his parents' death by being made the sole recipient of the family estate.

Even among urban families, where no such economic imperative reigned, adult children felt a heavy obligation to care for their surviving parents. Numerous children worked out the logistics of caregiving without the aid of Social Security and national medical entitlements. Surviving parents normally lived with a primary caregiver but also rotated among their other children. The children had an unquestioned duty to their parents, and the lines of caregiving were clearly delineated.

When I think about my grandparents and great-grandparents, the idea of removing them from home was inconceivable. Both sets of paternal great-grandparents lived to advanced ages and were cared for by my paternal grandparents. My father had fond memories of talking to his grandparents daily: All he had to do was walk down the long hallway of the large apartment to their separate quarters. Both sets of his grandparents died naturally at home of "old age." My paternal grandfather "dropped dead" at the relatively young age of fifty-seven, but my paternal grandmother lived into her eighties in her only daughter's home. When she grew senile and frail, her three sons contributed a monthly stipend for her medical care. My maternal grandmother also died young, but my maternal grandfather was lucky to have had four adoring daughters who spoiled him after he was widowed. He continued to live with his youngest daughter after she married, but he liked to circulate among his other daughters for weeks at a time. He helped raise his youngest daughter's children, and he was an integral member of her household until his sudden death at age seventy-four from a ruptured hernia.

It was not until the Medicare and Medicaid Acts of 1965 were passed that the idea of living with and being cared for by one's family changed. In one swift moment, the extended family was rendered superfluous as commercial nursing homes, financed by government contributions, took over the role of caring for the frail elderly. The cultural ties that bound multiple generations together in a single household rapidly attenuated, and the first Medicare generation to reach old age gained the dubious distinction of caring for itself.

Today, filial piety is nearly an anachronism, and ethicists argue about the moral obligations children should have toward their aging parents. The argument goes something like this: Children did not ask to be born and therefore do not have the same degree of commitment toward their parents that parents have toward them. Parents must raise their children and see them safely into young adulthood, but this does not necessarily obligate children to bear the burden of caring for a failing parent later. Because parents are simply discharging their normal responsibilities, the "parental sacrifice account" of filial obligation in which grown children "owe" their old parents care is nonsense (even though many grown children still subscribe to it). In *Am I My Parents' Keeper?* (1988), Norman Daniels argues that we cannot view children's obligations as equivalent to parental duties. We should not fall into the trap of appealing to the "traditionalist" view of a golden age of moral and emotional bonds as a signal for returning to outmoded values. Caregiving obligations were different in the "good old days," when parents died relatively young after brief illnesses. Long-term-care duties can now be so burdensome, he adds, that it would be imprudent to depend exclusively on individuals to care for their elderly.

What ethicists are trying to tell us is that we should not rely indiscriminately on implicit contracts to ensure that growing numbers of frail elders are properly cared for. Daniel Callahan, founding director of the bioethics research institute The Hastings Center, observes that some moral obligations *do* exist for family members to care for one another. But he also warns that "unlimited self-sacrifice on the part of the caregiver, in a time of rapidly increasing life expectancy and chronic illness, encounters heavy, and perhaps mounting resistance" (1987:101).

Most ethicists reject "reciprocity" as a moral validation for providing care. Do unto your children does not necessarily mean that children should later do unto their parents. The concept of reciprocity goes back to the *Commentaries on the Laws of England,* in which children were bound to their parents by principals of natural justice and parents who protected their helpless infants were entitled to be protected in their old age (Brakman 1994:27). Contemporary ethicists prefer the concept of gratitude, which implies an expression of appreciation to the formerly benevolent parent, without the aspect of repayment. Unfortunately, ethicists seem to be unaware of the importance of reciprocity in establishing and maintaining social relationships in many societies. "Reciprocity," as discussed in the anthropological classic *The Gift* (Mauss 1954), is the ingredient that binds together not only family members but also relative strangers. Reciprocity establishes an unspoken contract that is not broken until the favor is returned, and when it is returned, another contract is immediately established to sustain the ongoing relationship. One has the obligation to give and the obligation to receive. The point of reciprocity is purposely to maintain an imbalance that permanently binds one recipient to the other in a more profound way than mere give and take. Reciprocity, therefore, is not an unreasonable concept to express the ongoing mutuality and symbolic bond of parent–child dynamics, but it does seem to have lost favor in American society, where obligations between adult children and their parents are frequently considered incompatible.

People who look toward religion do not need inspiration from notions of reciprocity to validate parents' moral claims. Covenantal mutuality between the young and old is at the very heart of Jewish belief (Post 1991:22). Jewish law clearly states that children have two types of filial obligation toward their mothers and fathers: *service* and *reverent obedience*. The children must manifest their obligations through behavior—specific physical acts—not merely by expressing an emotional attachment. Judaism rejects the "social usefulness" argument concerning the vulnerable elderly, as does Christian social thought, which took up the moral tradition of generational social equality from the start. Given the Judeo-Christian emphasis on beneficence toward the most vulnerable members of society, many have questioned why these basic tenets have been forgotten.

Today, seven in ten care recipients suffer from medical conditions that are long term or chronic in nature (*Family Caregiving in the U.S.* 1997:14). Chronic conditions can turn caregiving into an endless nightmare, because the elderly are older, sicker, and frailer than ever before. Living with a chronic condition is like living with an uninvited guest who refuses to leave, no matter how many hints are given. Chronic diseases are incurable and relentlessly progressive. They sap one's strength even as one tries to manage them. These are just the physical effects. The illness is also the main element that segregates the sufferer from normal interactions with the outer world, taking on a dynamic of its own and tightening its tedious grip over every aspect of his or her daily life.

The chronically ill exist in a state of limbo. My colleague Robert Murphy, who suffered from the disabling effects of an inoperable tumor on the spine, described his feelings of alienation and sense of stigmatization in *The Body Silent*: "My identity has lost its stable moorings and has become contingent on a physical flaw. . . . The long-term physically impaired are neither sick nor well, neither dead nor fully alive, neither out of society nor wholly in it. They are human beings but their bodies are warped or malfunctioning, leaving their full humanity in doubt. . . . The sick person lives in a state of social suspension until he or she gets better. The disabled spend a lifetime in a similar state. They are neither fish nor fowl; they exist in partial isolation from society as undefined, ambiguous people" (1987:104, 131).

Chronic diseases have to be nurtured because they form a permanent part of one's life. One has to both monitor the illness and learn how to cope. All this takes up a lot of time and energy. In *Good Days, Bad Days,* Kathy Charmaz notes that chronic illness is "intrusive" because it forces its sufferer to make constant adjustments. The illness is like being on a roller-coaster—there are good days and bad days, depending on the "intrusiveness" of the symptoms (1991:42–49). When chronically ill people feel "well," they push themselves in the foolish attempt to persuade themselves that they are not actually ill. Then they become overtaxed and relapse quickly, only to be bitterly reminded of their illness by experiencing renewed episodes of pain and fatigue.

Perhaps the idiosyncratic nature of chronic illness defines its tyrannical hold over its victim. My mother was compulsively caught up in her disease, playing out her concerns almost surreptitiously. For more than a decade, she kept an accurate weekly rendering of her condition in her agenda. Noting the list of medications, the test results, and the ups and downs was her way to cope with the tribulations of her rare disease. Murphy observed that, although he tried not to brood about his disease, "it is always on my mind in spoken or unspoken form, and I believe this is true of all disabled people. It is a precondition of my plans and projects, a first premise of all my thoughts" (1987:104). Clearly, the disease becomes a silent partner in defining one's pursuits.

How many times have chronically ill people been asked by well-meaning observers, "What do you do with yourself all day?" Just going to the supermarket may constitute the day's major outing and consume all of one's meager resources. How many adult children wonder why a parent takes "all day" to accomplish a "minor" task because they are insensitive to the illness's dominant role in limiting a person's capacity to perform routine chores? The interrogators cannot understand how pervasive the consequences of chronic disease are.

Each modification of one's surroundings to eliminate physical obstacles, and each limitation of activities, is a reminder of one's condition. One is forced to simplify as the illness progresses. People give up cherished activities like driving and entertaining and differentiate themselves from the people around them by parking in special handicapped spots or sitting down in the supermarket. They may have to purchase adaptive devices to compensate for physical limitations. They may stop picking up relatives at the airport, stop going to the mall, and "forget" to walk or exercise. Sick people often cannot be bothered with such niceties as setting a pretty table or filling the house with plants, and they may dispense with common courtesies because they feel "entitled." Chronic sufferers may end up reducing their living space to a well-traveled path between one room and another or confining themselves to a favorite chair. Nothing is more painful than the day the chronically ill person realizes he or she cannot manage alone. Caregiving then becomes a question of not only helping the elderly run their households, but also of providing them with hands-on continuing care. The caregiver must come to accept that she or he may not be able to alleviate the suffering of an ailing parent who is on a downhill course. "Sometimes, it means sharing their suffering, helping them to shoulder the burden," notes Richard Gunderman (2002:42).

Paradoxically, technological advances, which seemed to offer so much promise for the elderly, have scarcely affected our ability to care equitably for those who have most benefited from them. We have yet to come up with morally comfortable solutions that will ensure the continuing well-being of our aging society and keep pace with the remarkable achievements of modern medicine.

Although the biomedical approach to medicine has dealt admirably with acute diseases, it has shortchanged the care of our senior population. According to a recent report on eldercare, "The gap is plugged by programs of long-term institutional care and informal home care that are at worst inhumane and niggardly, and at best starved for adequate funds and well-trained health care workers and social workers (*What Do We Owe the Elderly?* 1994:S11). Callahan posed the right question when he asked what the appropriate balance should be between the provision of acute health care and the provision of long-term care for the chronically ill elderly. He calls for a different type of medicine today—one that knows its limitations and focuses on the care of the chronically ill (1993:209).

Family members currently provide the bulk of long-term-care services to the elderly and underwrite some $38 billion of the $70 billion expended on long-term care. Recent projections suggest that these expenditures will more than double in the next twenty-five years to keep pace with the galloping growth of the senior population. Meanwhile, Medicare entitlements continue to rest on theories about aging that prevailed more than forty years ago. Families who care for ailing relatives at home rarely receive the benefit of community-based programs or services because of Medicare's skewed emphasis on acute-care reimbursements for inpatients. Compare our glaringly deficient programs with those in many European countries, where both home-nursing and institutional care are incorporated into comprehensive social-security systems that are financed by a percentage of the wage base assessed exclusively for eldercare. Germany, for example, has a universal, compulsory long-term-care program that is administered by a sickness fund whose contributions come from monthly deductions shared equally between employees and employers. The elderly are provided with nursing-home and home-health-care benefits, and family caregivers receive formal training and earn pension credits (Wiener and Cuellar 1999). Those who choose to stay at home (the majority) receive a monthly stipend; their caregivers are covered by social-security insurance and receive various supports, such as respite care. In contrast, the American system puts the onus of caregiving squarely on the patient's family. It fails both the recipient and the giver of care.

Who are the care recipients, and how are they cared for? A national survey of family caregiving shows that the mean age of care recipients is seventy-seven years and seven months, but nearly 25 percent are older than eighty-five. Sixty percent are female, and a little more than 40 percent are widowed. Some 22.4 million families provide assistance to an aging relative. Adult children constitute 37 percent of all caregivers, and nearly one-fifth of care recipients live with their caregivers. The majority of family caregivers devote an average of three hours each day to rendering care, despite such competing demands as paid employment. Forty percent of caregivers perform the equivalent of a full-time job and have borne the responsibility for an average of four-and-a-half years. Twenty percent of caregivers have been fulfilling this role for more than five years (*Family Caregiving in the U.S. 1997*).

Family caregivers provide an eclectic variety of services for the elderly, including assistance with marketing, shopping, banking, car repairs, housekeeping, cooking, assorted chores, doctors' appointments, and financial management. The next level of attention involves hands-on personal care, such as bathing, dressing, toileting, and administering medication. Another type of assistance falls within the rubric of nursing and may involve the performance of complicated medical procedures.

One usually takes on the role of caregiver spontaneously, without anticipating the enormous complications to come. Caregiving functions tend to expand almost insidiously as the care recipients grow increasingly infirm or have unexpected crises. Caregivers will go to considerable lengths to provide the necessary care at home, even if they have to hire full-time aides or appeal to the services of a case manager to coordinate the different types of care. Nursing homes, for the most part, are still considered places of last resort. Brakman concludes that, "when elder parents do take up residence in a nursing home, this is often experienced by the child and the elder as a moral, emotional, and physical failure" (1994:27).

Caregiving is overwhelmingly women's work. Women make up 77 percent of the adult children providing hands-on care and are likely to rearrange their professional and personal lives to manage the unpredictable needs of their parents. Caregiving takes an important place alongside women's other roles as workers, wives, mothers, and homemakers. The typical caregiving daughter is middle-aged and squarely "in the middle" in terms of the demands competing for her time and energy. Some 41 percent of caregivers are still raising children younger than eighteen when they first undertake the caregiving role. Women generally serve as primary caregivers to an older female relative; today, that relative is likely to be one's mother. In the past forty years, the proportion of fifty-year-old women with living mothers has risen from 37 percent to nearly 70 percent. It is common for a fifty-year-old woman to have a mother who is living but perhaps not well—that is, with a chronic illness or some frailty. This daughter may have put off childbearing in favor of career development during her thirties; now she finds herself the mother of children approaching adulthood while confronting menopause and her own eventual mortality. She may end up spending more years caring for an elderly parent than raising her children. For these women, the issues surrounding caregiving pose an enormous challenge.

Various researchers have commented that daughters look on caregiving not as a set of discrete tasks but as a diffuse responsibility that never ends (Brody 1981; Rutman 1996). Daughters feel intimately responsible for their parents' well-being and will go to great lengths to preserve the recipient's sense of dignity. They try to uphold an image of the parent as he or she was by presenting that fictional vision, as far as possible, to the public sphere. In *Who Cares for the Elderly? Public Policy and the Experience of Adult Daughters* (1991), Emily Abel views this act of protecting a parent's sense of personhood as a kind of moral guardianship. Daughters seem to have an intuitive, nonverbal engagement with their parents that allows them to translate their parents' feelings.

Why do middle-aged women have such a difficult time setting limits on their role as caregivers to their parents? First, these women traditionally have been raised to be nurturers and expect to make sacrifices. They learned this from their stay-at-home mothers, and even though women are now in the working world, shrugging off old values is hard. Daughters are still the ones who hold families together and embody the moral underpinnings of the family unit, even though the nature of family dynamics has clearly changed.

Caregiving is not something most daughters have to think about very hard. They just do it because they have to. Caregiving is often a natural, spontaneous act for one's parents. Daughters have an overwhelming desire to provide care when a parent needs it and do not expect anything in return. I have yet to come across a daughter who can proceed comfortably with her own life while ignoring the obvious needs of a parent. Take the case of Elaine Simmons, the visiting nurse who came to my parents' home for eighteen months to give Mother her Calcimar injections. Elaine held a full-time job while caring for a daughter with developmental difficulties and a husband brain-disabled in a freak accident. She also found time to be a caring daughter to an ailing father who traveled between his home up North and hers in South Florida. She coordinated every detail of her father's care for several years while respecting his wishes to retain a separate and distant household. Elaine was so good-natured and concerned about her patients that one would never know she carried such weighty responsibilities at home. She juggled her affairs so that each family member received attention without feeling slighted. Such intense caregiving seems to emanate from a sense of connectedness, according to Abel (1991:91), rather than from any notion of repaying a parent or canceling a moral debt.

Two of my closest friends cared for their fathers with such abnegation that they had to rework their professional lives. George Ann worked for a global nonprofit organization, a job that kept her traveling much of the year. When her widowed father broke his hip, she bought a house in Vermont, moved him in with her, and took a more sedentary job. Her father had emphysema and had been seriously depressed since his wife's death. George Ann saw him through congestive heart failure, several minor strokes, and many bouts of pneumonia, but she never considered putting him in a nursing home, even though her absent brother kept urging her to take the step. During the nearly four years George Ann lived in Vermont, her brother visited their father once. Two years after her father's death, George Ann still could not forgive her brother for his failure to participate in their father's care. By contrast, Carmen Nieves, a colleague in the Canary Islands, was fortunate to have both a brother and a husband to share in caregiving tasks. Nevertheless, she refused to

leave her father for more than a few days at a time, despite numerous professional invitations abroad. Her father suffered from
advanced Parkinson's disease and was eventually confined to a
wheelchair. Not only did Carmen Nieves cater to his bodily
needs; she also made sure he took part in the family's activities
by seating him in the front parlor, where he could greet and chat
with everyone who entered the house. He was a retired school-
master and enjoyed the comings and goings of his granddaughter
and her friends. Carmen Nieves's brother occasionally covered for
her when she went out in the evening; it was understood that they
would share the responsibility for their ailing father. The care was
accomplished in a low-key, unobtrusive manner, and her father's
death was a blow to the entire family.

Aspects of caregiving can be gratifying, but as the parent's
needs increase, caregiving takes over more and more of a daughter's life. Women may assume the tasks willingly when a parent
is relatively independent or step in for an emergency without
knowing what to expect in the future (Guberman et al. 1992).
Daughters are likely to take unpaid leaves of absence, reduce
their working hours, relinquish their jobs, eliminate their vaca-
tions, and abandon their social activities to keep pace with the
pressing demands of caregiving. But the progressive deterioration
of the parent cannot be stemmed, and in the end daughters often
feel frustrated and angry about their own powerlessness.

Caregiving is hard work. It is not something to undertake lightly
or to walk away from in the middle. It is not only physically taxing; it is emotionally wearing. Eldercare is also more complicated
than it was in the past and can involve multiple tasks over many
years. "It is hypocritical to envision it as anything but a hard,
bankrupting job," says Theodore Roszak. "The extensive care that
the frail and infirm require is uniquely the result of modern medicine. Nobody in any previous culture was expected to handle
demands of this magnitude and live a life of their own" (2001:121).
The caregiver must give unconditional support and function as the
parent's advocate without being patronizing. Many daughters have
likened the experience of caring for a frail parent to that of caring
for a growing child, because the daughter assumes the role of parent. Yet the experience is inherently different because the daughter is a witness to her parent's decline, and the result is not hard

to envision. What the daughter does to make an ailing parent more comfortable may ensure the status quo for a while, but it is never enough in the long run. Women tend to see the deterioration of a parent under their care as a personal affront and are burdened with guilt. It is hard for a daughter to act objectively amid such intense involvement.

Daughters who care for their mothers are particularly stressed because they identify so closely with their mothers' decline. Although their roles are now reversed, daughters continue to look upon mothers as the original nurturers. Daughters are not only constantly reminded of how their mothers used to be; they are also terrified of their mothers' infirmities, which "foreshadow" their coming old age. The anthropologist Robert Rubinstein, who studied the social context of caregiving by collecting daughters' narratives, concludes that, no matter how dependent mothers are on daughters, the relationship continues to remain one between a mother who has raised a child and her middle-aged daughter. This is the last chance for mothers and daughters to examine and work out crucial aspects of their relationship (1995:258).

When elderly people have both sons and daughters, the daughters inevitably end up as the primary caregivers. Sometimes, adult daughters share equally in the tasks of caregiving, but that is the exception rather than the rule. "Contingencies such as geographical proximity, gender roles, or interpersonal relationships conspire to make the burdens unequal, and often unfair, in practice," notes Harry Moody (1992:92). Sons who share in caregiving tasks usually expect their sisters to provide the personal care while they carry out the more "masculine" tasks related to managing the household.

Considering the broad range of caregiving duties performed by family members, the need to share the responsibility becomes obvious. Barbara Tarlow (1996) believes that the caregiving role should be negotiated among adult children because not everyone is cut out to be a good caregiver or is willing to make the necessary sacrifices. Good caregiving encompasses a number of indispensable qualities without which the experience can be transformed into a traumatic burden for all concerned. Some children may feel that a paid surrogate is an adequate substitute for personal caregiving. The neglected parent's emotional hurt is not easily forgotten. It is not uncommon for the elderly care recipient to feel abandoned when adult children are distant and uninvolved.

Men rise admirably to the occasion when daughters are lacking. Some of the finest stories in the caregiving literature are about men caring tenderly for their parents and feeling as much of a moral responsibility as women do. In *The Time of Their Dying*, Stephen Rosenfeld talks about the importance of investing time, unstintingly, in the care of a parent: "One must be there. Time and again I realized how futile it was to extract information or convey emotion at a distance" (1977:180). The journalist and writer Nick Taylor, who was sucked into the caregiving vortex as an only child, also experienced such sentiments. His memoir, *A Necessary End*, should be read by every potential caregiver because it depicts so nakedly his intense involvement with both parents as they declined. His caretaking career encompassed the period from 1983 to 1991. At first he felt he had to decide how much of his life he should sacrifice to care for his ailing parents. But then he plunged fully into the caregiving fray as he tried to deal with one crisis after another. His parents had retired to Mexico, and everything was fine until they both began to fall apart at almost the same time. The saga of his peripatetic movements began—back and forth and back and forth—in the pattern typical of the adult child who tries to put a stopper in the drain with each crisis-induced visit but finds that the drain is unplugged again before enough time has elapsed to resume his own life. Taylor had to relocate his parents to an assisted-living community in Florida and commuted between New York and Fort Meyers to deal with his mother's repeated strokes and father's subsequent cancer. He feared his parents' dotage, then their loss and a future in which the only two persons who had known him as a child were gone forever. No matter what he did, he never felt he had a handle on the situation, and he had no siblings to share his pain. He wrote the memoir (illustrated with old-fashioned woodblock prints his father had made) to keep them in mind and finally he realized that he was the embodiment of what his parents had brought into the world and that he was what he had to remember them by. "Ours is the tale of the end of the century," Taylor concluded, "anywhere children in the bloom of their lives must confront their parents' withering" (1994:28).

Tom Koch, the author of *Mirrored Lives: Aging Children and Elderly Parents,* cared for his father with total dedication. He became a frequent flyer between Vancouver and Buffalo, New York, "unable to stay in Buffalo and unwilling to stay away. Each new medical crisis returned me to Norm's house, and as he grew weaker, each new responsibility tied me closer to the world that Norm progressively relinquished. . . . I could not leave; it was impossible for me to fly that far knowing how tenuous was the balance in our Buffalo world. . . . This was the pattern, a gradual diminishment and a series of small incidents, as we waited for calamity to strike" (1990:173, 175). Koch's book illustrates how the strands of connectedness bind failing parents and caring children even closer together as their private world crumbles. Koch asked himself why he—and not his brothers—cared so intensely for his father. "It has to do with accepting his age and seeing my future in it," he surmised. "In short, my time is homage not to the husk that my father has become but to the man he somehow remains" (1990:156). Koch got so caught up in his father's care that he declined an important job offer and put off a major book project. After his father's death, he not only produced *Mirrored Lives;* he also started a project on family caregivers that resulted in *A Place in Time: Care Givers for Their Elderly* (1993). In the second book, he concludes that the crux of caregiving is not responsibility but compassion. Few family members are capable of such sustained compassion because the primary caregiver suffers along with the recipient and experiences, "once removed," the terrors and horrors of impending death.

In *Looking After,* John Daniel depicts the nitty-gritty of caregiving in frank, unapologetic terms. He was a reluctant caregiver for a mother who had moved into his home after she became increasingly forgetful. Daniel had conflicting feelings because she had never been a "mothering" type. He was annoyed and acted churlishly at times: "My mother had been a strong and vibrant woman. It grieved me to see her reduced to a stooped crone who dithered over vegetables at the store, who couldn't remember what she'd read half an hour before, who forgot to take the pills I placed directly in front of her at breakfast. It more than grieved me—it enraged me . . . because I was stuck with caring for a feeble old mother and didn't want to be" (1996:92). Yet he mourned his mother after she died and chastised himself. "In the time since her death, I've found myself saying, 'I'm sorry, Mama, I'm so sorry.' . . . I berated myself for not being strong enough to bear the modest office of caregiving. I blamed myself for my mother's irrevocable absence from the world" (1996:204, 214).

Researchers have consistently shown that family caregiving engenders family conflicts. Rare is the family that manages to stay together and act harmoniously under the multiple stresses of caring for failing parents. The national survey on family caregiving found that some 25 percent of caregivers report family conflict (*Family Caregiving in the U.S.* 1997:22). The conflict generally arises between the primary caregiver and the other siblings (Brody et al. 1989). Because most primary caregivers are women, sisters frequently find themselves on the outs with their brothers. "When caregivers are asked directly about relations with siblings," writes Amy Horowitz, "significant numbers do report deteriorated relations" (1985:210). Many siblings care deeply about their parents but do not engage in the actual care. Brothers may feel that hands-on care can be provided adequately by hiring outsiders, but daughters often believe that no outsider can care for their parents the way they do and are more sensitive to the fact that vulnerable parents may prefer their children's help. Brothers may act as though their sisters' careers are expendable or less relevant because they cling to the outmoded, sexist notion that men are the principal wage earners. Caregiving itself is devalued because it is an unremunerated personal activity—women's work—that receives little recognition beyond the family sphere.

Many wonder how much longer women can bear the emotional burden of caregiving. The responsibility is often imposed on the daughter with little discussion or planning, because girls have been socialized to "care" while boys are directed to "act." Despite the revolution in gender roles, people still assume that women will continue to provide the bulk of the hands-on care. Richard Martin and Stephen Post note that some women may have the inner resources to "shoulder this monumental responsibility" and may "live lives of significant self-abnegation," yet they question the ability of women to hold up under the increasing pressure (1992:62).

Explosions are likely to occur when the primary caregiver feels the effects of burnout and verbalizes her resentment to less involved siblings. A little more than half of all caregivers feel that other relatives are not doing their share. Caregivers are distressed not only by their siblings' lesser participation but also by their siblings' lack of emotional and instrumental support for their role as principal caregiver. The other siblings often take the caregiving sister for granted. Caregivers rightly feel that absent siblings are the least fit to criticize their efforts or offer unsolicited advice, especially when they are not there to witness the daily happenings. Absent children, however, may feel slighted by the primary caregiver because they are not consulted or kept abreast of changes.

The conflict is not actually between sisters and brothers but between the primary caregiver and his or her siblings. Koch's book amply testifies to the tension that can be generated among male siblings. Koch could not help but feel annoyed when one brother called to say he would visit their father for the weekend. It was his turn, the brother said. Koch commented with irritation, "His 'turn' would be mostly a holiday in which they would go out to dinner or visit the local art gallery, while mine had been a siege" (1990:76). How could his brother equate a three-day visit with his own months of constant ministrations? Koch was infuriated with his siblings. His brothers had asked for progress reports, which they interpreted as "dictatorial" because Koch included instructions for calling and visiting their father. His brothers were concerned at a distance: Two had not visited in months and the other in years. "They had not seen the evidence of his decline . . . and to me their distance meant they had abdicated the right to help decide his fate" (1990:118). What Koch resented most was the fact that his three brothers expected to continue their own lives without being restricted or inconvenienced. If Koch had not been in Buffalo, his brothers would not be able to enjoy such liberty. The tension escalated into "pitched battles," according to Koch. Four sons shared a father yet were like "islands on opposite sides of some temporal, experiential, tectonic plate that had shifted our lives, once anchored so closely, finally and forever apart" (1990: 179). And their father, the only link that joined their communal past, would soon be gone.

I empathized with Koch. I too had been guilty of sending letters to my brother that were actually thinly veiled lists of instructions, reminders to call our parents, and other admonishments. I felt I was fulfilling my duty as the primary caregiver, but he must have perceived the letters as meddlesome. A sibling who receives such a letter cannot help but resent its sender, even though that person is doing all of the hands-on care.

Numerous factors affect the quality of sibling relationships. First and foremost, siblings cannot afford to be angry with their parents, so they must take out their fear and frustration on one another. A failing parent is too often caught up in his or her own problems to focus on the undercurrents of care. Some siblings revive childhood rivalries and other old conflicts in the context of caregiving. Yet caregiving is sufficiently stressful to produce conflicts among siblings who previously enjoyed harmonious relationships. Adult children bicker about the type of care that is appropriate—should it be a nursing home or some sort of home arrangement? They squabble over the disbursement of the parents' funds—one sibling may feel that the parents' savings should be used to fund their care, another that those life savings are sacred and should be held for eventual inheritance. Parents who lived through the Depression may be loath to deplete the savings that took a lifetime to amass and worry that their medical expenses will leave nothing for the children. Siblings may have questions about inheritance and wills but feel that discussing such matters in the context of caregiving is tasteless. So they remain silent, and their silence breeds tension and taints their relationship. The possibilities for friction among siblings are endless. Primary caregivers may be so depressed and exhausted from sleeplessness, poor diet, lack of respite, and the endless routine that they cannot cope graciously with a difficult sibling. "Coming together to face a parent's illness requires an altogether different degree of cooperation and communication among siblings than organizing holiday dinners and family reunions," warn Nancy Hooyman and Wendy Lustbader in *Taking Care of Your Aging Family Members* (1986:45).

If filial obligations were shared more evenly and not simply left to dutiful daughters, families would be able to function as more effective caregivers to their parents. The burdens of contemporary caregiving can be extremely unfair, creating a new class of human casualties who will be unable to age successfully because of the disproportionate demands on their time and resources. "Increasing pressures on adult children to personally take care of their frail relative's every need is socially irresponsible," says Laura Olson in a detailed study of the political economy of long-term care (1993:179). The solution, she says, is to implement social policies that will address not only the needs of the care recipients but also those of the caregivers.

In a cogent summing up of the problem, Carol Levine notes that she eventually realized she had done nothing wrong in her caregiving. It was the system that was out of whack. "I feel abandoned by a health care system that commits resources and rewards to rescuing the injured and ill but then consigns such patients and their families to the black hole of chronic 'custodial' care" (2000:74). Only in the United States are family members inducted into a volunteer labor force because the health-care system, predicated on outmoded social policies, has not yet grappled with the issue of caring for our nation's oldest citizens. The void in long-term-care programs will only expand unless Medicare abandons its antiquated premises and comes to terms with the pressing needs of our rapidly aging society.

An equitable health-care system would empower potential caregivers by allowing them to choose to take on the caregiving role rather than forcing the role on them. In a timely essay on the institutional care of the elderly, Bela Blasszauer puts it aptly: "A society can, indeed, very well be judged on the basis of how it takes care of its elderly" (1994:14). Good care must be an ethical concern for everyone, and caring for the frail elderly must be the social responsibility of an entire nation.

CHAPTER FOUR

The Palms at Palm-Aire
"Everyone here is berserk."

JULY 6–AUGUST 17, 1993: 43 DAYS • "Nurse, nurse, . . . nurse, nurse," cried an elderly lady from her wheelchair. "Help! Help me, help me, help me!" came from a nearby doorway. A wiry old gentleman, partly nude, rushed up and down the hallway, trying to escape the ministrations of a male aide. One ancient woman clutched a teddy bear; another tightly held a stiff-sided old-fashioned pocketbook. Both ladies were heavily rouged— exquisitely made up, as if they were on their way to a gala—but in reality they were firmly wrapped in blankets and encased in wheelchairs. Two very elderly ladies, seated on a bench and chatting, peered up as I walked down the hallway. "Oh, look," one said to the other. "Look at her long hair, her skirt. Isn't she just gorgeous? It's Miss America." I smiled and said hello, but they didn't respond.

I had walked into what looked like a gerontological loony bin. Here were the human remains of decrepitude I had read about but firmly rejected in my career as a medical anthropologist, the stereotypic vision of the oldest old waiting silently in the corridors adjoining the nurses' station, staring into space, waiting to die, and so detached from the surrounding environment that most did not have the energy even to glance at me as I invaded their living space.

But this was not a gerontological warehouse. It was The Palms at Palm-Aire, a nursing home with one of the finest reputations in South Florida, where my mother was about to undergo physical therapy. When I entered The Palms the first time, I ignored the stench of stale urine in the air. I ignored the deep stains on the rug. I ignored the loud music reverberating through the hallways from invisible loudspeakers. I even managed to ignore the lineup of extremely old ladies who sat passively in their wheelchairs alongside the nurses' station. Most of all, I ignored my own feelings that even shabby Pine Manor across the road from Sacred Heart might be better. It was run-down and antiquated, the social worker kept saying. After all, didn't Mother's social worker know best? Mother needed good nursing care, and she needed to be near home so Dad could drop by. My feelings about The Palms were mixed from the start, but I was willing to give the place a try.

I could barely reconcile my initial negative impressions of The Palms with the very positive ones I had received from the personnel in the admissions office. The social worker, Peggy Jo, was patient and charming. I needed a sympathetic ear, and she seemed to have all the time in the world to provide it. Yes, some Medicare beds were available, but I would have to complete the paperwork before they could talk about admitting Mother. She spoke on the phone several times with Mother and came to the house to explain the admissions procedures to her.

"Mrs. Margolies, I understand you'll be joining us for therapy for a few weeks," she said. "I'm a good friend of your social worker. I'm here to help you. Do you have any questions you would like to ask me? Any concerns you'd like to express? Your daughter told me you're a very brave woman."

"Yes, but I'm very worried about entering The Palms. I'm worried about the therapy," Mother replied. "I'm afraid I'm not going to make it, and I'm leaving my husband at home. He's not well and can't be alone."

"Your husband can have meals with you, if you like. This is only a temporary situation, just for a few weeks, so you can receive your therapy and return home. I don't want you to worry. Your therapists will evaluate you when you enter and tailor a program just for you. You'll be able to work at your own pace. If you're tired, you can rest. If you need hot packs, we have them. We have very caring therapists."

"I know, but I'm also worried about being separated from my daughter. I know she has to go home. She's going home in a few days."

"I understand that your daughter will be back before you finish your therapy. Your daughter will be here when you need her. I'm sure you want to be able to function again at home. That's the only reason for coming."

"Yes, I do."

"Will you try your best? And, please, we want you to relax. Will you try?"

"Yes, yes, I will. I'm going to do my best. I know I have no other choice."

Later, when I went to Peggy Jo's office to pick up the paperwork, she commented, "I was charmed by your mother. Now I understand what you meant when we discussed her admission. I know we'll be able to help her. Don't worry. I'll be looking after your mother."

How could I not feel good about The Palms? Mother would be taken care of for a few weeks while she was finally exposed to the gentle but intense program of physical rehabilitation she desperately needed.

Mother's transfer to The Palms on July 6 went smoothly. I planned her move with attention to the details—a few pairs of running shoes for therapy, some shorts so her movements would be unrestricted, a sweatsuit, seven changes of clothing, matching hangers, drawer liner, a colorful quilt, photographs, a plant, some books, her diary and writing implements, hard candies to moisten her throat, and a new television set . Mother was temporarily placed in a double room near the nurses' station, but Pamela Peterson from the admissions office assured me she would be moved as soon as a private room became available. The rooms were The Palms's most attractive feature. Built to accommodate a wealthy clientele who bought into the continuing-care concept when it first arose, they were spacious and tastefully furnished. Not all the floor plans were exactly alike. Many residents had brought their own furnishings and transformed their rooms into an eclectic variety of homelike quarters away from home. I neatly hung Mother's clothing in the metal cabinet and placed her personal articles in the small dresser next to her bed. I carefully lined the larger dresser with blue flowered paper and put away her folded tops and undergarments. I then labeled all Mother's belongings with a black laundry marker, even though I had no intention of sending her clothes to the facility's laundry room, where they might be mishandled.

Mother received a lot of attention during the first twenty-four hours. Beth, the licensed practical nurse (LPN) in charge of her admission, reviewed Dr. Risden's instructions with me. I told Beth I had been giving Mother three respiratory treatments a day and that it was important to continue them. Did The Palms have a nebulizer? No problem; one would be ordered from Medicare. Beth also assured me she would contact a psychologist for a few sessions. The early-morning incident on July 4 had frightened me. I knew Mother was depressed, and instead of focusing on the task ahead, she kept asking rhetorically why she had been spared. Dr. Friedmann, The Palms's attending physician, arrived in the evening. A slightly built man with a cherubic head of thick hair, he looked as though he might have been a member of the high-school Shakespearean society. Mother liked him instantly.

"Why do you still have this Foley catheter?" he asked, looking at Mother, then turning and peering at me.

Frankly, neither of us really knew. "Mother left Sacred Heart with the catheter, and the visiting nurse instructed us to leave it in. As a matter of fact, she made a big point of measuring the daily urine output."

"Well, I definitely think it's time for this to come out."

Mother was delighted. She detested this appendage: It impeded her movement and pinched and pulled her as she tried to turn. The catheter had been left in for convenience, and the psychological boost of removing the odious object would be beneficial to her. No doubt about it, Friedmann's attitude instantly endeared him to Mother.

The next morning I found Mother dressed and resting comfortably on top of the bed. She had a serene expression for the first time since leaving Sacred Heart. The bustling attention of the previous day had energized her, and she looked ready to begin her therapy program in good spirits.

"Mother, Lunice will be coming in every morning to help you dress."

"I'm not sure I need a private aide."

"Promise me you won't dismiss her the minute I leave. Even if you think you don't need her, I'll feel better knowing she's by your side, at least for the first week."

"All right."

"I don't trust you, Mother. Remember, you gave me your word. Even if you think you don't need her—even if she just sits and stares at the walls—she stays. Lunice has been around a lot of nursing homes, and she'll be a big help the first few days."

"All right. I assure you. I assure you!"

"I'm going to come by later this afternoon with Kathy. It's important for you to start taking charge of your affairs again."

"No, I have enough to worry about. I don't want to be bothered. I don't want to think about bills."

"Mummy, you know Dad can't do it. We've already gone over a lot of things at home, but I don't want it to pile up while I'm away. Kathy will bring over the important mail for you to go over, and she'll help you by writing out the checks. All you have to do is approve and sign them."

"I'll give it a try."

I knew Mother had little desire to worry about household matters, but I sorely wanted to engage her interest again. I was convinced that by focusing on her life outside, she would be motivated to work hard.

Mother insisted that I stay for lunch. She raved about the home-style cooking, and I wanted to satisfy my curiosity. A low-salt but tasty bowl of chicken soup was followed by a crabmeat salad and a moist slice of lemon cake. The dining-room service seemed satisfactory. Many of the residents were wearing bibs and were helped by private aides garbed in distinctive purple aprons. Fortunately, Mother's tablemates were like-minded, alert people who were also there for physical and occupational therapy.

Despite my initial misgivings, I was confident that Mother would receive the attention she required. In fact, I felt enormous relief that she would be in a safe environment while she underwent therapy. I looked at her tranquil expression and was convinced everything was under control. It never occurred to me that Mother would not be fine at The Palms.

At home I set about dismantling the hospital equipment. I wanted to eliminate all traces of hospital gear and turn the room back into a den again. I realized what a mistake it had been to bring a big hospital bed into the house. It was difficult to crank up and down and was too high for Mother to transfer safely into a wheelchair, even with my help. Now the bed, the table, the wheelchair, and the nebulizer had to be returned immediately or

Medicare would charge Mother for another month's worth of hospital equipment. I could not take the nebulizer or wheelchair to the nursing home. They had to go directly back to the supply house, as the nursing home would be reimbursed for its own equipment requests.

Next I folded Marisa's clothes and packed them in large cartons that I stored in the closet. I told Fay she should give them to Marisa when she appeared. I knew she would surface as soon as I left town, and hoped it would be soon for Mother's sake. (Much later, Marisa admitted that she had called the house several times but hung up when I answered.) Dad was seething with anger and still wanted to burn her clothing. I felt that his anger would dissipate when he saw her again. They'll work it out, I thought. I was certainly too exhausted to deal with it.

I had planned to leave for the Canary Islands two days after returning to Caracas, but when I got home, I collapsed in bed and stayed there for forty-eight hours. I had been with Mother through her near-death experience and her arrival home, and through Marisa's disappearance and the hiring of a housekeeper whom I distrusted. Now the accumulated effects of a month's sleep deprivation hit me full force. I told Graziano I could not leave right away. I was too worn out and had to catch up with my own affairs. I was losing a grip on my own domestic matters and wondered how I could have managed without full-time live-in help. If it were not for Marisa's sister, Carlota, who had been with us since our son was an infant, I would not be able to go back and forth, leaving my husband to fend for himself.

The sooner I left, the sooner I could return. I was in a frenzy of indecision. In Caracas, I was only three air hours away from Mother; if I left, I would be six more hours away and would have to return to Florida via Caracas or Madrid in case of an emergency. For the past five years I had conducted a large-scale project on Canary Island migration to Venezuela and I was on the last phase. I had originally intended to leave for the island of Tenerife in early May; now it was mid-July, and I was afraid I would lose my grant if I did not comply with the award period. Worse yet, I had not seen sixteen-year-old Graz, who had stayed to complete the school year, in more than six months. Mother was definitely improving. I never would have left her if she had not been on the mend. She would be safe at The Palms. Nothing hinted otherwise.

I had trouble getting through to Mother right away. Not only was I back to the miserable phone service of Caracas, but when I finally did connect, no one answered. I was not concerned, because Noel and his daughter Allison had arrived right after my departure. Allison was shocked by Mother's fragile appearance, but Noel, who had last seen Mother at Sacred Heart when she was attached to a mechanical respirator, found her much improved. Noel, who spent most of his waking hours in hospitals, was not pleased with The Palms. The stench in the hallways turned him off, and the general atmosphere seemed detrimental to a rapid convalescence.

I finally got through to Mother from a phone booth at the airport while I waited to take off for Tenerife. Her voice sounded muted, but she was fine, she insisted. The food continued to be good, and she had enjoyed the weekend with Noel and Allison. She would soon be transferred to a private room and had started her therapy. There was little else to report. The situation was stable.

Graz had been waiting for me to arrive for more than a week and had moved from his schoolmate's home into the cozy cottage I rented while doing fieldwork in the Canary Islands. After neatly stocking the kitchen with groceries, he had set out a jug of red roses and a large plate of bananas, the island's principal export crop, on an old table in the entryway. He had barely assimilated the terrible news about his grandma and was having a hard time dealing with the first major counterpoint in his young life.

"Mommy," he said, "I don't know how to react or how to act. I can't believe all this has happened to Grandma. Nobody I love has ever been ill like this before. I want to speak to Grandma, but I don't know what to say."

"We'll call her tomorrow. Say exactly what you feel. Tell her you're thinking about her and that you love her. She always asks for you."

"I hope I see Grandma again."

"That's why I want you to come home with me. It's important for you to see her."

Graz's grandma held a special place for him. He was the child she had coddled and yelled at, listened to and advised, treating him in every sense exactly as her own. I had made a special effort to cultivate the relationship between my son and his grandparents by taking him to Florida during his school breaks.

We sat on the terrace behind the cottage. The hamlet was situated on a bluff overlooking the Atlantic and had changed little over the past century. Many farmhouses had been abandoned as people moved to the cities, but our modest cottage had been lovingly restored. I looked out over the rustling banana trees to the hazy horizon and inhaled the salt-laden air. If only I could hold on to this moment forever, the sense of serenity and happiness that entered my soul on being saturated with the sounds and fragrances of bygone days. I closed my eyes and, with my son by my side, napped peacefully for the first time in many months.

We flew to Lanzarote, the easternmost island of the Spanish archipelago, only 125 kilometers off the West African coast. I wanted to obtain a firsthand account of the conditions that had precipitated a mass exodus to Venezuela, depopulating the volcanic island. I called Mother from our hotel on the Teguise Coast.

Without doubt, her honeymoon at The Palms was over. The food was terrible, she was having vague stomach trouble, and the corridors were freezing. "I'm not going to make it through another week here," Mother said bitterly. "I'm going crazy, stir-crazy. The residents here are all berserk. I've never seen anything like it. There's nobody to talk to."

I was overwhelmed by Mother's outburst and not sure how to react. "How did everything change so quickly, Mother? Tell me, how is the therapy going?"

"That's one good thing. I'm actually enjoying the therapy and look forward to it every day. The girls have been giving me heat treatments, and my back feels much better."

"Do you feel that you're making progress?"

"Yes, definitely. As a matter of fact, Marisa has been practicing with me in the hallways."

"You mean Marisa has reappeared?"

"Yes, just a few days after you left. She came over to The Palms, sobbing and begging me to forgive her."

"Did you forgive her?"

"Of course! We'll have to let bygones be bygones. You were too harsh with her."

"You're right, Mother. I can't tell you how awful I've felt over this, particularly for you. I never should have criticized her. I wasn't my usual self."

"I don't think she wants to see you."

"It doesn't matter. What matters right now is her relationship with you. Did you ask Marisa to come by again?"

"No, she came and went."

"I'm sure she'll be back soon. But right now, you need to concentrate on the important things. Insist on speaking with the dietitian, wear your sweatsuit in the hallway, and most of all, concentrate on the therapy. I want you home as soon as possible. I'll call you again from Tenerife, and I want you to call me for even the smallest problem."

"I tried to call you to see how you arrived, and they refused to put the call through."

"What do you mean, Mother?"

"They said they would not put through any long-distance calls, that they don't make long-distance calls at The Palms."

"I've never heard anything so stupid. Who told you that?"

"The operator at the desk. I was having trouble dialing Spain."

"This is unbelievable. Call Kathy if you need to. Graziano will call you every day from Caracas. We've been having trouble getting through from this end, too. Nobody answers the phone, and when they finally do, they say you're not in your room."

"That's crazy. They know where to find me."

"We'll manage somehow, Mummy, and anyway, you'll be home soon."

When I got through the following week from Tenerife, Mother's litany of complaints continued. Now the focus was on Fay.

"You won't believe how this woman has humiliated and degraded me," Mother said. "When I asked her to take the laundry home, she threw my clothing on the floor, screaming at me that she hadn't been hired to wash my dirty clothing. I was a 'liar,' she said, because she hadn't been instructed to take home my clothing. Her only job was to take care of Dad."

"How dare she say that to you. I specifically told her she was to do whatever you asked." We went over these points, one by one, and Fay assured me she would carry out her chores responsibly.

"That's not all," Mother continued. "She parks Dad in the chair, never asks if we need anything, then walks out of the room to kibitz with the staff. She told Dory [one of the nursing aides] I was a 'witch,' 'a bad person,' and that I was just as mean at The Palms as I had been at home."

My face was heating up as I listened to this, but I tried to reply evenly. "How do you know that, Mummy?"

"Dory came in and repeated what Fay said."

"What did you do?"

"I wheeled myself out to the corridor and yelled at Fay in front of the entire staff: 'How dare you speak to the aides like that? How dare you come in here and bad-mouth me in front of the staff? Who do you think you are? You don't know anything about us, but you should have enough sense to realize that I'm very sick, and so is my husband. Don't you ever raise your voice to me again or speak to the staff about me behind my back.'"

"Mother, you should have fired her on the spot. She put on a good act when I was there. I spent hours going over the routine with her, from your laundry to the smallest details of Dad's food tastes."

"Dad hates her," Mother continued. "He went down the road the other day to Ann's house and started banging on her door. 'Ann, Ann, call the police,' he screamed. 'Get this madwoman out of my house. She's driving me mad.'"

"What did Ann do?"

"Ann was very alarmed. She tried to calm Dad down, then took him home and called me right away."

"Dad must have been disturbed by something Fay did if he had enough sense to go over to Ann's house. Maybe she yells at him and orders him around. Maybe she even forgets to feed him. Did you ask Dad about it?"

"Yes, but Dad just says he can't stand her and doesn't give me any details."

"Perhaps he can't remember them, but he clearly detests her. Get rid of her. There's no reason for you to put up with such nonsense. After all, you're the boss."

How could I handle this properly from the Canary Islands? This was a situation I had not anticipated. I had gone over all of the details with Fay, loaded up on her favorite food—anything to make her happy. We had been taken. The employment agency had sent us a person it had not properly screened. It irked me to think we were paying more than $3,000 a month for her to insult and intimidate my defenseless parents.

Now I understood why grown children encourage their parents to enter nursing homes. They cannot trust the hired help; they have no way to know whether their parents are being abused or intimidated. To complicate matters, the moment I left, Mother sent the one aide I trusted, Lunice, packing. Mother did not think Lunice had enough work to warrant her hanging around the nursing home all morning. Dad could not verbalize his fears to me. If it had not been for Mother, I would not have known about Fay. The experience marked a turning point for me: As long as I was there, things were fine, but when I left, everything disintegrated. I decided I would not leave Mother again until she was walking.

• • •

Although I was not a direct witness to Mother's five-week stay at The Palms, I was able to reconstruct the events, thanks to my extensive conversations with Mother and the ongoing surveillance of Marisa and Kathy, who were in and out of the nursing home nearly every day. Mother received a good deal of medical attention during her first week there, which led me to believe she would be adequately cared for. Her good-natured LPN, Beth, followed through on all of my requests and attended to others I had not even anticipated.

Although the therapy departments were located within The Palms, they functioned autonomously, with their own rules and staff. A person could have intensive therapy without staying at the nursing home, but most patients chose to reside there for convenience. Mother may have been depressed, but she entered therapy with the right mind-set. Her therapist noted that she was "highly motivated to recover and regain independence to go home." Five times a week, Mother received physical therapy that consisted of gait training with a rolling walker and transfer training from sit–stand and supine–sit positions. Mother tired easily and had to pace herself, but she was still able to achieve the objectives of the therapy plan by the end of a five-week period. Mother could manage an eighty-five-foot walk with a walker and was scheduled for physical-therapy discharge on August 16. In addition to her sessions, she practiced in the hallway with Marisa's help. However, the nursing-home staff soon put an end to this, insisting that Marisa was not a certified health aide and therefore not qualified to touch Mother. The staff was unwilling to risk an accident in full view of the nursing-home occupants.

Mother also made consistently excellent progress in occupational-therapy, practicing such tasks as dressing and grooming herself, maneuvering from the bed to a standing position, and setting up a food tray and feeding herself. By the end of July, she had met all of the short-term goals set for the period and required only "minimal assistance" to carry out the "activities of daily living," or ADLs. On August 1, Mother's occupational therapist noted, "Resident continues to exhibit a positive behavior and increased motivation to improve in all ADL functions toward independence, upon her wish to return to home and husband. Therefore OT recommends to continue program to maximize potential for self-care."

Back in the nursing home, Mother's progress was less impressive. Peggy Jo, the social worker who had been thoroughly briefed on Mother's health, summarized the care plan in general terms: "We will assist June in being free from discomfort, maintain her weight, maintain her appearance, increase her mobility, and encourage consumption of foods and fluids to induce healing and allow her to regain independence." After the first week, Peggy Jo barely entered the picture, but before bowing out, she characterized Mother as "demanding," "manipulative," and "particular," while giving lip service to her "frail and frightened" condition. Because of these disparaging labels, Mother earned a reputation at The Palms as a chronic complainer. In truth, Mother had simply voiced her opinions about her health so she could obtain the proper treatment. She could express her needs clearly, in contrast to the largely demented, disoriented residents of The Palms; therefore, she was depicted as a complainer. I doubt that many of the staff members could appreciate the discomfort and pain that were my mother's constant companions. They should have realized they were dealing with an acutely ill and demoralized woman.

Dr. Miller, a psychotherapist, came into the case at my request and had several sessions with Mother. He later told me that, although he found Mother "vital" and "cooperative," he was moved by her multiple health problems and emaciated appearance. Mother cried a lot. She told him she was depressed and felt she was on the verge of a nervous breakdown. She had been hallucinating and felt sorry for herself. Her enormous anxiety that Dad could not take care of himself was an ongoing theme. Dr. Miller advised her to bring Dad into The Palms if the situation became intolerable. But worst of all, Mother was angry that she had not been allowed to die. Dr. Miller wrote that psychological factors were affecting Mother's physical condition. It seemed to me that it was the other way around. No doubt Mother's medical complications had sent her into a fierce depression. Even the most optimistic person could not have escaped unscathed.

"Darling," Mother said during another conversation from Tenerife, "it hurts me to see how some of the aides treat the poor patients—particularly my roommate. They laugh at her; they don't come when she calls. It's a very sad situation."

"And how are your aides treating you, Mummy?"

"One is very young and sweet. She tries, and I like her a lot. But the other is rough. She's careless when she helps me into the wheelchair, and she keeps banging my ankles against the footrests."

"Well, tell her to be more careful, and if that doesn't work, complain to the nurse."

"I don't want to make it bad for her."

"Then try to work it out directly with your aide. Tell her you're in constant pain. She probably hasn't helped somebody in your condition before and may not realize she's being too rough."

"Believe me, I will. I've even sent Marisa to buy candies and cookies to give the aides. Anything to make life here a little more bearable."

Mother complained that she never had enough time to eat and that the dining-room staff took her plate away without asking whether she had finished. "They want the patients out of the dining room so they can clean up quickly," she said, "and it's fruitless to insist." Mother began to take her meals in her room, where she could eat at her own pace.

The Palms had started off with great fanfare—psychologists, podiatrists, speech therapists, and dermatologists—but the mechanism for rendering treatment soon bogged down. The well-intentioned care plan, begun so auspiciously and with such an impressive flurry of medical interventions, could not be implemented without hands-on coordination. Instead of improving, Mother's health deteriorated at an alarming pace.

Mother was making splendid progress with her therapy. Her morale improved as she became proficient with the rolling walker and was ambulating. But she began to suffer from bouts of diarrhea that sapped her strength. At first, I was not worried and assumed that the change in diet was responsible for her intestinal upset.

"What have you been taking for it?" I asked Mother.

"Nothing. They said they can't give me anything without the doctor's orders."

"Well, keep insisting. You can't afford to let this ride."

"They don't listen."

"Mom, have Marisa bring you Immodium and start it immediately. Call Dr. Risden if you can't get satisfaction from The Palms. After all, you have a right to speak to your physician without going through The Palms."

"O.K. I'll try to call Dr. Risden."

"Don't just try. Keep calling until you get him on the phone. Have you been watching your diet?"

"I stopped taking the Ensure. It upsets my stomach, and I've cut down on my food."

"No, Mummy, that's not the way to go. You need the Ensure. You have to have nourishment. You can't afford to lose any more weight. Talk to the dietitian about your stomach upset."

"No, it's impossible. It falls on deaf ears. I don't even think they have a dietitian. I told the aide I couldn't eat the lunch. It was some sort of crabmeat salad. I asked for dry toast and tea. You know what she said?"

"No, what?"

"She said they couldn't run a kitchen for just one person. They couldn't give me any special privileges. They refused to make me the toast and walked away. So I didn't eat."

"Mummy, I've never heard of such nonsense! You call the nursing home's director and give her hell. I swear, I'm going to call her and Dr. Risden myself from Tenerife."

"No, no, I'll call them today. I promise."

"O.K., Mummy. Remember, you promised. I'll call you back tomorrow."

But I could not call back the next day. After this conversation, further communication became impossible. I may have been in Tenerife, off the West African coast, but Mother was incarcerated in Outer Siberia as far as I was concerned. The telephone rang and rang, and when I finally did get through, I was given the old song and dance: Mother was unavailable, Mother was in therapy, Mother was not in her room, and so on.

Later I pieced together the full story. The nurse's notes corroborate what Mother told me. She suffered her first attack of diarrhea on July 8, and from July 19 she had continuing, escalating attacks through July 26. At this point, she began refusing certain foods, hoping that this would help relieve her stomach distress. The attacks continued, however, and it was not until August 8 that the doctor prescribed Lomotil. But the medication did not help, and Mother spent a wakeful night in pain. On August 9, the doctor ordered a stool specimen. It was collected on August 10 and resulted positive on August 11 for *Clostridium difficile,* a particularly virulent bacillus. Treatment with vancomycin began on the August 12 and was to continue for ten days. Only on August 14, after more than a month had elapsed, was Mother able to report that the diarrhea was coming under control. But the next day, which coincided with her birthday, Mother awoke feverish and achy. Despite her malaise, she made it to occupational therapy. On August 17, her therapist commented: "She has been doing well in all sessions, increasing her independence toward completion of OT goals. However the last 23 days resident suffered from a bad cold and had a small setback in function, bodily strength and weakness. Will continue to progress upon improved medical status."

I also learned that, whereas a healthy immune system can easily repel most bacteria lurking in institutions, the weak and the elderly are vulnerable. Resistant bugs are "hellishly" difficult to control, says the infectious-disease specialist Dr. Thomas Beam. "Resistant infections are present in every hospital and nursing home. . . . The only question is whether the institution is releasing that information" (as quoted in Cowley 1994:51). In Mother's case, the information was not released until after the damage had been done.

I was unhappy that I could not speak directly with Mother. If I could hear her voice, I would be able to gauge her well-being. I had spent nearly three weeks in Tenerife, extrapolating data from the emigration records. The tedious routine of copying hundreds of pieces of information into my notebooks was anesthetizing, but it did not relieve my constant anxiety about my mother. I had nothing more to do in the Canary Islands, and Graz and I were scheduled to fly to Caracas on Mother's birthday.

The situation at home had deteriorated rapidly after Dad ran to his neighbor's house. Fay complained to Noel on the phone that Dad was "impossible to live with"—he had tried to burn the house down and kept her up all night. "I suspect the truth is somewhere in the middle," Noel remarked, but I thought Fay's allegations were preposterous. Fay left by mutual agreement, and Dad moved into The Palms on July 28.

Mother was finally able to concentrate on her therapy because she did not have to worry about what was going on at home. She had admitted tearfully to the psychotherapist that Dad was not the man he had once been, and she wondered how he was being looked after in her absence. The sessions had helped her reflect on and clarify some issues. Mother was calmer and more relaxed with Dad at her side; she would not be separated from him again.

As soon as I walked in the door in Caracas, I called the nursing home to wish Mother a happy birthday. "Your mother is not in the room," the operator said.

"Go to her room and find her. I know my mother is in her room. I'm not hanging up until you connect me."

Mother finally got on the line. "I'm feeling somewhat better, even though I have a bad cold. What a birthday! They finally got around to taking a culture and prescribing antibiotics, and I think the diarrhea is finally coming under control."

"What did the culture indicate, Mother?"

"I don't remember what it's called, but I've never felt so humiliated in my life. I don't like the way they treat me here. You'd think I was a pariah: They've come into the room with masks and gloves and don't want to touch me. The aide was furious when I had an accident, and she yelled at me."

"She had no right to yell at you. You have an intestinal infection, and it seems to me they let it go."

"You're right. I've had diarrhea all month, and they just ignored it. Why do I have to be humiliated like this? If they came when I rang, I would never have had an accident. I tried to hold it in. But they just ignore the call bell. They always come too late. Not only that—they're dismissing me in therapy."

"But that's good, not bad," I said. "You've completed your therapy, and it's time to think about coming home."

"But I can't really walk yet."

"That's not what I heard from Graziano. You have the basics, and now you can practice at home."

"I haven't finished OT yet. I have another two weeks, and in the meantime they said I could practice PT in the hallways with a private therapist."

"I'll have a chance to see for myself. I'll be up in a few days, and we'll start planning your return home."

"I don't know if I'm ready to go home."

"I know you're afraid, but we'll work it out, even if you and Dad have to move to an apartment on the first floor."

"When are you coming?"

"This weekend. I just have to see what arrangements I can make for Graz's school, and then I'll be up."

"How's my darling?"

"He's fine. I expect to bring him with me."

But in truth, he was not fine. Not only were we returning to Caracas without having made any arrangements for the school year, but he had had an episode in Tenerife that frightened me. One night he awoke in a panic, calling for help; he could not catch his breath, and I had to use an asthma spray to normalize his breathing. In the midst of this attack, he confessed he was worried about a lump on the back of his neck. The hard, movable lump, about the size of a golfball, had been there for several weeks, but I had not noticed it because of his long hair.

"It's probably nothing serious, but we'd better have it checked out when we return to Caracas," I said. I did not want to think about the possible implications of the suspicious-looking lump. I wanted to take him to our family doctor before leaving for Florida.

I never had the opportunity. Marisa called me late in the evening on August 17. "I'm sorry I have to tell you this, Señora Luisa, but Señora June is in the hospital again. I just came from there."

"Oh, no, Marisa, not again. What happened?"

"Señora June had a temperature and cough and was short of breath. The nursing home sent her to the hospital at eight-thirty in the evening."

"I can't believe this. I never even got a call from the nursing home. Why didn't they call me?"

"I don't know. I have no idea."

"How is Mother?"

"She's perfectly aware of everything and very calm. The nursing home called the non-emergency ambulance to take Señora June to Coral Bay."

"Do me a favor, Marisa. Please go to the hospital tomorrow morning and tell Mother that I'll be on the earliest flight up."

This was the first time I had spoken with Marisa since she had left my parents' house. After we got over the initial awkward hump, though, we fell back into our old routine. Graziano had laid the groundwork by speaking with Marisa nearly every day while I was in the Canary Islands, and I was ready to forgive and forget.

• • •

I was relieved when I saw Mother. I had expected to find her half-conscious and heavily monitored when I heard the preliminary diagnosis of congestive heart failure; even though she was hooked to an external heart monitor in the telemetry unit, her color was good and she was in good spirits. She was tired but in a fighting mood.

Mother had had a persistent cough, a low-grade fever, and shortness of breath for a few days. A chest X-ray taken at The Palms showed bilateral pleural effusions. Dr. Friedmann was notified and ordered Mother's immediate hospitalization for probable congestive heart failure. She was "in no acute distress" when she was admitted, according to Dr. Friedmann, but he considered her prognosis "guarded."

"How did this happen, Mummy? I couldn't believe it when Marisa told me you were back in Coral Bay."

"I know. I can hardly believe it myself. I've had a cold and sore throat for nearly three weeks, and then the diarrhea. None of this would have happened if they had just paid attention to me when I complained. Everything was just left to linger."

"This whole business seems so unnecessary," I said. "I'm going to get to the bottom of it, not that it will change anything. And I'm not going to leave Dad at The Palms. I'm taking him home right away."

"No, leave Dad there for the moment. He loves the food, and you won't be able to take care of him properly. The only pleasure Dad has left is eating. He'll be all right. You're his lifeline now, but you need your rest, too. And I have to admit, it was a bad idea to share a room with Dad. I didn't get any rest at night while he was with me at The Palms."

"Well, I'm not convinced, but I don't think I'll have time to look for a new housekeeper. The thought of another Fay turns me off—I'm so burned up by that woman. I'll wait for a few days—at least, until you're out of telemetry."

I had had every reason to believe that Mother would complete her therapy quickly and return home. I never imagined she would pick up new ailments at The Palms that would lead her back to the hospital. I went to the nursing home the day after I arrived in Florida. It seemed odd that Dad, whose sole reason for being at The Palms was to accompany Mother, was now there alone. At the nurses' station, I was told that Dad was in the activities room. He was seated at the back of the group and had joined a sing-along.

When I tapped his shoulder, he turned around and greeted me with an enormous sigh of relief. I led him out of the room.

"Can you think of anything so senseless as to make me participate in a sing-along?" he asked. "My wife is in the hospital, very ill, and they make me participate in a sing-along."

"I know, Dad, I guess they're trying to distract you from your troubles."

"Do they think I'm in the mood to sing? They're ridiculous."

I went to The Palms each day, ostensibly to see Dad, and took advantage of the visits to chat with Mother's therapists and aides and observe the interactions between the staff members and patients. Marisa and Kathy had already given me a full report on what went on in my absence. Marisa had spent a good part of the day at The Palms, but the administrator did her best to bar her from the premises, insisting that she was not a licensed health aide and had no business pretending to be one. Kathy was annoyed with the way Marisa was treated and told me about a recent exchange: "One day I took over some checks to be signed, and all of a sudden this apparition appeared—the head gal, the nasty one. This small person walked up to Albert and took hold of his face in her hand, turning it from side to side.

"She said, 'You're not shaven.'

"'Excuse me,' I said. 'Who are you?'

"She didn't respond—just turned around and looked at Marisa and said, 'You're not allowed in here.'

"'Yes, she is. She's part of the family. And who are you?'

"Then she introduced herself and gave me the rundown on the rules. 'Marisa's here for TLC [tender loving care],' I said. That's what they need, since they're not getting the type of care they need here. And she's not being paid.' This woman didn't like me a lot. She didn't say much more after that."

Now I was determined to use my anthropological training to pinpoint the factors that had led to Mother's deteriorating health. I immediately asked for her medical records and was told that they were unavailable. Mother was the patient, and she would have to send a letter of authorization to release them.

"What are you up to?" Mother asked when I brought her the typed letter to sign.

"You have a right to see your medical records. I want to determine exactly what went on there."

"It's very simple what went on: They didn't care. They ignored my diarrhea, even though I kept telling them about it. It's a horrible place. I'd rather die than go back there. But don't do anything to hurt Dr. Friedmann. He's trying very hard."

"Mummy, I wasn't going to tell you because you have enough to worry about, but I'm going to find out what happened there, and then I'm going to give them hell. I'm ready for a good fight."

"Remember what I said about Friedmann."

"Don't worry. I know I have to be careful because of Dad, and I promise not to involve Friedmann. But the nursing home has to assume its responsibilities toward its patients. Thanks to them, now you're here."

It was hard to dislike Dr. Friedmann. He returned my phone calls promptly and answered my questions about The Palms without the slightest sign of impatience. When I asked him why Mother's colitis had been allowed to linger so long without treatment, he said he had not been informed about it. Still, the nurse's notes showed that he had telephoned in an order for medication to stem the attacks. Perhaps he did not remember or was unaware that Mother's problem was chronic. It seemed to me that the system in which the doctor telephoned his instructions and prescriptions and signed them later contributed to misunderstandings and poor communication. No doubt, Dr. Friedmann had been wise to admit Mother to the hospital, where he could monitor her directly.

When I obtained Mother's medical records, I found that they referred to her not by name but simply as a seventy-eight-year-old "female resident." In addition, personal attributes were recorded only when the staff perceived them as interfering with their jobs. As far as The Palms was concerned, my mother was a "demanding, manipulative, chronic complainer," just the type of troublesome resident they would prefer not to have around. But these were not her real characteristics; they were merely the staff's interpretation. The records included the doctors' consultation reports, progress notes, and telephone orders, as well as medication profiles, lab-test results, treatment plans, and progress notes from the rehabilitation department. A variety of assessments—

the nurse's admission assessment, a skin-rash assessment record, side-rail appraisal, "restorative" dining evaluation, pressure-sore identification record, and bowel and bladder assessments—completed the picture.

Some of the assessments seemed extremely derogatory. For example, the "restorative" dining evaluation consisted of a multiple-choice list of qualities that the assessor marked, yet all of the qualities were negative. Although the "restorative aide" noted that my mother needed help opening a milk carton, she did not record the reason—Mother's severely arthritic hands. Mother also "had an attention span of less than three minutes," but the aide might just as well have marked that Mother was "easily distracted from eating activity" or displayed "inappropriate social behavior," so ludicrous were the choices. The staff's attention to "B&B" (bowel and bladder function) appeared obsessive. The Palms kept a flow chart showing the state of residents' bowel and bladder habits, either "continent" or "incontinent," for every hour of the day.

Finally, the many pages of "Nurse's Notes" provided a running commentary on Mother's condition over each eight-hour shift. Some of the notes were subjective scribblings, some were simply incorrect, and others recorded procedures that had not been followed. Yet the mere act of listing them made them seem valid. For instance, the notes continually referred to my mother's "dentures" because, rather than asking, one of the aides decided that Mother's perfect teeth could not be her own. All of this seemingly purposeless record-keeping reminded me of George Agich's comment on the enormous amount of activity that goes on in the typical nursing home: "Much of this activity (charts, taking of vital signs, toileting, changing beds, and so on) is important and essential in the care of institutionalized elders, though it's often infused with meanings that are bizarre at best. Despite all the attention to physical well-being and the maintenance of the trappings of the hospital, such as uniforms, charts, and recording vital signs, there is little real therapeutic intent" (1993:550).

Why all the note taking? Was it simply written proof of the care rendered if the family or regulatory agencies requested it? The notes supposedly protected the interests of the nursing home, yet a careful reading revealed inconsistencies, deficiencies, and failures in the institution's care plans and showed the subjectivity of its assessments. As some observers have pointed out, this "official" record creates a type of documentary reality: When observations are consolidated into records, their social constructions are treated as reliable accounts, no matter how erroneous they are.

The therapists were delighted with my mother and tried to distance themselves from the nursing-home staff. Mother's occupational therapist had high hopes for her and admired her sustained motivation in the face of adversity. "Your mother is very emaciated," the therapist said when I stopped by the OT room, "but with a loose-fitting blouse and comfortable slacks she will still look very attractive. I wanted her to reach her limits, and that's why I approved another month's therapy. She was determined to regain her independence at home."

"What do you think went wrong?" I asked.

"I don't know, but I do know that your Mother had a bad cold and a setback last week. She was really too ill to do therapy."

"Do you think she'll make up for this loss once she's able to continue."

"Yes, but it will take a while. I'm sorry to have to tell you, I won't be here when your mother gets back. I'm moving [to another facility], where I'll have the opportunity to set up the type of rehab program I really want. I'll have the freedom to build a really good department."

"I understand. I'm sorry my mother won't be able to work with you again. She told me how much she enjoyed your company."

"Your mother was very lonely here. There was nobody to talk to, and she used to come to the rehab rooms just to socialize."

Next, I went to the social-service department to speak with Pamela, but she was gone. She, too, had taken a job at another nursing home. I told Peggy Jo I was unhappy with my mother's care and that I wanted an appointment with the administrator and the head of nursing to discuss what had happened.

"And in regard to my father," I continued, "I'm not pleased with how I found him the day after my mother was hospitalized. He was unshaved and disheveled. Why does my father look like a derelict? It's painful for me to find him this way. Is it asking too much that he be clean and presentable? You promised me you would look after my father personally if he were ever admitted."

Peggy Jo listened quietly. Finally, she replied, "I'll look into the matter, Luisa. I'll make sure your Dad gets the attention he needs."

Kathy's opinion corroborated mine. "June went in for therapy, and she ended up a very ill woman. How did it happen? Dirt and neglect. June had a chance. She always said the therapy was good, that the therapists were kind and did their job. But the lack of structure and order in the rest of the staff was astonishing."

Kathy minced no words: "I wouldn't send a stray dog to that place!"

Next, I called Dr. Risden, who had recommended The Palms. After I explained the events that had led to Mother's hospitalization, he said, "Well, I'll have to look into it. We certainly wouldn't want your mother to fall into the cracks."

"Dr. Risden, it's too late. My mother has already fallen through the cracks. You must not recommend The Palms to your patients, unless you want to finish them off."

"I can't understand. It has an excellent reputation, and I've sent many patients there."

"Dr. Risden, when was the last time you set foot in The Palms?"

"I have to admit, it's been a while."

"Well, how can you recommend a place unless you've been there recently?"

I was truly on a rampage that day. I felt like chewing Dr. Risden out for not following his patient into the nursing home. My wheelchair-bound mother had to make an office appointment and hire a nonemergency medical van so she could see her own physician. After all, he was the one who knew Mother's history.

"Dr. Risden, I would like you to attend to Mother at Coral Bay."

"I would be happy to," he answered, "but the matter is delicate, because Dr. Friedmann admitted her and is her attending physician."

"Well, I'll speak to Dr. Friedmann about it. Certainly, you can see a patient if the family requests it."

I asked Kathy to accompany me when I met with the administrator. Not only did I feel it was necessary to have a witness, but I knew Kathy's presence would make the administration understand that this was not a friendly social call. She was genuinely appalled by the conditions at The Palms.

"Don't worry, the woman and I detest each other," Kathy said. "She couldn't bear it that someone spoke up and told the truth. I'll be delighted to accompany you."

"Kathy, dress businesslike, bring your briefcase, and look as stern as possible," I said. Kathy could look frightfully formidable when she wanted to. She and I walked past the nurse's station and ran into Mother's physical therapist, who commented to the practical nurse on duty, "There goes a lawsuit. I see it in her face."

"I have a few issues I would like to air with you," I began, as Kathy and I sat face to face with both the administrator and the head nurse. "First, I'd like to know why you didn't call me when my mother was hospitalized."

The administrator calmly replied, "We usually don't call abroad."

"That's ridiculous," I said. "It was your obligation to call me. In fact, the 'Resident Rights' booklet you handed to my mother when she was admitted clearly states that you must inform a family member immediately of any transfer. You could have called my brother in Chicago. You had both our phone numbers on your admission sheet."

"How is June doing?" the administrator asked, ignoring my comments. "You know, we went to a lot of trouble to obtain very expensive antibiotics for her diarrhea."

"Did you?" I responded ironically.

Kathy interjected, "You are well aware that June was sick for over a month. Why did you get around to the antibiotics only last week?"

"June just told us about the diarrhea this week," the head nurse said.

"That's not true," I answered. "My mother has been complaining for more than a month. As a nurse, you know how debilitating diarrhea can be. And by the way, she picked up the *Clostridium difficile* here. I understand that it thrives in hospitals and nursing homes that are not kept properly clean."

"We did everything we were supposed to do," the head nurse said. "We followed all the correct procedures regarding your mother's treatment."

But that's not the way Kathy remembered it: "June said she had terrible diarrhea and had been complaining profusely over the fact that she was not cleaned promptly. When I started to question her, I was surprised at the number of days she had had diarrhea. I called in an aide on duty and said, 'Mrs. Margolies has been having a bad problem with diarrhea. Could you call her doctor? It should be looked into.' They just didn't care. There was no responding—they didn't pay any attention."

"On another matter," I said, "why wasn't my mother given her nebulizer treatments?"

"What nebulizer treatments?" the administrator asked.

"My mother was supposed to have three nebulizer treatments a day for her lungs. The medication was clearly listed on Dr. Risden's instruction sheet."

"Her physician did not order any nebulizer treatments."

"That's not true, I personally went over the list with her physician, and the nebulizer was on it. I wanted to bring the nebulizer from home, and you insisted that you would order your own. I see you crossed it off the list without the doctor's authorization."

"I'm sorry. No nebulizer treatments were indicated."

"I have a copy of the list Dr. Risden gave me. The nebulizer treatments are clearly listed."

We were going nowhere quickly. Clearly, we were receiving the stonewall treatment: Deny everything and claim to have carried out the appropriate procedures. Although I was still unsure about the organizational dynamics of the nursing home, I knew enough to realize that I was being deliberately misled. The Palms's obligation toward its residents was clearly set out in its "Resident Rights": to "care for its residents in a manner and in an environment that promotes maintenance or enhancement of each resident's quality of life." But the nursing home did not meet professional standards and failed to abide by its own guidelines, causing my mother grave harm.

Kathy got up to leave. It was pointless to continue. The damage had already been done. The staff had been neglectful. It was time for me to admit to myself that The Palms was poorly equipped to provide skilled nursing care and did not have the expertise to offer anything but routine custodial care.

After Kathy left, the atmosphere changed. The administrator and the head nurse had been defensive; now they tried to convince me of their good intentions. "I'd like you to realize," the administrator said, "that we've been extremely attentive to your mother. We even went out and ordered a very expensive medication. But, you know, your mother didn't get much rest after your father moved in."

"What do you mean?" I asked, wondering how my father could be responsible for my mother's stomach trouble.

"Your father needs to be watched constantly," the administrator said. "He's a very aggressive man."

I had to laugh. "Are you talking about my father?" I asked. "You must be confusing him with somebody else, because I've never heard anything so preposterous. My father is a sweet, gentle, quiet man. Where do you get off saying such things to me about my father?"

"Your father has severe brain damage," the administrator continued. "He has Alzheimer's disease. There's nothing you can do about it."

I did not know where she had gotten that idea. "Are you an M.D.?" I asked. "Did you give my father a neurological workup?"

"No, but it's obvious," she said. She also noted that Dad was "inattentive."

"My father is severely depressed, and he's worried about my mother, who, you may recall, is now hospitalized," I replied.

"Your father needs a full-time attendant. He went berserk when he arrived here. He ran out of the room naked and had to be sedated."

This was another event that Kathy had recalled differently. Dad's clothes that day were in "disarray," she had told me. "Nothing matched; he was unshaven; and he was becoming confused with the situation, because no one was paying attention to him."

"My father needed extra attention during his first few nights here, that's all," I said. "He was upset and disoriented. . . . You had no business asking the doctor to prescribe a sedative; it only made him confused in the morning. As soon as I can make the arrangements, I'm taking my father home, where he doesn't have to suffer these indignities."

I had had enough. Nearly a month in the Canary Islands had recharged my spirits, but now I was right back where I had left off. Also, my anger was rising. I had to get out of there, I knew, or I would explode. As I walked down the hall, Beth, the personable LPN who had attended Mother, called out, "Don't forget to say hello to June for me and tell her I hope she gets better soon." Some staff members were kindhearted, but this did not compensate for the poor performance of their supervisors.

Sadly, I was not quite finished with The Palms at Palm-Aire. Dad stayed on while Mother was hospitalized at Coral Bay because she wanted it that way. This gave me the opportunity to corroborate Marisa's and Kathy's accounts and see for myself the daily interactions between residents and the staff.

Nursing Homes Are Dangerous to Your Health

The Medical Model for Housing the Elderly

IN THE ENORMOUS corpus of literature I perused on the American nursing home, I rarely found anything positive. The early commentators who observed nursing homes in the 1960s—the decade in which the commercial nursing-home phenomenon exploded, thanks to the passage of Medicare entitlements—were particularly repulsed. Robert N. Butler, a geriatrician and tireless advocate for the elderly, concluded in *Why Survive? Being Old in America* (1975) that nursing homes had few nurses and could scarcely qualify as homes. Butler characterized the typical nursing home as a horror house for the frail elderly. Senator Charles Percy was equally revolted. Nursing homes are warehouses for the living dead, he wrote in *Growing Old in the Country of the Young:* "Stick a pin blindly into a list of all the nation's homes for the aged and you are apt to hit an atrocity. I have visited refugee camps in India and Pakistan where I found the refugees treated better than Americans in many of our nursing homes" (1974:83).

Even when Butler and Percy made their observations, the main purpose of the commercial nursing home was to profit. A nursing-home bonanza supported primarily by public funds was unacceptable to them in light of the deplorable conditions that ordinarily reigned. Butler decried the absence of comprehensive medical care and the glaring deficiencies in rehab services. Percy denounced the hiring of aides with no credentials, the use of tranquilizers to sedate patients, the numerous fire hazards, and the lack of regulations. Both Percy and Butler called for massive reforms that would allow nursing-home patients to receive the appropriate treatment under humane and sane conditions.

Percy was a prescient thinker. Thanks to his intervention, the Nursing Home Fire Safety Act, which provided firm directives on the installation of warning devices, and an omnibus reform bill were passed in the early 1970s. He also lobbied for services that would help the elderly remain in their homes when home-health-care provision was still in its infancy. He proposed direct cash payments and tax deductions for family members as incentives to care for their elders at home. This system of payments was enacted in Spain nearly twenty years ago but has yet to be taken seriously in the United States.

The modern nursing home evolved from the "mom-and-pop" operations that sprang up in the mid-1930s with the passage of the Social Security Act. For the first time in American history, people could afford to retire, live on their own resources, and pay for their own care. Nursing homes were still a relatively rare phenomenon during the Depression; most elderly people lived with their grown children, who cared for them when the time came. This was the custom until well into the 1950s.

The early nursing homes were family owned and operated. Each state had some form of aid for the needy elderly and reimbursed the homes for the cost of their care. The quality of these nursing homes depended on the goodwill of their owners, because the states did not begin to license them and enforce minimal standards until the late 1950s. Today, these family operations appear almost innocuous compared with the nationwide conglomerates that make up the nursing-home industry. The former owner of a nursing home for impoverished, inner-city "aged" in Cleveland whom I interviewed nostalgically recalled what had once been a hands-on business. His "rest" home was in a lovely Victorian mansion flanked by large shade trees. He was on the premises every day; his wife did the bookkeeping, and his elderly father helped, too. Residents lost their independence, he admitted, but were put on a regimen of twenty-four-hour care. Many of the inner-city elderly had lived in squalid conditions, and for the first time in their lives they were exposed to decent living quarters and a balanced diet. Good food was important to this former nursing-home owner; it was his job to give old people (who did not eat much, anyway) the very best. He had fallen into the nursing-home business by accident but made it his personal mission to run one of the best homes in Cleveland. Today, in light of the regimentation of the huge nursing-home industry, that objective seems quaint.

A study by the Bureau of the Census in 1939 showed that 1,200 nursing homes existed, with 25,000 beds. By 1954, nursing homes numbered 9,000, with 260,000 beds. Public policy played an important role in the growth of the nursing-home industry: Federal loans for the construction of privately owned nursing homes favored their expansion in the 1950s and 1960s. The enactment of Medicare and Medicaid in 1965 to provide medical coverage for the elderly and the poor, respectively, spurred the rapid growth of the nursing-home industry. By 1970, the number of nursing homes had burgeoned to 23,000, with more than 1 million residents. Public and private expenditures continued to rise, as well. The United States spent some $15.8 billion on nursing-home care in 1978. This sum had nearly quadrupled to $48 billion by 1990 and continues to spiral upward. By 2000, nursing-home care cost about $147 billion annually.

Various commentators have expressed ethical concerns about an industry that depends for three-quarters of its annual gross revenue on the federal government. By 1999, the nursing-home industry did $87 billion in business, of which 75 percent was funded by Medicare and Medicaid (Roszak 2001:80). The federal government both reimburses nursing homes for the cost of a semiprivate room and allows them to generate a profit by permitting a return on equity. The system encourages nursing homes to provide specialized services for which they receive reimbursements higher than for mere caregiving tasks that are labor-intensive, costly, and not likely to be recognized as a goal worthy of reimbursement. The result, contends George Agich, is that "the more an elder needs help with the activities of daily living, exhibits behavioral problems or requires more nursing procedures, the more the institution is reimbursed. Dependent elders are thus more valuable, from a reimbursement standpoint, than more functional elders" (1993:58).

Thanks to Medicare and Medicaid reimbursements, the nursing-home industry generates big bucks for its investors. Beds are in short supply as seniors compete for a limited number of spaces.

The *New York Times* notes that nursing homes have been able to pick and choose: By putting a lid on the number of Medicaid-certified beds (the average nursing home derives 60 percent of its revenues from Medicaid reimbursements), they are able to increase their profits by selling the remaining beds to a more affluent clientele that can pay its own way (Gilpin 1994:5). Growth in the industry has been aggressive. The large conglomerates that dominate the industry have absorbed small, independent operators across the country. Beverly Enterprises, the industry's giant headquartered in Arkansas, runs more than 700 nursing homes countrywide and rakes in annual revenues of nearly $3 billion (When a Parent Needs Care, Part 1, 1995:519). GranCare Inc., a California company, has grown rapidly not only within that state, where the number of facilities increased from eight to eighty-two, but also in the Southeast, currently its fastest-growing region. GranCare has spruced up its facilities to provide "transitional" care to recently discharged hospital patients and expanded into the distribution of pharmaceuticals and the provision of home-health-care services. GranCare recently merged with Living Centers of America to become one of the largest providers of long-term care in the country, with a total of 330 nursing homes and revenues of some $1.9 billion annually. During the bull market of the 1990s, shares in the sixteen publicly traded nursing-home companies increased by an average of 30–40 percent (Gilpin 1994:5). Stockbrokers advised investors to buy into the growing long-term-care industry as shares rocketed overnight, thanks to these megabuster deals.

Nursing homes are now ubiquitous, and the chances of ending up in one are nearly one in two. More than 40 percent of the senior population will spend some time in a nursing home, usually for short-term convalescence. The risk of ending up permanently in a nursing home rises dramatically with age. Some 15 percent of men and 25 percent of women older than eighty-five reside in nursing homes (Ouslander 1988:1559). Permanent nursing-home residents are not only very old; they are also typically frail, female (four in five), and sufferers of multiple chronic conditions. Elders alone and without family support to fall back on are at particular risk. They usually need help with daily activities and move into nursing homes when they can no longer manage at home. A precipitating factor often leads to institutionalization. Confusion, wandering, incontinence, and the growing need for extensive hands-on care are the key factors that lead to nursing-home admittance (Butler 1975:268). Or a crisis, such as the death of a spouse, alters the home environment so dramatically that the survivor can no longer manage at home.

Nursing homes have become "the normative final destination" for aging Americans (Rowles 1994:120). Seniors are actually geared to spend their final days in nursing homes, an alternative just as viable today as living with one's children was in the past. Aging parents refuse to be a "burden on their children" and hesitate to ask anything of them, even though they abhor the notion of ending up in a nursing home. Adult children are often the ones who exhort their vulnerable parents to enter nursing homes "for their own good," where they will be "safe" and "well-cared for," without having the vaguest idea of what nursing-home living is truly like. Pressuring a frail, sickly, aging parent to enter a nursing home is perhaps the greatest disservice a child can perform.

The arguments for entering a nursing home usually revolve around the issue of total care. Enter a nursing home and you will be protected from harm twenty-four hours a day in an environment where help is just a buzz away and your condition will be monitored around-the-clock. Nothing could be more fallacious than this stereotypical vision of what goes on in nursing homes. A vast chasm exists between what nursing-home policy specifies as its objectives and what actually occurs. Dozens of investigators have come away from nursing homes convinced that only a tiny proportion do what they set out to do.

The nursing-home model was formulated on the premise that people disintegrate as they age. Until recently, old age was erroneously equated with physical and mental deterioration, the loss of one's attractiveness, and the acquisition of negative qualities. The aging person, in a metaphorical transformation into a bodily machine, was thought of as some sort of object that deteriorated with advancing years. This senescence, or wear-and-tear, theory of aging, based on the idea of natural attrition, has found a comfortable niche in the nursing-home industry, which nurtures its continued existence. Much as hospitals were known fifty years ago as places of no return, nursing homes are now perceived as way stations of last resort. The distinguished gerontologist Harry Moody (1992) has appropriately referred to nursing-home placement as "the long good-bye."

Growing old inherently involves losses. As the aging lose their health, independence, spouses, and friends, they brood over the pervasiveness of the increasing losses. Being frail, infirm, and unable to care for oneself are fates worse than the final passage. But the fear of spending one's final days consigned to a nursing home is greater than the dread of ill health and increasing dependence. Institutional living has been identified as the principal factor associated with the wish to die among the elderly. Nothing compares to the impact of nursing-home residence on the vulnerable elderly. Those who remain at home, even the frail and failing, compare themselves favorably with the poor souls relegated to nursing homes. "We can only speculate on the reasons for the association," notes A. F. Jorm. "Perhaps placement in residential care is seen as . . . the end of a productive role in society" (1995:391).

The futility of nursing-home placement, the unspoken assumption that such a step is irreversible, has led to a widespread rejection of institutional care. Today's savvy elders are finally getting the message. Smart seniors are likely to say, "No, thanks. I'll think I'll pass." They know what goes on in nursing homes; they cannot help but read about the latest scandals in the newspapers. Well into the 1980s, the typical nursing home continued to provide "unloving care." Bruce Vladeck, whose *Unloving Care: The Nursing Home Tragedy* strongly condemned the nursing-home industry of twenty-five years ago, writes:

> The typical nursing home is a pretty awful place . . . even when it is clean and well lighted, staffed to minimally adequate levels, and provides decent food, adequate medical attention, and a full state of activities. It is awful because the circumstances, medical and social, of the people living there are extremely difficult to do much about, and because the presence of an adequate supply of individuals, motivated, educated, and trained to work effectively in such circumstances, is extraordinarily rare. Many nursing homes are no better than they have to be—quite a few are not even that good—and only a small fraction are as good as they can be. But even the best cannot escape the reality

that, although for many of their residents there is no other choice, they are institutions housing people with profound problems that are unlikely to get very much better. (1980:29)

A recent revisit to *Unloving Care* shows that the most flagrant abuses—the ones that used to make it into the muckraking media with surprising frequency—have been corrected. As a result of major legislation enacted over the years by federal and state governments and the passing of the Omnibus Budget Reconciliation Act of 1987, the quality of nursing-home care has improved dramatically. Residents' rights are clearly spelled out, and the Resident Assessment Instrument (RAI) was developed and implemented in 1990 to provide an accurate, standardized evaluation of the resident's health status. Every nursing home that receives state and federal reimbursements is now obligated to assess residents using the RAI on admission and periodically thereafter. The major screening instrument of the RAI is the Minimum Data Set for Nursing Home Resident Assessment and Care Screening, a diagnostic tool with sixteen sections that reflect different aspects of a resident's baseline condition. This instrument is used in conjunction with a set of eighteen Resident Assessment Protocols to provide sufficient information for the staff to develop written comprehensive care plans. Such regulations clarify the raison d'être of the thick medical histories compiled for each nursing-home resident today. Although the federal government stipulates the regulations for quality control, the implementation of those regulations is the responsibility of state officials. They are the only authorities authorized to certify and license nursing homes. State inspectors file an annual report that should be readily available in each nursing home for the perusal of residents and their families.

Various congressional committees tried to push through legislation in 1995 that would repeal many of the federal standards responsible for recent nursing-home reforms, bringing us around once again to a situation of no accountability by unscrupulous nursing-home operators. One wonders about the misguided efforts to slash the national budget by cutting the wrong corners. Senator William Cohen of Maine has said, "If we weaken federal enforcement, we will be sent back to the dark days of substandard nursing homes, with millions of elderly at risk" (as quoted in Carlson 1995:63). Fortunately, the move to slash the budget failed resoundingly; federal guidelines for conducting inspections were actually made more stringent, creating a backlash involving Vladeck, then the administrator of the Health Care Financing Administration in Washington, D.C.

As a result of new inspections that commenced in 1995, more than a quarter of Florida's 680 nursing homes, almost double the national rate, were found to be substandard. Beverly Enterprises, the nation's largest nursing-home holder, which controls 10 percent of the Florida market, was found to be particularly egregious. All four of its Broward County facilities received citations for flagrant violations. In 1997 alone, Beverly Enterprises generated profits of $5.28 per patient day, enough to erase the staffing deficits for which it repeatedly was cited (Harrington 2001:1454). But instead of providing high-quality care, fifty of Beverly's Florida facilities pleaded guilty to Medicare fraud and settled for $175 million (Lane 2001). Industry lobbyists contacted Vladeck to complain about overly zealous state examiners and to urge him to allow the facilities sufficient time to correct deficiencies before issuing a final grade. State ombudsmen, by contrast, felt that the crackdown would lead to improvements in facilities that consistently received poor marks. For them, it was inexcusable that investor-owned chains delivered considerably lower-quality care than nonprofit facilities. But the state of Florida has only 250 inspectors to monitor not only nursing homes, but also hospitals, group homes, and home-health-care agencies. The nursing-home industry had grown so rapidly that the job of properly inspecting and grading long-term-care facilities was becoming insurmountable.

High-quality care is still an elusive goal in many nursing homes. *Consumer Reports* rated forty-three nursing-home chains (and sifted through 6.5 million pieces of information) in a meticulous three-part series on eldercare. The magazine concluded that "the quality of care at thousands of the nation's nursing homes is poor or questionable at best" (When a Parent Needs Care, Part 1, 1995:518). Nursing homes accustomed to offering custodial care to frail elderly "residents" are inadequately prepared to treat the acutely ill "patients" who are now arriving on their doorsteps at an alarming rate as the result of early hospital discharges. Staffs composed largely of aides lack the training to recognize crucial signs indicating a resident's changing condition. Telephone orders transmitted by absent physicians to aides are a poor substitute for face-to-face contact between a doctor and patient. Geriatricians are well aware that the status of an elderly patient can change suddenly. Symptoms that may be innocuous in a younger patient can be life-threatening to a frail elder with multiple conditions and little resilience. Understaffing and a low nurse-to-resident ratio contribute to a syndrome in which symptoms are often dismissed as complaints and left to linger until they become unmanageable and an unavoidable cause of alarm. At this point, the "resident" is summarily discharged from the nursing home and sent to the hospital, where a medical doctor can properly monitor his or her condition. This was exactly what happened to my mother at The Palms.

Nursing homes also lack medical equipment. Portable X-ray machines must be brought in; lab tests must be sent out. This in itself may delay the reporting of results for several days. Nursing homes may not have the most basic medical supplies, such as oxygen, nebulizers, and ice packs. Try to get an aspirin if it is not on your order chart and see how long that minor request can take. As for dietary requirements, request a salt-free diet and you will find that it is impossible to get one, because nursing-home kitchens stubbornly insist on adding some salt to flavor the food. NAS, or no added salt, is the best you will do. Ask for a bland diet and you will discover that many nursing-home kitchens are little motivated to do the extra work involved in this particular chore.

The volumes of paper records generated by compliance with the new regulations may serve to protect the interests of the nursing facility, but they fail to fulfill their original objective of creating an effective care plan. (I doubt that anyone besides me systematically waded through the 176 pages of my mother's medical history at The Palms and came away with a clear notion of what really went on and what might have been accomplished under more propitious circumstances.) Each department generates its own treatment plan divorced from considerations of the resident as a person. Some of the plans are so general that they are meaningless (regain one's independence); some are patronizing ("graduate" to assisted care, receive bowel-and-bladder training, receive self-feeding classes); and others are so picayune as to be absurd (microscopic objectives regarding pressure sores) or too ambitious to achieve reasonably within the expected time frame (return to one's previous level of functioning within three weeks). Someone within a facility must be designated to prepare a concise program that can be implemented realistically. Unless assessments are integrated into some fundamental vision of what the comprehensive care plan should involve, the paper trail is worthless.

What factors have combined to allow such a situation to persist? *Consumer Reports* notes that some 40 percent of the facilities certified by the Health Care Financing Administration (HCFA) have repeatedly violated federal standards. But the agency's lax enforcement allows nursing homes to operate without taking corrective measures. Inspection reports, which are supposed to be prominently displayed in the nursing home, are rarely made available. *Consumer Reports* found that, as far as inspection reports are concerned, nursing homes fail to comply with both the letter and the spirit of the law. In a final condemnation of nursing homes' failure to improve, *Consumer Reports* cites the Texas lawyer David Bragg, who conducted an investigation for Governor Ann Richards in 1992 and blamed "industry influence on politicians, institutional lethargy of the regulators, and an apathetic public for the persistent deficiencies in nursing homes" (When a Parent Needs Care, Part 1, 1995:525). According to Bragg, if the same deficiencies in nursing homes had been found at a daycare center for toddlers, the outraged community would have lynched its owner.

Despite the increasing number of citations meted out for violations, effective compliance seems to elude state regulators. The responsibility for enforcing nursing-home regulations actually belongs to the HCFA, a division of the U.S. Department of Health and Human Services, which funds state agencies for conducting annual visits to Medicare-certified nursing homes. The economic sanctions are exceptionally high. Nursing homes with inferior grades can be fined into the six figures and denied Medicaid bonuses when they lose their superior rating. Doctors who habitually refer patients to a deficient facility are informed of the downgraded rating and are encouraged to look elsewhere. Yet a recent

Senate Special Committee on Aging report concluded that state regulators took a "lenient stance," even in the face of repeated, consecutive violations. Regulators routinely allowed nursing homes a 30–45-day grace period to correct the violation. Claims that the violations causing harm to residents had been corrected were often taken at face value, because the HCFA forewent a return visit. More serious sanctions, such as regular state monitoring and monetary penalties, were rarely applied (*California Nursing Homes* 1998). Only in 1998 were repeat violators finally marked for strict reviews that involved on-site visits every six months.

The boom years in nursing-home growth ended abruptly with the passing of the Balanced Budget Act of 1997, which set limits on specific Medicare reimbursements. The large chains that had expanded too quickly through acquisitions, and that had accumulated huge debts, were dealt an additional blow by the growing cost of liability insurance. By the year 2000, some 10 percent of the for-profit industry had filed for protection under bankruptcy laws (Weaver 2000:9). Understaffing and cost cutting led to a rising number of denouncements of the quality of care. A *Time* magazine investigation reported that, "owing to the work of lawyers, investigators and politicians who had begun examining the causes of thousands of nursing-home deaths across the U.S., the grim details are emerging of an extensive, blood-chilling and for-profit pattern of neglect" (Thompson 1997:34). One inspector cited before the Senate Special Committee on Aging told *Time* that she could not do a proper job because of "cronyism" between nursing-home operators and state inspectors (Thompson 1998:42). Case after case of abuses, ranging from inexplicable weight losses, advanced bed sores, undertreatment for pain, and the excessive use of restraints and sedatives, were reported nationwide. Bizarre occurrences, like the hatching of maggots in a resident's bed or death from ant stings, illustrated the Dickensian aspects of nursing-home care. In California, more than 3,000 suspicious deaths from treatable conditions like malnutrition and dehydration were eventually linked to inferior care. After a Sun Healthcare Group facility in California racked up dozens of citations that culminated in the death of two residents, the U.S. Department of Justice finally prosecuted a nursing-home chain

in 2001 for providing inadequate care (Heat Wave 2001). A recent
Special Committee on Aging report concluded that "the number
of homes cited for deficiencies involving actual harm to residents
or placing them at risk of death or serious injury remained un-
acceptably high—30 percent of the nation's 17,000 nursing
homes" (Aronovitz 2002:1).

The nurse-anthropologist Jeanie Kayser-Jones accurately captured
the medical dilemma of the modern American nursing home by
highlighting the problems of trying to provide sophisticated care
in a "low-technology" environment: "The nursing home is something of a paradox. Historically, nursing homes admitted people
who could be cared for largely by nonprofessional nursing staff.
However, since the advent of diagnostic related groups (DRGs) in
1983, nursing homes have admitted people in subacute conditions
who require care that can only be provided by professional nurses
and physicians" (1995:242). She notes that, without the right mix
of a skilled nursing staff, the daily presence of physicians, and
immediate access to diagnostic and pharmaceutical services, nursing homes cannot pretend to provide good acute care.

The cutting-corners approach to medical care has led many observers to conclude that nursing facilities are poor places to obtain
good health care. Medical care is "anemic," says Rosalie Kane,
the author of numerous articles on eldercare, because little nursing actually goes on in a nursing-home setting. Registered nurses
handle administrative duties, leaving the hands-on care to licensed
practical nurses and certified nursing assistants. Residents usually receive a daily average of seventy minutes of care from the
entire nursing staff and only five minutes from a registered nurse
(1995–1996:64–66).

The absence of registered nurses can have devastating effects
on the quality of patient care. A patient's condition can deteriorate rapidly, leading to hospitalization, when medical procedures
are not carried out in a timely manner. So glaring has the absence
of nurses in nursing homes become that the Institute of Medicine,
a nonprofit organization that provides advice on health policy
under a congressional charter, recommended that nursing homes
be required by federal law to have a registered nurse on duty
twenty-four hours "to lower the number of patient deaths and

hospital admissions" (Mitchell 1996). Federal health officials also recommended that new standards be imposed to insure that residents receive at least two hours of care a day from nurses' aides and at least twelve minutes from a registered nurse. These are not optimal amounts but minimal levels needed to protect patients from the consequences of understaffing (Pear 2000).

Nurses' aides make up some three-quarters of the nursing-home staff and frequently moonlight to make ends meet. Short-staffing creates a negative work environment, leading to rapid turnover, which has been estimated at 55–75 percent. Vast socio-cultural and ethnic differences may create a gulf between residents and aides that is unbridgeable without concerted efforts to achieve a sense of community that includes both staff and residents. In South Florida, the clientele tends to be middle-class whites from other regions of the country, whereas aides are predominantly female immigrants from the Caribbean. Although hardworking and family-oriented, these aides lack familiarity with American ways, and their paltry knowledge of the physiology and ethnography of aging handicaps them.

Caring for nursing-home patients is a demanding, "menial" job, and aides often take out their frustration on the recipients of their services. Most aides are neither monsters nor saints but fall somewhere in the middle, says the anthropologist Nancy Foner. She found that only a handful of aides were consistently abusive; the majority were capable of losing their temper, then expressing kindness a few minutes later. When they faced difficult, hostile patients, their compassion was tinged with psychological abuse that included teasing and joking at the resident's expense, glaring, or speaking gruffly. Aides also acted out more subtle forms of benign neglect by ignoring residents' requests, not speaking, and performing their duties sullenly or distractedly (1994:31–52).

In fairness to the lowest rung in the staff hierarchy, we must recognize that many nursing aides are caring, concerned people who try their best to carry out their jobs with pride. They provide the bulk of the hands-on care that so clearly affects the quality of the nursing-home experience, yet they often receive a minimal wage and may even be treated disparagingly by the supervisory staff. Theirs is not an easy lot: cajoling patients to eat, cleaning up messes and body fluids, lifting heavy patients, dealing with difficult patients, complying with tight schedules. The sociologist Timothy Diamond was realistic about the difficulties of patient care when he did undercover research as a nurse's aide: "The smells of urine and cleaning fluids, the nausea of cleaning up excrement-filled diapers and beds, the multicultural misunderstandings, the separate worlds of the senile" all caused him to view the position of nursing assistant with new respect (1992:xi). Diamond needed considerable agility, flexibility, speed, and patience to carry out seemingly simple tasks. He came to admire the ability of the seasoned nursing assistant to transform mundane chores into refined skills.

Worse than the problem of the quality of care, which can be remedied with time, effort, and sufficient resources, is the encroachment of nursing homes on the human spirit. Nursing-home patients are rarely happy and often wonder how they ended up in such a fruitless existence when they once lived by the rules (Gubrium 1993). Only the demented manage to be oblivious to the goings-on around them. MUZZLED IN A NURSING HOME, THE SPIRIT IS EXTINGUISHED is the arresting headline of a timely *Los Angeles Times* article that dealt with the consequences of treating frail, old bodies as negotiable entities. "There's no room in these corners for free spirits—people unwilling to do what they're told, when they're told. Freedom is too much of a threat to efficiency and profit margins," said Mike Ervin, the disability-rights activist who wrote the article. He called for equitable alternatives like home care to replace the "nursing-home prison." "Suppose you had no control over your most basic life decisions. Someone else would determine when and even if you got out of bed, when you went back to bed, what and when and if you would eat, with whom you would associate. That's life in a nursing home. It is this systematic denial of rights, even without the endemic abuse and neglect, that makes living in these institutions dismal" (1994:B7).

A few residents fortunate still to have their wits about them have documented conditions in the typical nursing home. Who on the outside could avoid feeling indignation and rage at the pitiful cries for help from those imprisoned in a living hell? Take, for example, the notes scribbled by Anna Mae Halgrim Seaver and found by her son after her death in a nursing home. They illustrate the frightful assaults on her autonomy, individuality, and sense of self-esteem:

> This is my world now. It's all I have left. You see, I'm old. And I'm not as healthy as I used to be. I'm not necessarily happy with it but I accept it. Occasionally, a member of my family will stop in to see me. He or she will bring me some flowers or a little present, maybe a set of slippers—I've got 8 pair. We'll visit for awhile and then they will return to the outside world and I'll be alone again. . . .
>
> Why do you think the staff insists on talking baby talk when speaking to me? I understand English. I have a degree in music and am a certified teacher. Now I hear a lot of words that end in "y." Is this how my kids felt? My hearing aid works fine. There is little need for anyone to position their face directly in front of mine and raise their voice with those "y" words. Sometimes it takes longer for a meaning to sink in; sometimes my mind wanders when I am bored. But there is no need to shout. . . .
>
> Something else I've learned to accept is loss of privacy. Quite often I'll close my door when my roommate—imagine having a roommate at my age—is in the TV room. I do appreciate some time to myself and believe that I have earned at least that courtesy. As I sit thinking or writing, one of the aides invariably opens the door unannounced and walks in as if I'm not there. Sometimes she even opens my drawers and begins rummaging around. Am I invisible? Have I lost my right to respect and dignity? What would happen if the roles were reversed? I am still a human being. I would like to be treated as one. . . .
>
> A typical day. . . . The afternoon drags into early evening. This used to be my favorite time of the day. Things would wind down. I would kick off my shoes. Put my feet up on the coffee table. Pop open a bottle of Chablis and enjoy the fruits of my day's labor with my husband. He's gone. So is my health. *This is* my world. . . .
>
> My children put me here for my own good. They said they would be able to visit me frequently. But they have their own lives to lead. That sounds normal. I don't want to be a burden. They know that. But I would like to see them more. One of them is here in town. He visits as much as he can. (Seaver 1994:11)

Fictional accounts of life in nursing homes also convey that sense of helplessness. The elderly Caro Spencer, the protagonist of May Sarton's *As We Are Now*, laments, "I am in a concentration camp for the old, a place where people dump their parents or relatives exactly as though it were an ash can. My brother, John, brought me here two weeks ago. Of course I knew from the beginning that living with him would never work" (1973:9). She continues, "I am learning that any true cry from the heart of an old person creates too much havoc in a listener, is too disturbing, because nothing can really be done to help us on the downward path. So, mentioning the horror of growing old alone becomes an intolerable burden. There seems to be only a few responses possible. One is the dreadful false comfort of the cliché, 'It can't be as bad as all that' or 'things will surely be better tomorrow, dear.' I suffer excruciatingly from endearments that are casual and perfunctory, because I am so starved for real feelings, for love itself, I suppose" (1973:73). The despondent Spencer was so disturbed by being placed in a nursing home by her family that she gave up all hope of leaving. She stored her copybooks in the refrigerator to protect them, then set the trash cans and curtains on fire, literally going out in a blaze of righteousness, determined to end her suffering.

Nursing-home residents are not the only ones who feel outraged. Relatives often bristle at the indignities heaped on the victim merely for being institutionalized. For years, Elaine Marcus Starkman had provided hands-on care to her mother-in-law, Maury, with increasingly conflicting feelings. She resented the burden at the same time that she felt an obligation. Eventually, Maury was institutionalized. Despite the excellent reputation of the nursing home in which Maury was placed, Starkman was incensed by the conditions. "She continued to hold her head high, refused to cry out about her indignities, unlike the others," Starkman writes. "During our visit, Maury was upset that her stockings and panties were placed in a community drawer, and the aide put her in adult diapers. . . . 'This isn't a charity ward,' her son insisted, 'We pay for better care. She doesn't need diapers; they can use underpants if they watch her and toilet her every two hours'" (1993:82). On her mother-in-law's one-year anniversary at the nursing home, Starkman lamented, "Where do I escape to? To a friend's, and what did we talk about? Her mother' s savings drying up from payments to a convalescent home, her brother's lack of involvement. A predictable American family pattern by now" (1993:96).

Cultural anthropologists bring a unique approach to the study of nursing homes by basing their interpretations on observations extending over many months. Apart from conducting research, anthropologists have lived in nursing homes as patients and worked in them as nurse's aides. The real tragedies of the modern nursing home, according to their in-depth studies, are not the blatant abuses that proliferated before federal controls put a stop to them but the subtle and more difficult to document abuses of benign neglect and disrespect. The routine is all-encompassing, thanks to bureaucratic measures designed to make the nursing-home experience as banal as possible.

This "tyranny of regulations" makes it hard for nursing-home residents to live from day to day on their own terms. Not permitting anything to interfere with the bureaucratic goal of running the nursing home is more important than meeting residents' personal needs. Daily routines are broken down into a number of discrete tasks that must be carried out and charted in the resident's medical records. In fact, it does not really matter whether the job is actually done as long as a paper record shows that it was. The result is that, "at every level of the nursing department, efficiency and organization are valued over compassion to residents" (Foner 1994:67). Accomplishing these tasks depends on a hierarchical organization in which a large number of aides perform menial tasks while the more complex, medical tasks fall into the hands of a small number of qualified personnel. Because the supervisory staff is divorced from hands-on care, it has little appreciation for how the daily regimentation destroys the last vestiges of residents' autonomy.

Nursing homes are typical examples of what Erving Goffman called "total institutions." Some institutions, such as colleges and summer camps, segregate their members into age-graded units in which peer contact is most important. Others, such as prisons, monasteries, leprosariums, and nursing facilities, exert bureaucratic terrorism over their residents and deny them latitude in their daily lives. The anthropologist Jules Henry (1963) observed that nursing-home residents become "symbolic prisoners." They are rarely consulted about their own care or the details of the daily routine. Residents are told whom their roommates will be, what time they may eat, when they must arise, and when they should go to bed after a day of structured activities. Every moment of their lives is accounted for.

Social scientists concur that American nursing homes "depersonalize" and "dehumanize" their residents by devaluating them: ignoring their wishes, neglecting their needs, disregarding their privacy, and failing to acknowledge their unique personalities and former roles in life. By exercising control over their powerless "children," the staff can carry out its routine jobs more effectively. One does not have to give detailed explanations to dependent children or allow them many choices. That would simply confuse them. In turn, residents are reluctant to complain, correctly surmising that they will feel the repercussions immediately in the type of care doled out by the aides. They are often so intimidated that they fail to exercise their rights and may not even know or remember what these rights are. An aide's ability to retaliate by making life miserable is a powerful mechanism that encourages residents to remain silent.

Residents of total institutions may react to their loss of autonomy and privacy by languishing in passivity. "Stripped" of their homes and familiar surroundings, deprived of such simple pleasures as outings and owning pets, and denied the ability to conduct their personal affairs, residents often feel hopeless, angry, and bitter. In the best scenario, they may compensate for their loss of control by forging new relationships inside the institution. This was the case of Joe Torchio and Lou Freed, nursing-home roommates described in Tracy Kidder's *Old Friends*. Proximity bred a close and tender friendship as the two commiserated about their poor fortune. They comforted and looked out for each other and demanded no more than the other could give. Indeed, Lou became more important to Joe than Ray, Joe's former "friend for life." Ray found excuses to put off visits to the nursing home, even though the facility was spectacular. "After every visit Ray would go home and mix himself a stiff martini," Kidder writes. "Visiting Linda Manor distressed him, partly because he would imagine himself there and also because he had imagined a rich old age for Joe, filled with literature, and he thought of Joe's life and of its ending here as a tragedy" (1993:318). Old friends from the outside often find it too difficult and time-consuming to retain meaningful contact. For all but the strongest, the nursing-home resident is a reminder of what one could become.

In the worst possible scenario, residents respond to institutionalization by falling apart. Their health disintegrates, and they may become passively defensive by refusing to eat or cooperate with the staff. The anthropologist Maria Vesperi, who worked as a nursing-home aide to get an insider's view, depicts the horrific decline of eighty-nine-year-old Mrs. O'Rourke, who had been placed in the home because her family could no longer supervise her wandering. They thought she would be safe, but instead of supervising her, the staff controlled her wanderings by prescribing powerful sedatives that only made her unsteady on her feet. The staff then tried restraining her with a Posey belt (a type of straitjacket for hospital patients). After a week at the home, notes Vesperi, the unfortunate woman "was under 24-hour sedation and daily physical restraint" (1983:227). Mrs. O'Rourke reacted by becoming incontinent and refusing her food. She rummaged through her roommates' drawers at night, creating a general commotion, swore, and made obscene gestures. Unless they were aware of the circumstances, most people would come to the logical conclusion that Mrs. O'Rourke was acutely disturbed. Other studies also show that the functional status of the frail elderly declines when they enter an institutionalized environment and rarely returns to its former level. "Institutions are not healthy places for the elderly" is the shameful indictment of a health-care bureaucracy that focuses on the patient's concerns only in the last instance (Polich et al. 1993:255–256).

The nursing-home environment creates a vicious cycle in which the patient's mental status deteriorates as he becomes attuned to a limited set of acceptable behaviors and activities. The nursing-home "specter" creates a type of "mindlessness," Betty Friedan notes in *The Fountain of Age*. "Older people who accept their 'deteriorated' status may indeed be reduced to mindlessness; given no opportunities for new and challenging experience, they sink into brain-numbing passivity" (1993:88–89). Friedan is vehemently opposed to nursing homes because she feels that the vital stuff of life is snuffed out once one is consigned to a place where "care" terminates not in life but in death. Nursing homes, no matter how well they are run, are still institutions that constrain autonomy. Even the best nursing home cannot serve as a surrogate for a family's care.

The old-fashioned nursing home oriented to the custodial care of a frail, predominantly demented clientele is on the way out. Nursing homes have already begun to reinvent themselves to survive.

Just as the banking and insurance industries began to duplicate the services of brokerage firms in the 1980s, the nursing-home industry is waging a turf war with hospitals and aggressively competing to meet the needs of a sophisticated and diverse consumer market. To succeed, nursing facilities must rethink their underlying philosophy. Despite the negative stories that appear in the press, Americans still believe that the modern nursing home can play a role in providing care for some segments of society. The trend is to move away from custodial to sub-acute and skilled nursing care in special units. Early hospital discharges have led to a need for intermediate-care units where patients can continue convalescing before going home. Nursing homes are able to offer specialized care comparable to hospital care at significantly lower costs. Other creative solutions and alliances will surely arise in response to modifications in the health-care system and the growing dominance of managed-care plans. The new nursing home may become not a place of no return for the sickest, frailest members of the elder population, but a sound mix of specialized care units for patients with different needs.

Although the nursing home of the future is still in the making, the results are beginning to have an impact on the quality of care in many parts of the country. A fine example of the revolution under way in the nursing-home industry is the Jewish Home for the Aged in Miami. The Jewish Home is no mere nursing home but an attractive campus with clusters of buildings and living spaces designed to serve a heterogeneous clientele. Rehabilitation, acute-care, and Alzheimer's units are housed in separate buildings with their own staffs and tailored programs. It has responded to consumer demand by building an assisted-living division modeled on the concept of independent living in individual apartments, and has made a real effort to reach into the community by running a day-care center for the frail elderly, a home-care service, and a volunteer program whose elderly participants are often older than many of its residents. The Jewish Home also publishes a newspaper that circulates throughout Miami's metropolitan area. The home has tried to instill pride and loyalty in its corps of aides by offering incentives to improve the working environment. Further, the facility is attractive, with pastel walls; wood floors; subdued lighting; cheerful, spacious rooms; well-appointed common areas; and lush landscaping. No dazed residents line up against the walls, and there are no freezing corridors, repugnant odors, stained rugs, slippery floors, loud music, or plaintive cries for help—that is, no dismal, sterile environment that reeks of death but is still considered adequate in many nursing facilities throughout the country.

Ultimately, the process of reinventing the nursing home will be predicated on our ability to appreciate that frail elders have an inherent right to receive good medical care while being treated as competent human beings. What is the point of extending life if a living death confronts old people as they await their last days in a place of no return?

CHAPTER FIVE

Coral Bay II

"You're ready to leave.
Your condition is stable."

AUGUST 17–SEPTEMBER 3, 1993: 17 DAYS • Mother was receiving excellent care at Coral Bay and was being thoroughly tested. No doubt about it; I was there to confirm it. I asked Dr. Friedmann whether he objected to calling in Dr. Hafner, the cardiologist who had pulled Mother through her crisis at Sacred Heart. Perhaps he would be able to offer insight into her repeated bouts with "congestive heart failure." Not at all, Dr. Friedmann responded; he was amenable to all suggestions. Dr. Friedmann coordinated nearly daily chest X-rays, frequent blood counts, a pleural-fluid cytology, microbiological analyses of the sputum, an anti-nuclear antibody test for rheumatoid activity, and liver, gall-bladder, and pancreatic ultrasounds, all under my watchful eye. He was determined to get to the bottom of the pleural effusions.

The results were inconclusive. The bilateral pleural effusions persisted, but the pulmonary vascular markings did not appear to be congested, again casting doubt on the initial diagnosis of congestive heart failure. Mother's white-blood-cell count was elevated and, together with the mysterious fever, led Dr. Friedmann to diagnose probable bronchitis. Mother was pleased with the attention but tired of the constant testing. When somebody called to ask how she felt, she routinely responded, "I'm coming along. I could be better. They're experimenting on me here, doing their best. They're trying to determine what I have. They're working on it."

I was still upset by Dad's admission to The Palms during my absence, and walking into an empty house was disconcerting. I was surprised to find the house in disarray—it looked as though a bumbling thief had ransacked it. I dashed off a letter to the manager of Helping Hands, the employment agency that had sent us the incompetent housekeeper. You can imagine my state of mind:

This letter is to follow up on our recent phone conversation. I would like to strongly repeat that Fay _____, who worked in my parents' home from June 29th to July 29th, should not be employed by your agency. She's an incompetent housekeeper and does not have the patience to work with the frail elderly.

My error in dealing with your agency was in trusting the word of the social worker who recommended you. I was not as careful as I should have been in insisting on written references that I could personally check. You read Fay _____'s recommendations to me over the phone. When I asked her for written ones, she told me that her previous two clients had died (in her arms no less). I shudder to think what could have happened if she had continued to work in my parents' home. I don't think your agency should vouch for an employee's character unless you actually knew her. This was not the case.

To mention just a few basics, . . . Fay intimidated my father by yelling at him and barking orders in an officious manner. Within two days, he ceased to be Mr. Margolies, but was Albert. "Albert, sit down," "Albert, come here," Albert, do this, do that, drink your tea," and so on. In fact, my poor father fled to his neighbors and asked them to call the police to get Fay out of the house. She neglected his personal needs. When friends came to the door, he was unshaven and his clothing was dirty. He lost more than ten pounds under her "care." Fortunately she left before my father became her next victim! . . .

I am not interested in listening to any excuses this person might have. She is not qualified, and she cannot be trusted to be alone with an infirm person. As an agency that purports to specialize in caring for the elderly, there is no excuse for a situation, such as the one I have described, to have developed.

The only response I received was a check to cover the charges for Fay's long-distance phone calls. I should have followed through with a consumer agency but let it ride. I should have sued Helping Hands, but I had more urgent matters to attend to.

Mother was right. I was too busy with her to get in touch with another agency and start looking for a good housekeeper. I thought I had done my homework before. I had amassed several burgeoning portfolios with the names and descriptions of home-health-care agencies in the area. It had been an enormous job, and I had done it on my own, following up on contacts through the hospitals' social-service departments, looking through the phone directory, and making dozens of cold calls. It was all so risky, even though I had gone about it methodically. There were thousands of home-health-care agencies in South Florida. How does one distinguish one from another? One thing I did know was that nobody could come close to taking Marisa's place. I had asked her to come back to the house, but she now had a boyfriend and her own life to lead. I knew I could not take care of Dad and attend to Mother's needs at the same time. I did not think it was appropriate for Dad to spend his entire day visiting the hospital, and I certainly could not leave him at home by himself. For the moment, he would have to stay at The Palms.

The visiting hours in the Coral Bay telemetry unit were peculiar. They were long enough, but they never coincided with meal-times. Although Mother assured me she was eating properly, I was not convinced. By her third day in telemetry, Mother had lost her rosy color and seemed to be spending more and more time napping. Whenever I arrived, she was asleep. She opened her eyes only when I called her and seemed to have little interest in being aroused. I could not break through to her and was alarmed by her somnolence. On the fourth day, Mother slept around-the-clock. I was unaware that a new term to describe her condition—"cachexia," or extreme wasting of the muscles in the upper and lower extremities—had entered her medical records. I did not need to read Mother's chart to understand that, in the four days that had elapsed in telemetry, Mother was being consumed. I was horrified when I took a good look at her skeletal body. Her face had not changed much, but she had two bony protuberances around the knees, and her once sturdy thighs were now about the same thickness as my upper arms. I shook Mother awake.

"Mother, I think you've lost a lot of weight since entering the hospital. You're all bone. Why?"

"I haven't had much of an appetite. In fact, the food repels me, and it's too much trouble to eat."

"Haven't the nurses been helping you with your meals?"

"Well, one or two did at the beginning, but I've been too tired to eat. I can't cut the food, and it's too much of an effort."

"Mummy, if I had only known, I would have insisted on being with you at mealtime. You assured me that you were eating, and I believed you."

"As a matter of fact, I don't plan on eating anymore. This is as good a way to go as any."

I paused and took in my mother's words. Suddenly it dawned on me that she had not eaten any meals since she had arrived at Coral Bay and intended to starve herself to death. I did not know Mother was "markedly cachectic," but it was obvious that she was giving up without a whimper.

"Mom!" I called. "I think I know what you're about, and I don't approve. If you're going to stop eating, I'm not going to stick around and watch it. I'm not going to stay here for this. It's too painful. Mummy, you have to start eating, or you're going to snuff yourself out. Dad needs you. This is not the way to go about it. Now, decide."

"Darling, it's not that I'm doing it on purpose. I'm just not hungry, and it's too much trouble."

"Mom, I don't care. You have to eat. We've been through this before. I don't care if you're in the telemetry unit. I'm going to speak to Dr. Friedmann about this and make sure I'm allowed in at mealtimes."

"That won't be necessary."

"Mummy, you know I don't trust you. Do you know what they told me? You weigh less than seventy pounds. You've lost nearly half your body weight. You can't go any lower than that if you expect to stay alive. I'm not going to watch you drop any lower. You've reached your limit."

"Well, I'll try, though I'm not hungry."

"Very well, and I'll help you. I'll be here at every single meal from now on."

This was the first time I actually felt that Mother was nearing death. She was not attached to any lifesaving devices, and there were no life-threatening circumstances such as the heart-block crisis at Sacred Heart. But Mother's listlessness was a potent factor. She no longer cared and was quietly committing suicide. Close your eyes and drift off to endless sleep, soothing sleep, painless sleep. Why come back? To be humiliated by people like Fay or face a future in a place like The Palms? Too much of an effort to try and walk again, better to just let go. This scenario was running through my mind as it must have been going through Mother's. I knew her too well. I would not let her do this. Not yet.

I almost felt I was sitting vigil by Mother's bedside, so uninterested was she in her surroundings. I felt helpless. For the first time, nothing I said had an impact on Mother's behavior. I used to be able to spur her on, and her condition would improve, but now she was going downhill fast, even though none of her doctors could pinpoint the cause.

Suddenly, Mother awoke from her lethargy, opened her eyes, and looked at me. "What's the matter, darling?"

"Mother, everything. It just depresses me to see you like this. It's ironic that the minute you finish your therapy, something happens, and you're back in the hospital again." I had a headache and a bad sore throat and had put on a surgical mask before entering Mother's room. "I almost feel like crawling into bed myself. That's how sick I feel."

"Then I'd have you here around-the-clock," she quipped.

"Frankly, Mummy, if I had a choice, I'd prefer to be in a Venezuelan hospital. First, the nurses are much kinder, they call their patients "mi amor" or "mi cielo," and they're more considerate. But it's not the nurses I'm thinking about. A family member is always invited to stay overnight, and all the rooms have couches for that purpose. You don't have to run back and forth, and the patient feels she's being accompanied. They call it the 'companion' couch. It's just—"

"You mean, it's just more compassionate," Mother interrupted.

"Yes, that's exactly what I mean."

"Well, next time I get sick, I'll have to do it in Venezuela."

I was glad Mother had tried to make a joke. I felt better immediately.

• • •

While I was with Mother in South Florida, Graziano and Graz had driven to Coro, Venezuela's oldest colonial city. Graziano's voice was panicky when he called me on Sunday evening to ask about

Mother. Graz had been listless throughout the trip and had started vomiting earlier in the day, as they drove home.

"Does he have a temperature?" I asked.

"No, just a splitting headache."

"Then give him some Tylenol and put him to bed. He'll probably be better in the morning."

Graz got on the line. His voice was even more strained than his father's. He did not have a specific complaint—just a bad headache and extreme fatigue.

"Honey, I'll call you back in the morning. I'm sure you'll feel better after a good night's rest. I'm having a rough time with Grandma right now, so I'll get back to you in the morning."

Graz was vibrantly healthy and never had headaches. I was sure he would be over it by the morning.

Mother was at her worst on her seventh day in telemetry. She was so weak I could barely arouse her from her self-imposed sleep. It came as a shock when the nurse informed me that Mother was ready to be moved to a regular room. Are they crazy? I thought. While my mother is slowly dying, they're telling me her condition is stabilizing. Mother had not been detached even once from the oxygen supply that ran from a wall socket to her nostrils via a thin, flexible plastic tube clipped over her ears. There had been no significant changes in the bilateral pleural effusions, and she was still running a temperature. Yet she was being booted upstairs, where she would no longer be closely monitored.

"Get ready," the nurse commanded Mother as she was about to begin picking at her dinner. "You're moving upstairs."

"Just a minute," I said. "The dinner tray just arrived. We'll move upstairs after dinner."

"I'm a very busy person. Get your mother's things together. She's moving now."

"No, she isn't! I'll get her things together, but she's going to finish her dinner first."

The nurse left Mother's room in a huff. What's the matter with her? I wondered. She returned with a companion, and together they transferred Mother to a cart and covered her with a blanket, piling her plastic urinal and other hospital appurtenances on top of her legs. Then they left, and Mother and I waited in a strange state of anticipation for almost an hour.

The nurse was not apologetic when she finally reappeared, and she pushed Mother's cart through the hallways with obvious annoyance. "If you don't mind, I'll just leave her here," the nurse snapped as she handed Mother's medical records to her new nurse. She had done her duty, and without a word of acknowledgment, she left Mother's room. The new nurse and I looked at each other conspiratorially as we worked in unison to make Mother comfortable. I was glad Mother was out of the telemetry unit—no point in being monitored for a phantom heart condition. Dr. Hafner had again insisted that Mother's heart was not the issue; he had seen the test results and reconfirmed that she had a strong heart.

"Do you mind if my mother is moved to a private room?" I asked her new nurse.

"No, not at all, but this is just like a private room. Nobody's scheduled to be admitted here, and you can sit on the other bed. Why go through the extra expense?"

The floor was very quiet. It was still summer, and a lot of the rooms were empty. I hoped a roommate would not invade Mother's semiprivate room. The woman across the hall had closed her door and placed a sign outside, requesting that the staff knock before entering. Now I closed Mother's door; I wanted privacy for my mother and myself. I was sure she was not going to survive the night, and I did not need strangers witnessing her passing. Mother was too debilitated to lift her head off the pillow. She was not in any obvious distress, but I had never seen her so listless.

Mother perked up briefly that evening, just as I was preparing to leave. She was pleased with her new nurse, Laura, who was solicitous and soft-spoken. She had warmed Mother's blanket in the microwave and asked whether Mother needed anything before she went off duty.

"You really lucked out in the nursing department. It's been a while since you've had such a 'warm' person for your nurse," I punned.

"Yes, you're right, but there's something about her I can't put my finger on. Let just say she's been around and leave it at that."

"It's strange you should say that, Mother. She went into nursing late, but aside from that, I don't get the feeling she's been around."

But Mother was right. When I told Laura that I lived in Caracas, not South Florida, she was surprised. "You must be joking. I lived in Caracas, too," she said, "but some fifteen years back. I wasn't a nurse then. I worked as an office assistant for a very prominent otolaryngologist. As a matter of fact, we became 'good friends,' if you know what I mean, and I accompanied him to Tokyo and other cities for medical conferences."

I could not believe what I heard. Not only was this physician a close friend but Graziano and I had mistakenly blamed his ex-wife for breaking up their marriage. She was the flighty one, and he was the saintly doctor. Now it came together, and I finally understood why the wife had been so furious during the divorce proceedings. When I told Mother the story, she had a good laugh.

"You see," she said. "I told you this woman has been around."

Mother was languishing, not just ailing, I told Graziano when I called Caracas, and I was troubled by her emaciated condition. Graz still had a violent headache, and it had gotten worse. Graz could scarcely speak when he got on the line.

"Where exactly does your head hurt you, honey?" I asked.

"All over, but I feel the throbbing right where the lump is, and I can't bend my neck."

"My God! You mean the lump on your neck?" I had pushed the matter of the lump to the back of my mind during the dreadful week with Mother. "Do you have any other symptoms?"

"I'm so nauseous I can barely sit up."

"Graz, I don't like what I'm hearing. Did you tell Poppy all this?"

"Of course, and Poppy's already made an appointment with the doctor for tomorrow morning."

I could not get Graz out of my mind all night. The situation reminded me of Graziano's bout with encephalitis fifteen years earlier. I called Graziano back at 5:30 A.M. "How is he?" I asked.

"He's about the same. We were up in the night. Nothing I gave him seems to have helped."

"Graziano, you have to get him to the emergency room immediately. I think he has encephalitis or meningitis. Go to the hospital right now, and call his doctor from there. Don't wait for his appointment."

Graz's doctor performed a lumbar puncture and by evening had determined that Graz had viral meningitis. Mother was hospitalized with severe cachexia and seemed to be fading away, and now Graz had a virulent brain inflammation. Was God putting me through a test? I knew I had to get back to Caracas, but I also knew I could not leave Mother. If I left her alone, she would simply slip away. She now weighed sixty-four pounds and had started consuming her own muscle tissue to compensate for the loss of body fat. There was no way I could leave her. Now that she was on a regular visiting schedule, I intended to monitor her meals.

I called my brother. "Noel, Graz's fever has just been diagnosed as viral meningitis, and he's in serious condition. I need to return to Caracas right away, even if it's only for twenty-four hours."

I was waiting for him to offer to cover for me, to fly to South Florida to be with Mother. "Well, that's too bad, " he said. "I understand. I understand if you have to leave."

"No, you don't understand. I cannot leave Mother alone right now. Her condition is too delicate."

Despite the empathy, Noel did not make the offer, and in truth, I did not feel anyone would watch over Mother the way I could. Mother needed my exclusive attention, and I expected to orchestrate every single aspect of her care.

Graz was out of danger, Graziano reported the next morning, and would not suffer any permanent damage. The meningitis had been caught in time. Graz would have to spend a few more days in the hospital, but his doctor expected no further complications. I told Graziano that I would stay with Mother. No matter how much it pained me to make the decision, I could not leave her alone. Graz had Graziano, but Mother had only me.

More and more, I thought of Mother as two separate entities— my wonderful mother with the vibrant personality and my sick mother trapped in a failing body. With the exception of Laura, the staff treated Mother as an impersonal body that required custodial care. A routine of sorts evolved. She was plopped into a Geri chair—sort of an upholstered highchair for adults—after breakfast and stayed there until just after dinner. The Geri chair was originally used for difficult patients but is now a convenient device for chronic-care patients. The patient can neither escape nor fall out and is comfortably surrounded by a tabletop roomy enough to hold a meal tray and assorted belongings. The patient is also sitting up to ingest food, which is healthier than being prone, and the foot stool and headrest can be adjusted, allowing the patient to change positions.

I shuffled back and forth between Coral Bay and The Palms in a stultifying attempt to attend to both parents. In the morning, I stopped at the nursing home to check on Dad and make sure he was properly groomed. Then I headed to Coral Bay, having worked out a circuitous route with little traffic, arriving just in time for Mother's lunch. After lunch, I retraced my path to The Palms to pick up Dad and take him for his afternoon visit with Mother. I usually brought up a tray from the hospital cafeteria for Dad's dinner, and while he dined I helped Mother with hers. Once I was satisfied that Mother was properly tucked back in bed, Dad and I headed to the nursing home, where here, too, we underwent the nightly ministrations. Between The Palms and Coral Bay, I was scarcely at home. I usually stopped at the supermarket in the evening to stock up on frozen dinners. I popped one into the microwave when I got home, ate it while I watched the news, and drifted off on the living-room couch. When I managed to muster the strength, I forced myself to work through the Medicare statements that piled up like dirty laundry.

Mother and I conducted a silent battle over food. She had no appetite and was still uninterested in eating, and I was just as insistent she finish her meals. The staff made a fuss over her cachectic condition, and they were right to be concerned. Dr. Risden stressed that any weight loss was significant because Mother had been a "frail, thin woman" all her life. She had lost more than ten pounds at The Palms, and the additional weight loss in the telemetry unit made the situation precarious. Sherwin Nuland notes that severely cachectic patients are so "profoundly" weak they cannot breathe and cough effectively, increasing the possi-

bility of inhaling vomitus and contracting pneumonia (1994:218).
I no longer bothered to bring homemade goodies, because I knew
Mother would not eat them. But I spoon-fed her each morsel on
the hospital plate, because I was determined she would receive
the required minimum calories. I had to stand over her, as well,
while she slowly sipped the Ensure or she would not bother. I
even held the can for her. The process was tedious. Sometimes it
took a few hours to finish a meal, and then we were almost ready
to start over again.

"Mummy, it's painful for me to see you like this. I need to see
you get better."

"I don't want you to have to see all this. But I just don't have
an appetite."

"Forget the appetite. Forget the 'experiments' you keep telling
everyone about. Let's concentrate on simple things, like finish-
ing your food."

"They're driving me crazy with their experiments, waking me
up at 4:00 A.M. to weigh me."

"Just tell them no. They don't have to weigh you every day.
All they have to do is look at your legs and they'll know whether
you've gained weight."

"I'm worried about Graz. Is Graz all right? Noel told me Graz
had meningitis. Did I hear properly?"

"No, you must have confused it with Graziano's bout with
encephalitis. Graz is fine, just fine."

This was the first time I had lied to my mother. I did not want
to worry her and did not tell her that Graz had been hospitalized.
She would have insisted I return to Caracas. It had not occurred
to me that my brother would tell Mother. I had assumed he would
collaborate in the subterfuge.

I understood the importance of Mother's body weight, but the
methods used to measure Mother's food intake and to weigh her
were downright silly. The sling scale that the early-morning staff
used was very inaccurate. Every day, according to this scale,
Mother's weight fluctuated over a five-pound range. The weighing
was supposed to be coordinated with her food intake. The nurses
glanced at her tray after she finished and noted on a chart taped
to the bathroom door the food items consumed. They frequently

included as "consumed" items that Dad or I had nibbled; at other times, they did not make the necessary notations. I did not see the point to all this activity, although I was frightfully aware of the importance of building up Mother's body weight.

• • •

While Mother had gained a reputation at The Palms as a troublemaker, Dad was quickly identified as the one with the short attention span. The real reason Dad had entered The Palms was that he could not care for himself at home, but his official admission slip mentioned atrial fibrillations, angina, his pacemaker, and his risk of congestive heart failure. Dad was supposed to be a heart patient, yet the nursing staff rapidly labeled him "demented." The staff noted that he was "confused" upon admission, was "incapable of understanding his rights and responsibilities," and had "diminished cognitive status." Dad was not considered a candidate for physical or occupational therapy; his care plan was confined primarily to helping him "exercise his memory by asking him to remember his room number." Dad was defined as an easily distracted person with a fifteen-minute attention span. When I ran into Brenda, the social director, she had no compunction about telling me that Dad had advanced Alzheimer's. "Not to worry," she chirped cheerfully. "There's nothing you can do about it."

When I mentioned to Mother that I could not stomach Brenda's chipper, condescending attitude, Mother countered that Brenda had to act that way—it was part of her job to motivate the residents to participate in the scheduled activities, even when they weren't interested. Months later, when I saw Brenda in a local TV spot hawking the benefits of a foreclosure company, I could not help but recall her versatility as a lay diagnostician.

Although Dad was happy to be reunited with Mother when he entered The Palms, he was unduly worried about her condition. No staff member associated his fears about her recovery with his aberrant behavior. Dad was upset and had a hard time sleeping. He kept covering and uncovering Mother, waking her up in the process, and wandered into the hallway, where he promptly got lost. He also tried to get dressed in the middle of the night and attempted to fit into Mother's shorts when he could not find his own closet. Dr. Friedmann prescribed Restoril for Dad's "insomnia," although this drug is counter-indicated for elderly, debilitated patients. Restoril produces vertigo and can also cause confusion, drowsiness, and lethargy.

The nurses' evaluation noted that Dad was on medication that would require increased safety precautions. According to his care plan, he required twenty-four-hour supervision because of his wandering and poor trunk control. Despite these directives, Dad was not receiving the attention he required. He was always alone when I went to The Palms, and I usually found him roving unsteadily down the hallway. Dad's bathroom reeked of urine; it evidently was not being cleaned every day. He continued to look as though he had slept in his clothes even after I complained to Peggy Jo. Each day, a schedule was posted at the nurses' station, listing the patients who were to be bathed and have their nails cut. Dad's name regularly appeared on the sheet, but this did not mean he was actually showered. Someone was shaving Dad, though. His face was filled with razor nicks, and half of his luxurious mustache had been carelessly trimmed away.

Then there was the matter of the wandering clothing. Although I had taped instructions on his bathroom door indicating that Dad's clothing would be washed at home, his soiled clothing was gone whenever I went to collect it. It rarely returned, and I had to make a daily trek to the laundry room and the unclaimed clothing room to search for his missing garments. Some of them surfaced, but the rest seemed to disappear into thin air. I finally caught on the day Dad's colorful quilt disappeared from his bed. I knew I had seen it from the corner of my eye and walked into Ben's room across the hall. Ben was a hyperkinetic Alzheimer's resident in his upper eighties who liked to streak down the hallway nude. Dad's quilt was on Ben's bed, and Dad's missing glasses were on Ben's nightstand. I furtively riffled through Ben's drawers and discovered Dad's briefs and some of his best cotton shirts. I felt sorry for Ben, who had once been a prominent lawyer and mayor of his hometown and was now too far gone to feel his own humiliation. News of his past achievements was prominently displayed on the wall above his dresser. His drawers were disheveled and filled with faded undergarments and cheap polyester shirts that had lost their shape. No wonder he was attracted to Dad's clothing, which had not been subjected to the merciless wear and tear of institutional laundering.

Dad calmed down while Mother was hospitalized, but every day at The Palms brought a new irritant. On his fifth day of solitary confinement there without Mother, he fell out of bed and was found sitting on the floor at 6:30 A.M. The aide helped him up, but he was unable to stand on his own. She cleansed the cut on his hand with hydrogen peroxide and helped him back into bed. Someone from the nurses' station called me at 8:00 A.M. and told me Dad had fallen. I rushed over and found him curled in a fetal position on top of his bed. His hand was thickly caked with dried blood and had turned an unsightly shade of deep blue.

"Dad, how did this happen?" I asked.

"I don't know. I got up to go to the bathroom, and the next thing I knew, I was sitting on the floor. I kept shouting for help because I couldn't get up."

"Did they come right in?"

"No, I was shouting for a long time."

"How do you feel right now?"

"Everything hurts, and I can't move my right arm."

"You must have broken the fall with your arm and hit your hand against the bedframe. I think you should stay in bed today and just rest."

Nobody had looked in on Dad since the aide had washed his cut several hours earlier. I was alarmed about the swelling and discoloration moving up his arm. I washed the cut thoroughly with soap and water, covered Dad with his comforter, and walked to the nurses' station.

"I'm surprised to find that nobody has been in to check on my father since he fell early this morning. You know he's on Coumadin [a blood thinner], don't you?" I asked angrily. "And he shouldn't be on Restoril. It only confuses him and affects his balance. My father needs an ice pack immediately, and his hand needs to be X-rayed. It's grotesquely swollen."

"We don't have any ice packs here," the aide said lackadaisically.

"Well, improvise!" I retorted.

"We did call his cardiologist and are waiting for instructions."

"You don't need instructions to apply an ice pack, for heaven's sake."

A nursing home without an ice pack? I turned around and walked out. It was easier to go home and get an ice bag from Dad's drawer than to discuss the merits of applying ice with an indifferent aide. When I returned, I reminded the aide that she had to refresh the pack after I left. I told Dad I would be back after visiting Mother, and he dozed off with the ice pack on his hand. By late afternoon, his hand was noticeably swollen, and the aide reapplied the ice pack—my ice pack—to his hand. When I returned, the portable X-ray ordered by the house physician still had not arrived. The aide claimed that Home X-ray had been called at 5:00 P.M., but by 9:00 P.M., when I decided to leave, the equipment still had not appeared.

The following morning, the aide informed me that my father had been uncooperative and had refused the X-ray.

"What time did they arrive?" I asked.

"They came about 10:30."

"At night? Do you expect any normal person to allow a stranger to wake him up late at night for an X-ray? It's unbelievable that you would disturb my father's rest. I insist you call them back this morning."

It was not until the end of the second day that Home X-ray finally got around to returning. By this time, Dr. Hafner had assured me that the marked discoloration was a side effect of the Coumadin and would fade. Another day went by before the results became available. Dad's right hand was not fractured or dislocated, but I already knew that, because the swelling was beginning to subside.

I did not realize how common falls are in nursing homes. Some 30–50 percent of nursing-home residents fall each year. Most falls seems to occur in the patient's room or the bathroom, and about half are related to getting in and out of bed or a wheelchair and getting on or off the toilet. Various factors conspire to make the nursing home a dangerous environment: insufficient supervision of the patient because of low patient-to-staff ratios; design faults, such as slippery floors and poor lighting; and the use of psychotropic drugs such as tranquilizers and sedatives.

It was obvious to me that Dad had been written off at The Palms. Not only was he not considered a candidate for physical or occupational therapy, but he was not even exposed to an ordinary exercise program that might improve his balance. In fact, there was no exercise program to speak of. Residents were not allowed to use the pool available to the assisted-living division and were rarely taken outside for walks. The residents got entirely too much rest. Dinner was served at 5:00 P.M., and patients were bedded down two hours later, when it was still light outside. Dad's "wandering"—his only form of exercise, as far as I could determine—was treated with sedatives that only made him shakier. His walking ability deteriorated rapidly at The Palms. When we went to visit Mother, I had to support him under the arms, or he would slide to the sidewalk. Taking him to the hospital every afternoon and bringing him back late stopped his wandering, and his ability to walk began to improve. I knew, though, that I had to get him out of The Palms, where he was at recurrent risk for falls.

• • •

Mother's new rheumatologist, Benjamin Klein, was unfailingly courteous and conscientious. He made his rounds near dinnertime, when we were all assembled around Mother's bed. He greeted Dad with a handshake and took the time to engage him in idle talk. He was equally solicitous of Mother but could not hide a note of concern. Dr. Hafner had advised Dr. Klein that Mother's ventricular function was normal, and he would now try to find the cause of the repeated pleural effusions. While he awaited the results of the pleural fluid cytology, he told Mother that if the effusions were stable and were caused by her rheumatoid arthritis rather than by congestive heart failure, they would just need to be watched.

But when I followed Dr. Klein to the hallway to voice my concerns about Mother's worsening condition, the story was different.

"Your mother is a very sick woman, you know. Her sed rate has shot up, and she may even have vasculitis."

I knew that an elevated sedimentation rate was an important indicator of Mother's chronic inflammatory disease, but vasculitis, an inflammation of the blood vessels, was one complication

I had not thought to worry about. "Surely, there's something you can do. My mother is getting weaker every day," I said. "And something new keeps cropping up—her hairline's receding; her face is shrinking in; yesterday another tooth fell out; and she can't seem to last a few minutes without the oxygen tube. Her white count keeps rising, and now she has thrush."

"Your mother is a seriously ill woman," Dr. Klein reiterated. "I don't mean immediately or tomorrow. She's in no imminent danger, but her condition is very advanced. Maybe she can live like this another six months, at the most."

"You know, Dr. Klein, I appreciate your telling me this. I appreciate your frankness. You're not telling me anything I don't already know. I know my mother's condition is very serious. I know all the nuances. I've been following them constantly. But surely there's something you can do. What about increasing her prednisone? My mother has always responded well to it before."

"That would not be good. There are too many pernicious side effects," Dr. Klein answered. He paused and then said, "But we'll give it a try. I guess we have nothing to lose. I'm going to increase your mother's dose to 60 milligrams for the next few days, starting tonight. And I'm going to order some therapy for her, starting tomorrow afternoon."

"Thank goodness! I don't think I could watch my mother spend another day in that Geri chair."

"Don't get your hopes up too high. Remember what I said about the long-term prognosis."

I was upset when I went home that evening. Dr. Klein was sincere and had spoken the truth. How much longer could Mother withstand the escalating crises? They were taking an enormous toll on her overall health. Her weight now hovered around sixty-five pounds. The six-month prognosis kept reverberating in my mind. I was grateful for Dr. Klein's frankness. Not one of Mother's doctors had had the guts to tell me she was approaching the end. Each and every one had focused on her immediate condition and disregarded the long-term picture.

The next morning, Mother had clearly rallied. The intravenous infusion of a high dose of prednisone had served as a magic bullet, and Mother was sitting up in bed when I walked in. Her black mood had lifted, and she had eaten her breakfast without being prodded. She continued to improve as her appetite, aided by the steroids, came back. Dr. Klein had clearly saved Mother's life. She was delighted with the thought of resuming therapy, which gave her an incentive to get out of bed and start moving. Her face was radiant when she succeeded in walking down the hall with a walker. But mine must have registered dismay, because Mother had shrunk noticeably during this hospital stay. I had never seen her so tiny and frail. A nurse approached me as Mother turned around and walked in the other direction. She put her arm around my shoulder as I tried to contain the tears.

"I know what you're thinking," she said. "I lost my own mother just a few months ago. Your mother is a determined woman, but the body can go just so far. I really feel for you."

I smiled at Mother as she slowly walked toward me again. Maybe she would pull through after all. Dr. Klein was pleased that afternoon when he made his rounds.

"Mrs. Margolies, you've surprised us! You're getting better. You're clinically better. If you keep this progress up, you'll be ready for discharge in a few days."

Mother nodded her head in agreement, but I could tell that even she was unprepared for this positive turn of events. Mother was growing stronger, but on the fourth day of therapy she called me at 11:00 P.M.

"Mother, what a surprise. Why aren't you asleep?"

"I can't sleep. I spoke to Dr. Klein at length. He came in late this evening, and I haven't been able to sleep since he left."

"Tell me what's the matter."

"Everything's the matter. I've just had terrible news. There's nothing that can be done for me. It's the condition. I don't have congestive heart failure. The doctor said that the fluid in the lungs is from my rheumatoid arthritis. They're not going to get better, and the effusions are not going to go away."

Mother was sobbing as she told me this. I, however, saw a tiny window of hope. I had never been able to accept the diagnosis of congestive heart failure. It just did not make sense in light of her healthy heart. Every time I thought of congestive heart failure, I envisioned sinister consequences for Mother. "Mom, maybe this is not such bad news," I said. "Your rheumatoid condition can be treated. It can be brought under control. Maybe you're just experiencing a flare."

"No, this is the end. He was very clear about that. Nothing can be done."

"Mummy, please, maybe the end will come in six months, a year, two years from now. You're definitely improving; you're getting ready to leave the hospital."

"No, we've talked about this before. I know when my time has come. How much can a body take? It's something we all have to face eventually. It's my time to die. I'm being realistic. It's nature taking its course."

"I know," I said, "but not yet."

"This is just like Mamma. Mamma had congestive heart failure, but now I think it wasn't that."

"Mummy, it's completely different. Your mother was not treated then. It was 1939; there weren't even any antibiotics. Whatever she had simply ran its course. Remember when people went into the hospital and never came out?"

"Listen to me carefully. I want to be buried in my rose chiffon suit. I've always loved that suit. And I want you to go over the burial papers this week and make sure you have everything in order. And I want you to have your blood checked. This disease runs in the family."

I listened quietly as Mother became pragmatic. (She never thought I could collect my own diseases or any from Dad's side.) I was genetically disposed to come down with an autoimmune disease. My aunt Myra had died relatively young of systemic lupus erythematosus, and her daughter died of the same disease in her mid-forties. Two male cousins had contracted Crohn's disease, an inflammatory bowel disorder, as young men. Both of Mother's two remaining sisters suffered from rheumatic conditions, and my maternal grandmother seems to have ended her life with pulmonary fibrosis and rheumatoid-induced congestive heart failure.

Much later, when I conducted my research, I realized that the clue to Mother's strange, recurrent episodes with congestive heart failure lay in her history of chronic autoimmune diseases. It was not until I had collected and analyzed Mother's old medical records that I learned she indeed had a history of fibrotic disease of the lungs associated with her mixed connective-tissue disease. The term "fibrosis of the lungs" cropped up continually. In fact, the etiology of the current episodes of congestive heart failure was buried in her hospital record of June 1, the day of her near-death crisis with heart block. The first specimen of pleural fluid collected indicated a "chronic active inflammation." But only Dr. Hafner picked up on it, insisting more than once that Mother's heart failure did not stem from coronary disease. Temporary conduction abnormalities are not uncommon when a rheumatoid lung is stressed, leading to heart block and left ventricular dysfunction. Had I only known that the stress on Mother's body after the hip fractures had triggered a severe flare, leading to recurrent pulmonary edema and so-called congestive heart failure, I would not have taken her home and acted as if her "temporary" crisis were over. I would have insisted that the underlying rheumatic condition be treated aggressively. Now it was too late for that.

• • •

This time, I was not going to leave anything to chance. Mother was improving, and Dr. Friedmann said she probably would be able to leave Coral Bay right after the Labor Day weekend. On Wednesday, September 1, I told Mother I would be visiting nursing homes the next day and would not be in to see her until late evening. I knew she would rather die than return to The Palms, the catalyst of her present difficulties. I was merely biding my time with Dad. Wherever Mother went, he would follow. I had removed most of his belongings from The Palms, bringing him a fresh change of clothing every day. For all practical purposes, I had already moved him out of The Palms.

Although the social-services director at Coral Bay gave me a list of nursing facilities in Broward County, I decided to start farther north, in Palm Beach County, and work my way southward. I visited eleven nursing facilities in all, beginning with Victoria Park in Boca Raton, which is famed for offering fresh popcorn daily. I told Victoria Park's marketing director, Karen, that I was interested in a Medicare bed for Mother after the holiday weekend, and she promised to call me as soon as she spoke to the social-services department about Mother's discharge.

From Victoria Park I proceeded south to The Forum, whose nursing home is set back from an artificial lake and surrounded by willow trees—a lovely and low-key setting. The rooms had a homey feel, and the large dining room was suffused with sunlight. I was particularly impressed with the cozy dining alcove reserved for patients who needed assistance with their meals. It was lunchtime, and the Parkinson's patients seated in the charming room were being helped by their wives. This tableau of elderly women feeding their ailing husbands was strangely comforting.

This was the place for Mother, I decided. The subdued tone was just right for her quiet temperament. Further, when I discovered that the admissions director was a renegade from The Palms who soundly bashed it, I knew the place was right. The Forum could accommodate Dad in the assisted-living section right away, but no Medicare beds were available for Mother in the nursing division. The Forum would let me know.

My next stop was Royal Court East in Pompano Beach. This facility was highly recommended by the Medicare social worker and had one of the best reputations in South Florida. Its proximity to home was an advantage, but the lobby was detestable. Some misguided decorator had tried to convey Southern charm via scenic wallpaper, a soaring ceiling, fake potted plants, and pseudo-baroque furnishings. Inside, the dingy "bar," drab dining room, and narrow hallways illuminated with harsh fluorescent tubes were deserted. The small rooms sorely needed paint and were furnished with cheap institutional pieces that had seen better days. The admissions director was eager to place Mother in a Medicare bed, and Dad could enter the private wing for only $95 a day. All would be arranged instantly, I thought, if this woman had her way.

"Don't call the hospital, please," I said. "I don't know yet when my Mother will be released, and I'm here only to familiarize myself with Royal Court."

"Don't worry, don't worry," she answered. "I won't do anything you don't want, but I would appreciate it if you would let me know soon one way or another."

I would call her as a simple act of courtesy, but I would never send my mother to such a dismal place. My rule was simple: I would not permit Mother to go anywhere I would not go myself.

As I left, I glanced across the road at Royal Court West, the sister facility for Alzheimer's patients. It had barred windows. The husband of one of Mother's hospital roommates had died there.

After Royal Court, my sense of well-being sank. I continued to Park Summit, a complex in western Coral Springs owned by the Marriott consortium, which also owns The Forum. Park Summit was based on the same model as its more elegant sister—independent living, assisted living, and skilled nursing. The nursing facility was on an upper floor of the high-rise and had only twenty or so beds. The place was spotlessly clean, bare bones in style, and harshly institutional. The patients obviously had grave problems and were there for the long term. It looked like a place of no return. I did not envision Mother there.

Heading east, I visited more facilities in Pompano Beach. I was demoralized and did not even bother going to the admissions offices. The thought of one more conversation with an admissions director was unbearable. I just walked in and strolled past the nurses' station, as if I were going to visit a relative. It did not take me long to case the place. How many people were at the nurses' station? Were a sufficient number of aides wandering around, or were they scarce? Did the patients look well cared for? Were they neatly dressed, or were they left in bed? Were they sitting alone in the entrances and staring blankly into space? Were the rooms clean or shabby? Did the hallways smell of urine? The faintest whiff turned me off, because it meant that the staff was not maintaining cleanliness. Who knew what toxic microbes might be lurking? Mother could not afford to pick up another bug in a new nursing home.

I even visited John Knox, a Christian nursing home affiliated with the well-known John Knox Village, which received most of its patients from within its retirement community. This home was also spotlessly clean, but the residents seemed to be long-timers receiving custodial care. They were mostly female, very elderly, and lined up in a row along the sides of the recreation room, staring listlessly into space. This place definitely would not do. Mother needed a more energetic facility where she could get therapy, have meaningful communication with her fellow patients, and leave in a few short weeks.

By now I was in a foul mood. At the next stop, I went directly to the therapy room. After all, if Mother's primary goal was to receive good therapy, wasn't that where I should start? There, the physical therapy room resembled a storage closet more than anything else. Chairs and tables were haphazardly tossed along one side of the room. No therapists or patients were in sight. Every facility certified by Medicare is required to have a therapy room, but this was one example of a nursing home that complied in name only.

I arrived at LovingCare, at the southwesternmost tip of Broward County, at 6:00 P.M. or so. The neighborhood, in heavily populated Lauderhill, was congested, but the nursing home was situated on a quiet residential street that looked as if it had been transformed recently from a cow field. Still, despite its impersonal air, the nursing home seemed acceptable in a crunch. The director, a youngish woman, was personable, and a Medicare bed was available immediately.

From LovingCare, I drove directly back to Coral Bay. It was dark, and Mother had already dined. "Well Mom, I really missed you," I said as I entered her room. "This is the first day in a while that I haven't been with you. I visited eleven nursing homes today but couldn't finish. Time simply ran out."

"What did you see?"

"I feel you will find what you need at either Victoria Park or The Forum. They're different from the others. The level of care seems to be about the same at both places, but I prefer The Forum. I like its ambiance better. The nurses at The Forum were holding a staff meeting when I arrived. They seemed genuinely concerned about their work. LovingCare will do in a pinch, however. I didn't find anything there to actively dislike, but The Forum is my first choice."

"Dr. Friedmann was in a little while ago and said that I will be ready to leave tomorrow."

"But tomorrow is Friday, the day before a holiday. No beds are available over the long weekend. And you're not ready. You need to gain some weight before you leave the hospital. I can't believe it."

"Well, you'd better believe it. I'm being discharged tomorrow."

"I'll call Friedmann and speak to the social-services department early tomorrow. I won't allow them to discharge you unless you can go to the right nursing home. It's going to be a big problem. Nothing is available until after Labor Day. Why didn't he let us know earlier? It's not right to just spring this on us. He definitely said, 'after Labor Day.' "

"Call him if you want, but he said I'm ready to leave tomorrow. Anyway, I want to leave. They're not doing anything more for me here."

"Mother, you'll get better care here than in a nursing home. It's incredible—a Friday afternoon before a long holiday weekend."

But it was true. Dr. Friedmann was discharging Mother before rather than after the long weekend. I knew she was restless and wanted out, but I was determined to find the right place. I needed more time.

The next morning I went directly to the social-services department. "How did it go yesterday?" Ilene, the department head, asked.

"I visited eleven nursing homes, working my way down from north to south. Between these and what I'd seen before, I have a pretty good notion of what's out there. Frankly, I found the whole experience demoralizing. If I hadn't taken notes after each visit, I wouldn't be able to distinguish one place from the next."

"Have you come to a decision?"

"Yes, I would like Mother to go to The Forum, and if that's not available, then Victoria Park. I couldn't in good conscience allow my mother to spend even a day in some of those other places. A few of them did not even have decent therapy rooms. And some were simply depressing."

"What did you expect?" she asked, smiling. "Nursing homes are depressing, yet they're also necessary."

"Would you like to stay in one of them, Ilene?" I asked. "You know, it only takes a little imagination and some sensitivity to make a facility palatable. How can anyone recuperate in a place that's depressing? To quote one of the residents at The Palms, 'It's the pits!' "

Ilene looked bemused. "The Palms has one of the finest reputations in Broward County."

"Oh, Ilene. When was the last time you set foot in The Palms? Before you recommend a nursing home, you should at least visit it once in a while—better yet, spend an entire day there. The neglect at The Palms is outrageous. Yet the abuse is so subtle you would have to be there day in and day out to appreciate it. Most of the patients are so out of it they can't speak for themselves. When Mother spoke out, even to get a Tylenol after a two-hour wait, she was labeled a troublemaker. Don't ever send anyone from Coral Bay to The Palms. Remember: It's the pits!"

"That's why I don't like to make personal recommendations," Ilene said. "It's our policy to give each family a list and let them make their own decision. I'm only trying to help you. By the way, Royal Court called yesterday afternoon. What should I tell them when they call back?"

"Tell them no. I specifically asked the admissions director not to call you, because I wasn't really interested."

"It's a good nursing facility, Luisa."

"If it's so good, why are so many beds available? The answer is no, absolutely no."

I reiterated that I wanted Mother to leave the hospital *after* Labor Day. Dr. Friedmann had insisted Mother needed those extra days, and now he was giving us less than twenty-four hours' notice. I went to Mother's room and called The Forum and Victoria Park. No beds were available that day, and nothing would be available until Tuesday, at the earliest. I was told to call back after Labor Day; new patients were not admitted over holiday weekends. Then I called Dr. Friedmann. He gave me the usual runaround. His hands were tied with the hospital committee; there was no justification for holding Mother over the weekend.

I went back downstairs and told Ilene that nothing was available. Consequently, Mother would go directly from the hospital to Victoria Park or The Forum on Tuesday.

"Luisa, let me clarify something for you," she said. "Your mother is being discharged *today*. She should leave before dinner. It's not advantageous for you to insist that your mother stay on. It will cost you thousands of extra dollars, because the hospital has agreed that her allotted days are up. As long as a nursing-facility bed is available somewhere in Broward County, your mother has to leave. She can move into one of the facilities that has beds available, such as LovingCare, and when the weekend is over, she can be moved to another facility. She may even decide she wants to stay at LovingCare."

Her smile was beginning to wane and so was my patience. Somewhere in my papers was a reference to patients' rights concerning premature discharge. Ah, yes, it was a statement from Sacred Heart Hospital, but I was so tired from my tour de force the day before that the details escaped me. Ilene's adversarial attitude was nearly the final straw.

"Ilene, you and your hospital don't have my mother's best interests at heart. She's an extremely ill woman, and it would be criminal to move her twice when there is absolutely no reason she cannot stay through the weekend. You know better than I do that nursing homes don't admit patients on Friday evenings. You don't care about the patients here. You care more about your rules and regulations." I was about to cry. "I can't discuss this with you anymore. You're unreasonable. You don't give a damn." I turned around and walked out, determined not to show any more emotion in front of a stranger.

"I'll make some more calls and let you know later," Ilene said. "Will you be in your Mother's room?"

Mother seemed oblivious to the little drama swirling around her. She wanted to leave and was convinced she would be the victim of benign neglect if she insisted on staying. She was probably right. I had seen the level of care plummet instantly once Sacred Heart decided that Mother had exceeded her allotted time.

I had spent the entire day in fruitless efforts to postpone Mother's discharge. It was nearly dinnertime when Ilene's assistant appeared at the door. "I've spoken with Victoria Park, and they're willing to give your mother a private room for a few days," she said. "When a Medicare bed becomes available, she can move."

"That sounds fine. Let me discuss it with my mother, and I'll meet you at the nurses' station in a few minutes."

I returned to Mother's room. "Mom, this is the best solution," I said. "They really want you out of here today, and Victoria Park looks like the right place."

"How much does a private room cost?"

"About $200—more economical, believe it or not, than a semi-private room at Coral Bay. And anyway, I'm treating you. All you have to worry about is getting better."

"No, I'd rather spend the money on a private-duty aide to help me. I'll go to . . . What's the name of that place?"

"LovingCare?"

"Yes, LovingCare."

"Can I trust you, Mom? Remember when Lunice followed you to The Palms. You dismissed her the first day. At Victoria Park, you probably won't need a private aide."

"No, let's do it this way. Let's just get going."

At the nurses' station I said that my mother would be leaving after dinner and that the van should pick us up at 6:30. But no sooner had I returned to Mother's room to help her with dinner than the van appeared. We were told that if we did not go downstairs "immediately," the van would charge us for a double run. Marisa had just arrived, and we decided to wrap up Mother's dinner and leave right away. Marisa accompanied Mother in the private van while I followed in the car with Mother's belongings.

I could not relax when I finally got home and riffled through the files until I located Mother's Sacred Heart discharge papers. I should have asked Ilene for a copy of the patients' rights document, but I had been too befuddled to do so. Its basic message is that, according to federal law, the discharge date must be determined *solely by your medical needs,* not by Medicare payments. If you think you are being told to leave the hospital too soon, you have the right to ask a hospital representative for a written notice of explanation, called the "Notice of Noncoverage." This notice explains that Medicare will no longer pay for your hospital stay. Then you have the right to request a review by a Peer Review Organization (PRO). However, the PRO will review your case only when the hospital and the doctor disagree. If the hospital and the doctor agree (as they usually do), the PRO will not review your case before the Notice of Noncoverage is issued. Once the Notice of Noncoverage is received stating that the physician agrees with the hospital's decision, the patient must request a review from the PRO by phone or in writing by noon of the first work day after receiving the notice. The PRO must also ask for your views on the case, and once it notifies you of its decision, you have the right to request a reconsideration.

As long as you are knowledgeable enough to request a review, the hospital cannot bill you until the day after you receive the Notice of Noncoverage. I had made an egregious mistake at Mother's expense. I should have requested a review. It would have been impossible for the Notice of Noncoverage to reach us until after the Labor Day weekend, at which time Mother would have left for the nursing home of her choice. And the hospital could not start billing us until the day after Mother received the notice. So the hospital would be responsible for the few extra days not covered by Medicare. Mother was a liability by now. According to the hospital, she was well enough to leave, but she was far too sick to be discharged to her home. Damn Ilene and the interests she represented. She knew the procedures, and she knew Mother could not be served with a Notice of Noncoverage until after the Labor Day weekend. Mother had the law on her side. I should have taken a firmer stand, but I had allowed Ilene to intimidate me. I was vulnerable and the hospital had bullied me into accepting Mother's discharge against my better judgment.

Enough Is Enough
Prolonging Living or Prolonging Dying?

THE MAJORITY of American elders can now expect to die protracted deaths from chronic conditions. The ethicist Margaret Pabst Battin has called the pattern in which death comes after a long downhill course a new epidemiological reality (1994:13–14). Frail elderly patients are kept alive for long periods of time, and "even when it seems the person can decline no more and still remain alive, further losses are possible" (Sankar 1994:109). Congestive heart failure seems to be the new buzzword for describing the cardiovascular disorders that commonly befall the frail elderly in the last years of their lives. The aged heart is unable to pump enough blood to meet the body's needs, and its ability to respond to stress is impaired. Congestive heart failure, like Alzheimer's, osteoporosis, osteoarthritis, and adult-onset diabetes, is a discrete geriatric syndrome. One in four persons older than sixty-five will suffer from congestive heart failure. The intensive-care units in hospitals across the Sunbelt are filled with elderly patients who are in and out every few months with repeated episodes. These patients are stabilized and sent home but are expected back with another relapse.

I can think of many caregivers within my circle of friends and colleagues whose parents were repeatedly pulled back from the brink of death. My friend Linda's father had been on life-support systems more than a half-dozen times. His process of dying took a few years and prevented him from enjoying the last part of his life. He survived one particularly lengthy stay in the ICU after suffering cardiovascular complications, only to leave the hospital enfeebled and heavily dependent on a walker. When I asked Linda why her family agreed to the use of a ventilator during his final crisis, she said they had no way to know whether he was actually dying. He had come out of crises before, and they gambled that he would come out of that one.

Protracted dying means that one dies in progressive decrements, that we die "too long." According to Walter Bortz, this is not the natural or "dignified" death we hear so much about but "a slow, downward spiral wherein each day is paler and gloomier than the one before" (1991:284). *Dying* rather than *death* is the real villain for Bortz. Protracted dying robs the patient of his or her last vestiges of self-esteem. When it occurs in an impersonal hospital setting, it isolates patients and makes them dependent on the technological wizardry of the medical staff. In a study of behavior and attitudes during the final phase of life, Mary Louise Nash concludes that protracted dying is incongruent with the notion of "dignity." Patients feel a sense of powerlessness and loneliness while they cope with pain and the physical losses brought about by their illnesses (1980:69).

The sociologist David Wendell Moller (1990) points to a curious paradox vis-à-vis the dying patient: Although medical technology has created expectations of omnipotence, patients and their families feel powerless because the dying process has been usurped by the institution. The patient is managed as a series of discrete medical interventions. When death comes knocking at the hospital door, the physician ignores it, because bureaucratic procedures and technical virtuosity have subsumed the humanitarian tasks of providing comfort and support. Life must go on, even in the face of death.

How do we know when someone is dying? This is the big question for which medical science has no definitive answer. The day it finds one, the care of our graying society will be revolutionized. Bortz tells a story about one of his patients, an eighty-eight-year-old woman admitted to the emergency room in "respiratory arrest." He instructed the staff to proceed "full code" ahead. They had to break her ribs to get her breathing again, but they saved her life. Bortz felt she would be able to weather the crisis brought on by her high blood pressure. Her health was stable, and her high blood pressure was easy to control. She returned to her home and husband after six weeks in the hospital and lived a good life before she died suddenly more than a year later (1991:291–296). Bortz knew he had made the right decision because he was familiar with his patient's medical history and her way of life. Hers was a life worth living, despite her advanced age.

Sara, a social worker and one of my friends in New York, spent ten years directing social-service programs at a hospital in Wyoming. When I asked her whether she had participated in bioethical decision making, she told me the following story. She had been a great admirer of a prominent specialist at her hospital until an episode involving her mother dampened her enthusiasm. Her mother had come to Wyoming for a short visit but stayed on because she was not feeling well. She was admitted to the hospital at which Sara worked and was diagnosed with terminal colon cancer that had metastasized to her lungs. The specialist refused to treat her, claiming that at nearly ninety she was very old and would die soon anyway. She would be dead within eight hours without treatment, he said, but nothing could be done. It would be a terrible death. Sara appealed to another staff physician, a surgeon, who agreed to operate. He removed large sections of the colon, performed a colostomy, and inserted a feeding tube into the stomach. Sara was furious with the first doctor. "You don't know my mother," she told him. "She's not like any other eighty-nine-year-old. Just a year ago, we were traveling around Europe together, and there's no reason why she can't be alive a year from now." No procedure was performed after the initial surgery, and Sara's mother received no chemotherapy or radiation. She lived for ten more months—"quality months"—with little pain. As the end approached, Sara administered tiny amounts of morphine to alleviate her mother's pain, and she died quietly at home, holding Sara's hand. Sara had advised her mother to risk the operation: "If you come out of it, there's a good chance you'll be better, and if you die during the operation, you won't know what happened and will have avoided the terrible suffering predicted by the first physician." Sara told me the story to illustrate one of the bioethical issues that arose at the hospital: to treat or not to treat in light of a patient's advanced age.

Who was right—the physician who refused to treat the patient because of her advanced age, or Sara, who felt that her mother could enjoy a few more months of life? Sara, certainly, if you look at her mother's personal history. But the physician who tried objectively, perhaps coldly, to assess the elderly woman's chances of recovery probably has some champions. There are no easy answers. Both stories show how important it is to have a good grasp of the patient's medical history and to know something about the patient's lifestyle. My mother was lucky that one of her attending physicians had known her for many years and knew about my parents' devoted relationship. Further, my mother was alert and agreeable—a cooperative and charming patient—which made it easy for her medical team to keep trying, despite her poor long-term prognosis.

Age is a significant factor that must be considered when evaluating a patient's medical history. The older we are, the closer we are to death and the more likely we are to suffer from multiple debilitating conditions. And the older we are, the more vulnerable we become, because our dwindling reserves make it more difficult to bounce back from one crisis to the next. Beyond these elemental facts, we enter a vague world of medical uncertainty in which the outcome is hard to predict. Chronological age becomes just one more component in the total picture.

The problem is not simply one of chronological age; it also involves the technological aggressiveness with which modern medicine is now practiced. The "medicalization" of life and death has brought the era of natural death to a close, thanks to the transformation of doctors into technicians. Ivan Illich was the first to lament the depersonalization of medical treatment in *Medical Nemesis* (1976). The ethicist Daniel Callahan has described the pursuit of medical technology to the limits as "brinkmanship," in the "gambling effort to go *as close to that line as possible*" before withdrawing treatment in the misguided effort to combat death and hold it at bay just a little longer, no matter what (1993:41). The problem with technological brinkmanship is that it makes it extremely difficult to determine when a person's death is imminent. It deforms the dying process, in Callahan's opinion, by drawing out and exacerbating the frail, debilitated period of the twilight of our lives. Paradoxically, the same medical technology that has contributed to our longevity is making it more difficult to enjoy our old age and die when it is our rightful time. Callahan cogently argues that modern medicine should not be used to extend lives endlessly, but our ambivalence about such matters, and our difficulty in coping with the new realities of death and dying, have contributed to the status quo. The ideology of "automatic therapy" aimed at prolonging life at all costs is pursued with such zeal that it prevents doctors from perceiving when it is better simply to let nature take its course (Avorn 1986:295).

Ethicists also remind us that, even though death has been relegated to the sphere of technology, it is actually a spiritual crisis concerning the manner in which patients face the end of life. The bioethicist John Hardwig notes that, although his discipline has a lot to say to physicians and other health-care professionals, it has ignored the dying patient. He believes that patients who do not complete advance directives or who find the proxy decisions irrelevant are actually reacting to this emphasis on medical treatment. Treatment and technology seem to have become the mantra for end-of-life care, he says, when the real focus should be on the spiritual crisis that dying patients and their families face (Hardwig 2000).

An important caveat here: We should not dismiss technology to a point at which we lament the disappearance of the family doctor and the era in which compassion and a doctor–patient relationship compensated for the paltry offerings of scientific medicine. Anthropologists who have conducted fieldwork among the "primitive," the poor, and the disfranchised peoples of the earth are painfully aware of what happens without the benefits of modern medicine. In societies whose members lack access to preventive medicine, most die prematurely from endemic and infectious diseases; few people survive to old age. My colleague Melvin Konner, who did extensive fieldwork in the Kalahari and then entered medical school in his fourth decade, says that he "revered" the technical capacity of modern medicine and felt scorn for the critics who belittled it. Yet his previous grounding in the cultural context of health and disease allowed him to "question the supremacy of technique that has, in the eyes of some critics, rendered American medicine a spiritual wasteland and its practitioners impotent to confront matters of life and death other than with a test or drug or scalpel" (1987:361).

Ron Carson has called for a return to tradition when it comes to considerations of death. In our culture, he said in a poetic paper delivered to the American Gerontological Society in 1994, the inevitability of our demise is a brute fact, and there is nothing worse than death. We empower modern medicine to conduct an all-out assault to defeat death. But modern medicine can keep death at bay only so long, and we must eventually relinquish control and incorporate the important detail of our own mortality. If we were to look for comfort in traditional practices, such as the comings and goings of the family and friends who surround a person dying at home, we would put ritual back into death rather than isolating the dying person in a strange place. Then, perhaps, we would replace the terror of unbearable dying with a feeling of solidarity and support.

Why is it so difficult to die at home these days? I had my first fieldwork experience in the 1970s in a small highland town in central Mexico. The people in the town died at home, held their *velorios* (vigils) at home, and marched through the streets, accompanied by the entire populace, to the cemetery. The sequence of ritual events was carried out in full sight of the community. Nothing to hide, nothing to fear—death was an integral part of life. Until recently, these kinds of death experiences were the norm throughout the rural world. My colleague Ruth Behar notes that, in the northern Spanish village where she conducted her fieldwork, an impending death was announced with solemn strokes of the church bells. "In the company of Christ, the priest, kin, and neighbors," she writes, "the person could 'die well,' taking leave of life in the grace of God. . . . Now it is a sign of status, being modern, to die in a hospital" (1991:354–356). Sadly, this is progress—to die in a distant place and return to one's hometown encased in a coffin, ready for a quick burial.

In the modern hospital, it is hard to know when a patient is dying and harder yet to let him go. "No one person attends to the dying patient," says David Thomasma. "Different services are stacked up like planes at a busy airport, waiting to attend the dying person. . . . There is little possibility to maintain the personal and social ritual of dying" (1991:105). I am reminded of the story of a father and son who faced the father's bout with pancreatic cancer. Both were physicians and the son was also the director of resuscitation research at Columbia University's medical school. The father whispered, "Norman, I have been a surgeon for almost fifty years. . . . In that time, I have seen physicians torture dying patients in vain attempts to prolong life. I have taken care of you for most of your life. Now I must ask for your help. Don't let them abuse me. No surgery. No chemotherapy." The son gave his word and thought he had made this wish for comfort care clear to his father's physicians. But the son's directives fell on deaf ears. As soon as he left, the medical team began performing one procedure after another, including elaborate diagnostic tests and futile surgery, for which Medicare later reimbursed them (Paradis 1994). Tragically, the father was released from suffering only by death, and his family was unnecessarily traumatized for years. The social relationships and personal rituals that are familiar to anthropologists because of our "low-tech" methods of conducting research were patently absent in this typical hospital death. The late Norman Cousins was wise to point out, after his own recovery from a massive heart attack, that the problem is not the technology but the "impersonalization" that accompanies its application. The patient is sent forth to do battle and exposed to endless rounds of mysterious procedures without the necessary psychological supports (1983:145–151).

A more subtle but serious consequence of technological brinkmanship is the deterioration in the quality of our lives that it brings about as the end approaches. It insures that our final years will be characterized by debilities and our final days by pain and suffering. A seeming success is but a temporary reprieve in a downward spiral that terminates in death. "More often, death is the outcome of a long and difficult struggle with a disease that generates first one unpleasant variety of refractory symptoms, then another," says Ronald Koenig. "These impositions diminish and adulterate the quality of day-to-day experience until there is little that can be relished or enjoyed and there is little hope that the balance can be returned even to a tolerable level of comfort" (1980:9). In *Choosing Medical Care in Old Age* (1994) and *Lifelines* (2001), the geriatrician Muriel Gillick drives home an important point: Each debilitating event reduces the person's level of functioning because of his or her dwindling physiological reserve. Each step in the downward decline toward frailty leaves the patient weaker and more dependent. Gillick notes that the organs can work well enough to keep a person going under ordinary circumstances, but a medical crisis can quickly change the picture from slow decline to swift descent. Gillick tends to be more cautious than the general practitioner, because she recognizes that uncertainty is built into the outcome of geriatric patients and that frailty always culminates in death. "Precisely because the frail person often does not have a single uniformly fatal diagnosis," she writes, "families often do not appreciate how tenuous their relative's existence is and fail to prepare for death" (2001: 186). Families must bear in mind that, by saving a patient through technological sleight of hand, they are only postponing the inevitable outcome.

On several occasions, Mother's internist Dr. Risden had reminded me how difficult it was to determine her outcome. I had brought this issue up with him because I never felt confident about her prognosis from one crisis to the next.

"It is hard to know the outcome," he advised. "Your mother is unusual—a very strong woman who's determined to get well. But the elderly don't bounce back like younger people; they have little resilience. They can be coming along fine [in the hospital], and then a minor crisis occurs and completely changes the prognosis. That's the problem with the elderly that sets them apart—they're a constant challenge. The immediate post-op period is the honeymoon, but after a few days complications set in. That's why the postoperative period is so critical for any surgery, not just for hip fractures."

"I guess your job is to save the patient," I said, "and when you're in a hospital setting you don't think about the ethical issues."

"True, but maybe someone should think about setting limits. The lawyers seal the fate of the health-care system, and the control over one's patients has been taken away from the physicians. There are all sorts of legal constraints, and the system obligates you to do everything possible."

How can a frail, chronically impaired patient marshal his or her meager energy? Each person has limits. How far the medical team should go must depend not on its own criteria but on the patient's convictions about what he or she wants out of the final chapter of life. We each have our own threshold for tolerating pain and emotional distress. The patient is often the one to let us know when enough is enough. Kathy's mother, for example, reached her mid-eighties in good health, then seemed to fall apart suddenly.

She bounced back and forth between home and hospital for several months, and finally had to have kidney dialysis. This required thrice-weekly visits to the hospital's outpatient division and constant adjustments in medication.

"How much longer can my mother go on this way?" Kathy asked rhetorically when I called to inquire about her mother.

"I think the only one who can answer that question is your mother," I said. "She will let you know when she's had enough."

Sure enough, Kathy's mother tired of the time-consuming routine after a few months and told her doctor the quality of her life had declined to such a point that it was no longer worth living. She asked to be relieved of the dialysis treatment. The physician explained what would happen if the treatment were terminated, and she courageously—but realistically—refused to back down. Her kidneys failed four days after she rejected the treatment, and she died at home in her daughter's embrace.

Sometimes the patient's spokesman has to be the one to let go. My Uncle Sidney, Aunt Gussie's husband, suffered a massive stroke after enjoying a long life of apparent good health. He was convinced that a scenario like Mother's repeated hospitalizations and Dad's plunging health was not for him. He preferred an abrupt end. "No heroic measures," he told his wife and clearly specified in his living will. Despite his directives, he was put on life support when he was admitted to the ICU. He stayed there until his son, a neurologist, caught a flight to Miami and persuaded the hospital staff to remove the respirator. Uncle Sidney lingered for another day before he passed away. My aunt was at peace with this decision, because she knew Uncle Sidney did not want to stay alive as a helpless invalid.

What Callahan and other ethicists are asking us to remember, and to accept graciously, is the biological inevitability of death. The acceptance of death as part of life can be liberating, says Jerome Groopman (1997:135). Once we erase the illusive boundaries, death will be as natural when it comes as was life when it began. None—not one—of our technological pyrotechnics will alter death's course. But doctors are not supposed to err. Young doctors in particular regard death as a medical failure and are often determined to do "battle" beyond the call of good sense. Their mission is to conquer death. Grown children, too, can be incorrigible. We so push our parents to fend off the enemy that we fail to see death from the perspective of those approaching it. We allow medical advances to come between our dying parent and ourselves and end up defensive rather than supportive.

I refused to face my mother's impending death. I feared it and did my mother a terrible disservice by denying its existence. We talked, but I participated reluctantly. Coming back from the brink once was enough for Mother, who was not suited to the role of martyred survivor. She hated the thought of leaving a life she had embraced with such verve, but she had made her peace with its finite nature. She, and others of her generation, could accept what we are loath to acknowledge simply because members of that generation are so close to the end of their natural life span.

Not everyone has to die an undignified death. Our final passage is not necessarily wrought with thorns and throes. I remember Rose Epstein, who was in her late sixties when my parents met her in New York. For more than twenty years, they watched her grow steadily more infirm. She did not have a specific disease or syndrome; she seemed to be suffering from the cumulative effects of advancing age. She usually stopped by our apartment when Mother returned from work. Mother watched over her like a "mother hen," and when Rose missed a day, Mother checked on her. One week, Rose missed two days. She failed to respond to the bell, so Mother knocked, but Rose still did not answer. Finally, Mother called Rose's daughter, who also had been trying to reach her mother. Rose had been watching television after dinner when she died quietly. I remember feeling shocked at the time. Rose had had no opportunity to say a proper goodbye. But when I compare her death with my mother's protracted dying a quarter century later, I see how fortunate Rose was. She drifted off gently without having to endure any heroic measures to prolong her life. I thought of Rose often during the months I cared for Mother.

Doña Calle, a dear friend, was the matriarch of a huge extended family composed of six sons and daughters, twenty-two grandchildren, and a growing clan of newborn great-grandchildren. She grew up poor in a peasant family on the island of Tenerife. Her young husband was unwilling to share their parents' fate and emigrated to America to seek his fortune. Doña Calle raised the children in his absence and invested his earnings in land and housing. Theirs was the first generation to leave a small stone hovel behind and dwell in decent quarters on the town's main street. Doña Calle outlived her husband by many years and never once removed her black shawl, black kerchief, and black woolen stockings. Although Doña Calle had rheumatic pains and assorted ailments, her hands worked and her eyesight was good. She spent her afternoons embroidering lacy tablecloths in the Canary Island tradition, using reading glasses and a very large needle. She was one of my best informants; we both enjoyed the interviews I conducted while she sat in front of her embroidery frame. I crossed the ocean to attend her ninetieth birthday party, an extraordinary event put together with much fanfare by friends and relatives from all over the island. When I was ready to leave for home, she told me she would not be seeing me again. This was her usual lament, so I hugged her and told her to take care of herself.

"No, no," Doña Calle insisted, smiling sweetly. "I will never see you again. My body is old and tired. This time I mean it."

Sadly, Doña Calle was right. She did not reach her ninety-first birthday. One dreary midwinter day she caught a chill and told her daughter she was too tired to embroider. She then said goodbye to her favorite granddaughter and went to her room to take a nap. She never woke up. Knowing her body was wearing out, she willed herself into a permanent sleep. It was fitting. She died at home in a way that allowed her family to mourn her loss as the culmination of a long, well-lived life.

When I learned that my friend Emmanuel, a physician, had also died at home, I knew he was fortunate to expire among his own things, in his own bed, and accompanied only by his family. Emmanuel was approaching eighty and had suffered from an incurable cancer for nearly ten years. He had endured surgery, chemotherapy, exploratory surgery, and more chemotherapy. Nothing helped. Finally he said, "No more." He told his oncologist he wanted to live his last years as a normal person. He knew his tumor was evolving very slowly and that the chemotherapy would not cure him. He did not feel that a remission was worth it if he again had to cope with the consequences of an aggressive course of treatment. I first met Emmanuel at an international aging conference in Acapulco, where he congratulated me on my presentation on productive aging. He was already quite ill but continued to attend professional meetings, travel, visit museums, and dine out. During his last year of life, he traveled to France, Greece, and Israel and spent many weekends at his farm in upstate New York. He also had time to orchestrate every detail of his death. He gave away his medical textbooks because he thought the task would be intolerable for his wife. He prepared his papers and specified his last desires. He left his son a list of the people he wanted contacted when he died, and that is how I learned about it.

Rose, Doña Calle, and Emmanuel: They knew that time was running out. All three marshaled their physical and emotional resources to confront the end, but each played out distinctive patterns of withdrawing and saying good-bye. They were fortunate to have died at home, unencumbered by life-sustaining medical apparatus. They showed little ambivalence. They were cognizant of life's final event and knew when it was time to leave.

What shall it be—accept or fight? When do we know when to let go? When is enough enough? This is the philosophical dilemma that now occupies the medical profession, ethicists, philosophers, and many more. The subject of how to manage one's last years and one's last illness takes up thousands of pages in the medical annals, but it is yet to be satisfactorily resolved.

CHAPTER SIX

From LovingCare to Victoria Park

"Yes, we have a Medicare bed."

SEPTEMBER 3–SEPTEMBER 19, 1993: 17 DAYS • While Marisa helped Mother settle into her new room at LovingCare and unwrapped her cold dinner, I approached the nurses' station with her medical records and discharge orders from Coral Bay. The nurse's aide seemed amiable, and I cautioned her: "Two things are important. First, my mother's steroid injections. She's coming down from a very high dose and must be closely monitored until she reaches her maintenance level. Second, her Ensure. She's supposed to receive three cans of Ensure Plus daily. You'll notice from the medical chart that my mother weighs about sixty pounds. She must have her liquid nutrients."

"Don't worry; I'll take care of everything," the aide assured me. Then she led me to Mother's room and carried out the usual admissions workup. She asked Mother detailed questions and followed up with a superficial examination of her body. The long diagonal mastectomy scar, now faded and benign-looking, never failed to impress observers that Mother was still around nearly a half-century later. The nursing-home staff were needlessly concerned that Mother would be unable to tolerate an IV needle in her mastectomy arm. "Her arm will not swell," I kept telling them. "My mother had a mastectomy when she was thirty-two years old. Believe me, that's the least of her problems."

My second impression of LovingCare was even less rosy. True, the facility had admitted Mother at the last minute, but it was also filling a Medicare-certified bed. Mother's semiprivate Medicare room was cramped. There was just about enough room for two beds, two nightstands, and a dresser, but not for the wheelchairs, walkers, and other medical gear patients needed. Mother's wizened roommate was childlike and seemed desperately frightened. She probably suffered from some sort of dementia and was crying because she could not open her milk container. I helped her with dinner while Marisa finished serving Mother the warmed-up meal from Coral Bay. Then I put away Mother's few items of clothing and soothed her itching back with body lotion. It was late. I could do nothing more that evening, yet I was reluctant to go. I felt uneasy about leaving Mother without a phone. It would take a few days to install, and by then Mother would be out of LovingCare. Marisa promised to return the next morning so Mother would not be alone. Mother now insisted that a private aide was unnecessary. She would just get in Marisa's way. I told Mother I would be back after lunch with Dad. I had spoken with him on the phone but had not been to see him for two days. I felt neglectful. Because of the nursing-home visits and my attempt to abort Mother's discharge, my poor father was on hold.

The logistics of admitting Mother to LovingCare had exhausted me, and I overslept the next morning. I woke up in a panic at 10:00 A.M. When I called the nurses' station, I was told that Mother was resting comfortably. But when I hung up, Kathy called. "Luisa, I tried to get you all yesterday afternoon," she said. "The Palms called to let me know your father has been wandering around all day in his pajamas."

"Kathy, why didn't they contact me?" I asked.

"They tried to reach you first, and then they called me."

"Kathy, I took three changes of clothing to The Palms the day before yesterday. I know Dad's slacks are not dirty. I know what they do with the stuff. They just roll it in a ball and throw it in the hamper."

"Well, that's what you should expect from The Palms, Luisa. Don't worry about it. I just called to tell you to take over a fresh change of clothing."

But I decided not to take any more clothing to The Palms. Beth, the LPN, was at the nurses' station when I arrived. "Your father is fine. He's waiting for you—and by the way, he's still in his pajamas." I nodded and hurried down the east-wing hallway, walking right into Dad, who was headed toward the nurses' station. He was disheveled: One leg of his pajamas was rolled up, and the other hung down. He had not shaved in the two days since I had last seen him, and he had a sour odor.

"Dad, remember, I told you that Mother was being discharged from the hospital. She's in another nursing home because she didn't want to come back to The Palms. We're going to visit her after lunch, but I can't take you there in this condition."

"Well, let's go home," he said.

"O.K., Dad, but it's lunchtime, so we'll stay for lunch. Let's put on your old clothes, and after lunch we'll go home to shower and change before visiting Mother."

This was going to be a delicate balancing act, trying to stay abreast of Dad's needs and care for him without ignoring Mother. I was annoyed at The Palms's staff for neglecting Dad's physical needs. The rudiments of hygiene seemed to me to be the least I could expect. Dad had always been fastidious about his appearance, and seeing him in this condition irritated me. By the time we got home, Dad was exhausted and needed a nap. It was clear we were not going to make it to Mother's by noon. I was worried about her lunch. However, I could not take Dad to visit Mother looking like a bum. Dad napped in his rattan chair as though he had never been away. Then I took him into my bathroom—the one with a walk-in shower—stripped off the wrinkled clothing, and soaped him down, making sure to wash his ears and fingernails, which had been neglected at The Palms. I combed Dad's heavy eyebrows and thick mustache, powdered him, brushed his teeth, shaved him with an electric razor, and dressed him in a new striped cotton shirt and freshly pressed slacks. Dad was beginning to look like his old self again. His beautiful mustache had been clipped in a grotesque way a few weeks before, and it was finally growing in. By the time I deemed Dad presentable, it was past 3:00 P.M.

We arrived at LovingCare at 4:30, near the dinner hour. Mother was frenetic. "Where have you been?" she asked. "I was so worried about you."

"You're right to be worried, Mother, especially when I told you we would be here at noon. But I had to take care of Dad. Can you imagine—Dad didn't have a stitch of clothing, and we had to start from scratch. So I took him home for a shower and shave."

Mother was amused by my explanation and happy to see Dad, who sat down by her side and took her hand. But her displeasure with LovingCare was impossible to hide. She had not received the

Ensure—not even one can—and she could not swallow the lunch of baked beans and a cut-up hotdog.

"Did you eat anything at all?" I asked.

"I had the milk, but even then I had to wait a long time, because I couldn't open the container," she answered. "They walk in and throw the tray on the table and never ask if you need any help. And they don't wait long enough for you to ask for it. In fact, they don't even bother to glance at you."

"This is ridiculous." I said. "You have to eat, and you must have the Ensure. You can't afford to lose an ounce. You can't miss even one meal."

I went to the nurses' station and asked the aide why my mother had not been given a bland diet, as indicated on her chart.

"She had a bland diet. That's as bland as we get here."

"No, my mother cannot swallow. She needs a pureed diet. Please look at her chart. Before I left yesterday evening, you promised you would bring her the Ensure on schedule, yet she hasn't had one can all day. She should have had three by now. Her condition is extremely delicate, and you must follow the hospital's instructions."

"I'll bring the Ensure in a few minutes."

"No. I want the Ensure now—and with some ice, please."

She looked at me blankly and told me to get the cup and the ice myself from the kitchenette off the nurses' station. I did not mind but wondered how Mother would get her Ensure if I were not there. It was now almost dinnertime, and the Ensure would fill her up just before she had to eat.

When I returned to Mother's room, she chided, "I can't stay here over the weekend. I can't stay here alone. I'll die. There's no attention. I was wet most of the evening and couldn't reach the cord. I couldn't reach the water. It's the usual story: I told them about all these things, but nobody listens. The food is impossible. It doesn't look like anything I've ever eaten before. And they're not very nice. The woman in the next bed has been calling for help all day, and they just ignore her. They run in and out of the room and don't give you the time of day."

I had heard all this before. LovingCare was neither better nor worse than any other place Mother had been in. The lack of attention to the patient's immediate needs and the inaccessibility of the call button and the water pitcher were common enough, but the food issue was another matter entirely. Mother could not afford to skip a meal or miss a serving of Ensure. Her life depended on it.

"What should I do, Mother? Marisa didn't show up. There's no phone, and I was sure she was with you while I went to collect Dad. Shall I get a private aide in for the weekend so you won't be alone? I agree, the situation is unbearable."

"No. I don't want a private aide."

"Mom, didn't we agree on a private aide? Instead of a private room at Victoria Park, you wanted to come here for a few days and have your own aide. Are you worried about the cost? It's only for the weekend, and your rider will cover most of the expense. That's why you have the rider, for occasions like this. I don't think you've ever used the rider."

"Let me think about it, darling."

"O.K. We'll work something out. Maybe I'll call Victoria Park in the morning and see if I can get you a private room just for the weekend. I think we made a mistake by coming here. I'm sure you'll get much better care there. You can't afford to wait through the weekend under these circumstances."

By now, Mother's roommate had received her dinner tray, but Mother's had not arrived. Outside her room, I could hear the dinner cart being pushed up and down the corridor. I looked out. All the trays had been distributed except Mother's.

I went back to the nurses' station to advise the staff that my mother's tray had not appeared. I was assured that the tray would be sent in immediately. Fifteen minutes went by, and I presented myself at the nurses' station for the third time. "Is there a problem with my mother's dinner?" I asked. "The trays are already being collected, but my mother never received her dinner."

"Well, your mother is on a pureed diet, and we don't have any pureed food here."

"Are you telling me you have no provisions for a pureed dinner? This is a nursing facility, is it not? Please go to the kitchen and ask them to blend whatever was on the menu."

The nurse's aide disappeared and returned a few minutes later to tell me that the only pureed dinner the facility could provide was a scoop of cottage cheese. The kitchen was closed for the night, and hot meals could no longer be prepared. I took the cottage-cheese platter to Mother's room and told her I would go for take-out. Dad was growing restless and did not want to sit any longer. Yet we could not leave until the food issue was resolved.

On the way to LovingCare, I had noticed a Chinese restaurant and decided to bring back dinner for three. Dad had been pacing up and down the corridor, but now he disappeared. I went to retrieve him and saw that he had turned the corner and was shuffling down the hallway toward the room.

"Dad, come back with me to Mother's room. I'm going out for Chinese, and I want you to stay with Mother until I return."

"I'll come with you."

"No, Dad. It's important for you to stay with Mother. Mother needs you."

Dad sat down again at Mother's side, obviously more restless than before. He began unlacing his shoes and pulling them off his feet. One shoe fell to the floor, and he started tugging on the sock to take it off, as well. "No, Dad, put your shoe back on. It's not time for bed yet."

"Well, are we ready to go?" he asked.

"We'll go after dinner, Dad. Remember, I'm going out for Chinese, and we'll go home after dinner."

I was in a sweat as I walked out of LovingCare. Dad's actions were bizarre, and Mother could not stay there. The combination was intolerable. I crossed the busy intersection and walked across a fake moat into the Chinese restaurant. The place was crowded; I had forgotten it was Saturday evening. The pleasant din typical of large Chinese restaurants, the pungent cooking odors—the normality of the scene—was jolting. My eyes welled with tears. How sorry I felt for myself and for my parents. Just a few months earlier, we had been just like the people in this crowd. We had dined at a similar Chinese restaurant in a most unremarkable way, and I had taken that dinner for granted. It was unthinkable that that would be the last time. I had to wait for the food and wandered into a bookstore that was going out of business. My eye immediately fell on a bargain in the family section: *Taking Care of Your Aging Family Members.* I grabbed the book and rushed back to pick up my order.

Dad was not in the room when I returned, and Mother claimed he had gone for a walk. In the hallway I found Dad being escorted back to the room by one of the aides.

"You cannot allow your father out of the room," she said. "He's been wandering up and down the hall, into the other rooms, and annoying the patients. They don't like that."

"Frankly, my father has every right to walk up and down the hallway. He's not bothering anybody, and as a matter of fact, you have plenty of your own patients who wander in and out of the rooms, annoying others. One comes into my mother's room every few minutes, and I don't see any staff members escorting her out. My father probably couldn't find my mother's room. All you had to do was walk him back without making such a fuss."

"We have enough work with our own patients. I can't worry about your father."

"You don't worry about my mother, either, and she's a patient here. You even forgot to bring her dinner. And now, if you'll excuse me, I went out to buy dinner and don't want it to get cold."

We were all pleased with the Chinese meal. I settled Dad into the chair once again and set the tray on his lap. I had ordered won-ton soup for Mother and added several teaspoons of rice, creating a nutritious if unorthodox meal in a nursing-home facility. I went to Mother's bathroom to dispose of the paper containers, and when I returned, Dad was gone again. He was pushing the food cart, filled with discarded trays, up and down the corridor. Dad had a pleasant expression on his face and ignored my entreaties to return to the room. I grabbed his hand, but he pulled away, determined to fulfill his mission.

"Dad, come back to Mother's room. We're leaving, and it's time for you to say goodbye to Mother. Come now, before the nurse's aide sees you out here again."

Dad followed me reluctantly. I had never seen him like this before—restless, bored, wandering aimlessly, oblivious to his own wife. I imagined that it was a manifestation of "sundowner's syndrome," which I had learned about while reading up on dementia. The syndrome is well named: When the sun goes down, the sufferer's personality changes, and he acts in ways that are not only inappropriate but also unlike his usual behavior.

Maybe Dad was just tired or confused by Mother's move. He was ready to leave.

Mother was amused. "I see Dad doesn't want to be with me," she teased.

"We have to leave, Mother. I have to get Dad back to The Palms and into bed. I think all these changes are a strain for him. Truly, I can take care of you, and I can take care of Dad, but both of you together is a real challenge."

Mother smiled. "Go! Take Dad back to The Palms. And then go home and get some rest. I'll see you in the morning."

"Don't worry, by tomorrow I'll find a solution to the Loving-Care situation," I said. "I'll work it out somehow."

I told Mother I would stop at Victoria Park the next morning and come directly to LovingCare without Dad. I was determined to get her out of there, no matter what.

Traffic was light on Sunday morning, and I arrived at Victoria Park by 9:00. The admissions office was closed over the Labor Day weekend, but the receptionist told me to wait in the nursing director's office. If Victoria Park would not take Mother, I thought, I would take her home for a few days. This would not be easy without a wheelchair and hospital equipment, but if I could not manage alone, Marisa would help me. We were both more practiced now, and I was confident we would be able to care for my frail mother.

The head nurse, Diane, arrived. She had a dour expression and a serious demeanor. I explained that my mother had been discharged from Coral Bay earlier than I had expected and was waiting for a Medicare bed at Victoria Park. In the meantime, she was in a Medicare bed at LovingCare. I tried to remain calm as I recapitulated the events of the past thirty-six hours at LovingCare. I explained why my mother's condition was so delicate.

"This is a holiday weekend, and we normally don't admit patients under these circumstances," Diane said after listening to my improbable story.

"I understand." My heart was racing. "But this is an emergency. I'm asking you to admit my mother into a private room. We should have done this in the first place, but she was adamant about waiting for a Medicare bed. Now I realize that we made a terrible mistake, one that could have disastrous consequences. I'm asking you to make an exception, because my mother will not survive the weekend there. As a matter of fact, if you can't admit her now, I'm taking her home. She can't stay at LovingCare another minute. Can you imagine—a skilled nursing facility where they forget to feed you and then give you the runaround when you remind them."

"I'll be back in a few minutes," she said. "I don't even know if a private room is available."

When Diane returned, her expression was hard to decipher. "We have decided to admit your mother to the private unit. I don't know when a Medicare bed will become available—probably Tuesday. We'll know on Monday after the first discharges. As soon as a bed becomes available, we'll move your mother. How long will it take you to bring her?"

"About two hours," I answered. "I'm going directly to Loving-Care to pick her up."

"Don't forget to bring your mother's medical records and her discharge sheet. We'll need them to admit her."

"I took them to LovingCare with her and hope I don't have any problem retrieving them."

"If you have a problem, you must at least bring the discharge sheet with the medication instructions."

"O.K. If I can't obtain her records, I'll pick them up on Monday directly from the medical-records department at Coral Bay. And, thank you. I can't tell you how grateful I am. I'm so relieved."

"And another matter," she continued. "Don't forget to bring your checkbook. We'll need a deposit of $1,000 before admitting your mother to a private room."

"As a matter of fact, I have my checkbook with me."

"How are you going to bring your mother?"

"I'll bring her over in our car. I'm sure I can manage without special transportation."

"Fine, we'll be waiting for you."

I stopped at The Palms before heading for LovingCare and was pleasantly surprised to find Marisa there, shaving Dad. He was always happy when Marisa was around. She pampered him and knew exactly what he liked. I asked her to stay with Dad for a few hours, because I would probably be busy most of the day with Mother's transfer.

"Marisa, I'm so glad you're here," I said. "It was sweet of you to check on Dad. I don't want to sound like I'm complaining—I just want to know what happened to you yesterday."

"I couldn't come yesterday, I went to the ballgame. Colombia was playing."

"Well, Mother waited for you all day, and I arrived late because there were problems with Dad. You have every right to go to the game, but don't tell Mother you'll be in to see her unless you're sure you can make it. She was very disappointed. You have to keep your word with the elderly. It's very important."

Marisa looked abashed. "I hadn't thought of it that way, Señora Luisa. I promise to handle this differently from now on."

"Thanks, Marisa. I know that if there were a phone, you would have called Mother."

She nodded. I had to be careful with Marisa. She was attuned to the nuances of my voice, which tended to reflect my general state of disenchantment not with her, by any means, but with the situation in which we were all captive participants. Marisa and I had made our peace, and I was not about to jeopardize it.

"Dad," I said, "I'm moving Mother to a better place and won't be back to see you until later this evening. Do you think you can manage?"

"Yes, I'm fine. Don't worry about me. But why are you moving Mother? Where is Mother? In Coral Bay?"

"Dad, Mother was discharged to a nursing home called Loving-Care. Remember? Yesterday we visited her there, and we had Chinese food together in her room."

"If you say so. I don't remember."

"Dad, we had Chinese take-out because they forgot to bring Mother's dinner. Imagine if they forgot to feed you here at The Palms."

"That's not good," he said.

"Right. So I'm moving Mother to Victoria Park, a nursing home in Boca Raton, where she'll get the proper attention. She needs skilled nursing care, and she's not going to get that at The Palms, either."

"So why am I here?"

"You're here because you were keeping Mother company when she was here. As soon as Mother's settled at Victoria Park, you'll move there with her or come home."

"I'll come with you now."

"No, Dad. You stay here with Marisa. Once Mother is settled in, we'll go over together."

Mother looked serene when I arrived at LovingCare. She was dressed in her sweatsuit and was seated in a wheelchair. Maybe the move was not necessary after all, I thought briefly. But I could not back out. The arrangements had been made, and I had already written a check.

"Well, how's it going ?" I asked after kissing Mother. "I see from your face it could not have been so bad this morning."

She looked up at me inquisitively and said, "They came for us last night."

"Who came for you?"

"They did; the nuns! They came for Dad and me. They were lined up in a row like little Indians and asked, 'Who is going to go first—you or your husband?'"

My heart pounded. "Mother, what do you mean?"

"They came to take us to the land of the dead. The holy angels came for our souls. They were whispering among themselves, 'This one is going to die; she won't last the night—she hasn't eaten and weighs only sixty-five pounds. A person who weighs that little is finished, can't possibly survive.'"

"But, Mother, you're here, talking to me. You're alive. Nobody came for you last night. And Dad is at The Palms this very minute with Marisa."

"I saw the nuns, and I'm ready."

"And what did you tell them—you or Dad?"

Mother looked at me without responding. She was clearly at peace with herself. The frenetic unhappiness of the evening before had vanished.

"Mother, you must have had a dream, or maybe you were half-awake. The nuns in white—they must have been the nurses' aides. And maybe they were commenting about your weight. They probably thought you were asleep. How stupid of them."

I could see she was not convinced. It was not like Mother to have such a dream or a vision. She must have been reacting to the meal incident.

"Mother, I've just come from Victoria Park, and the arrangements are all made. I'm taking you there right now."

"Are you sure? How are we going to pay for it?"

"It's only for a few days, and remember, I'm treating you. It's not much more expensive than The Palms. You need to be pampered a little bit, and you'll get the attention you need."

"What about Dad?"

"Dad can go into the assisted-living wing upstairs. He won't be able to share your room, because the Medicare unit is separate. Anyway, it's probably best for you to have separate quarters. Dad feels frustrated when he can't help you, and you need your rest. Dad can move in right after the Labor Day weekend. Karen, the marketing director, said that admitting him will not be a problem. Victoria Park has space available in assisted living right now."

I explained to Mother that I had to stop at the nurses' station before we could leave. I approached the desk with trepidation. I had not seen these staff members before. "I just wanted to let you know that my mother will be leaving in a few minutes. Are there any special procedures that have to be followed?"

"Your mother is leaving? But she just got here. She can't leave. Why does your mother want to leave? Is there a problem? Doesn't your mother like it here?"

Why go into the whole story? I thought. "No, my mother wants to go home. She's been hospitalized for a long time and wants to be at home with her family. My father's health is delicate, and he can't make the long trip as frequently as he would like."

"Well, your mother can't leave. She has to be discharged by the doctor, and the doctor is not on call today."

"I understand that it's a holiday, but you can page the doctor. I am definitely taking my mother home in a few minutes."

"No, you'll have to speak to the doctor first. I'll call him now."

But the doctor was not at home and could not be paged. I dreaded to think what would happen in a real emergency. The aides did not know what to do; they obviously did not have a precedent to follow. "Listen," I said. "I will take responsibility for my mother's departure. She's my mother, and furthermore she's leaving of her own free will. There's no way you can detain us. This is not a prison. I do need her medical records, though."

"No, we can't do that. The medical records are part of her chart and have to stay here."

"Can you photocopy them?"

"No, we can't. The office is closed."

"Then I must have the discharge sheet from Coral Bay. You really don't need that anymore."

The aides gave me the discharge sheet, and in return I had to write and sign a release taking all responsibility for my mother and absolving LovingCare of any eventual medical complications. It was inconceivable that anything bad would happen to Mother between LovingCare and Victoria Park. Nothing bad ever happened when she was with me. I prepared her things. She had very little, because I had taken enough only for the weekend. I left the paraphernalia that accumulates during institutional stays—the cup, water pitcher, grooming supplies, rinsing tray and washbasin, all paid for by Medicare—behind. We already had a large collection at home in assorted colors, and she would undoubtedly receive another new set at Victoria Park. I wheeled Mother to the car. Nobody offered to help us or escort us out. In fact, no one bothered to look up as we rolled past the nurses' station, in full view of the aides. The private guard at the front door, unaware of the drama inside, offered to help me transfer Mother to the car. I declined but asked him to take the wheelchair, the nursing home's property, back inside. I knew how to transfer Mother, thanks to our therapy sessions. I propped her head and sides with pillows and placed another one under her feet.

What a relief! I never imagined I would have to kidnap my own mother. The tension of my visit to Victoria Park and altercation with the LovingCare staff was draining, but what a feeling of liberation to be out of there. What frightened me most about LovingCare, I think, was the passivity of its patients. They were clearly very old, very sick, or both. Many had Alzheimer's disease and wandered, confused, up and down the hallways. For example, the woman across the hall appeared to be in the last throes of Alzheimer's. She was bedridden, and at mealtime an aide had prodded her roughly, propped her up, and poured a can of Ensure Plus down her throat with a funnel. It upset me to see that the last vestiges of this woman's dignity had been stripped away and she did not even know it. How can people in that condition demand to be treated with the respect they deserve? All it takes is one small accident, one split-second incident, to destroy one's capacity to function autonomously. The nursing home did the rest. The standardization at LovingCare, a national chain, also turned me off. The facility had no personality and no individuality, and the rooms were too small to squeeze in two patients with their assorted gear. The food was nutritionally inadequate, and the staff showed no compassion or real concern about meeting patients' needs. The aides certainly could not care less, and I had not seen a single registered nurse while Mother was there.

I looked at Mother. The normality of our momentary situation was excruciating. She and I were finally sitting side by side in the family car, with no intrusions or hospital gear to disturb us. I felt a yearning for past times, normal occasions. Why don't we go shopping? I thought. To hell with Victoria Park and the past five months. Only six months earlier, Mother had accompanied me to buy a washer–dryer to ship to Venezuela. Her posture and balance had been fine. In fact, she had walked more energetically than Dad, who had no muscle condition to impede him. I snapped out of my reverie. Mother was in a sweat and sliding down the seat toward the floor. I pulled onto the grass shoulder and went to her side of the car. Her heavy sweatsuit was drenched despite the air conditioning, and she had no control over her body's relentless march downward.

I moved into the back seat and put my arms under Mother's shoulders, gently pulling her back from the edge. "Are you all right, Mother? Are you sure you can continue?"

"Yes, go on. I'm a little short of breath, but let's go on."

"It's probably from nerves, from all the excitement of leaving. You'll feel better as soon as you're settled in."

When we arrived at Victoria Park, I left Mother in the car for a few minutes while I went to the reception area. I ran back out, fearful that Mother had slid to the floor in my absence. Within a few minutes, two smiling registered nurses, immaculately

groomed and wearing jaunty starched caps, came to greet Mother
and help her into a wheelchair.

"Welcome to Victoria Park, Mrs. Margolies. We've been waiting for you," a nurse said. "Why don't we go upstairs while your
daughter parks the car and brings up your things?" Then one of
the nurses looked at me. "Do you need any help?"

Mother and I exchanged glances. It was the first time in months
that she had been greeted graciously and treated like a real person, not just a sick body whose mind might be dulled and unresponsive. By the time I got upstairs, Mother was resting on top
of the bed. The nurse explained that it was the practice for all
patients to be dressed during the day. Those who needed to rest
did so on top of the covers, fully clothed. Today was an exception, though, because of Mother's trip, and I retrieved her pajamas from her overnight bag. As the nurse removed Mother's
drenched sweatsuit, I thought about the contrast between Victoria Park and the other nursing facilities I had visited.

● ● ●

If I had to rank Victoria Park as a skilled nursing facility on a scale
from one to ten, I would give it a ten for effort. If one needed to
be placed in a nursing home, this was the ideal choice. First, Victoria Park was beautiful—a two-story, sprawling, Mediterranean-
style building set amid several acres of ponds, lawns, and mature
oak trees. It had a spacious and tastefully furnished reception
area. One moved from the reception area directly into the atrium,
a two-story common area for patients that served as the nerve
center for the entire facility.

Originally, I viewed the atrium as a frivolous addition to a
nursing-home environment, perhaps because I was uncertain of
Mother's outcome. She certainly did not need an ice-cream parlor, for instance. She was too sick for such amenities. Now I realized that the atrium was cleverly contrived. It not only looked
out on a pleasant terrace with umbrella tables, chairs, and potted plants; it was designed so that everyone had to pass through
it on the way to the other wings. The atrium was furnished simply with park benches situated strategically to avoid obstructing
the traffic. The activities room, beauty salon, barber shop, den-
tist's office, ice-cream parlor, "pub," dining room, and physical-,

occupational-, and speech-therapy rooms led off from the atrium. All communities, no matter how artificial, need a common space in which their members can come together and partake in shared ritual activities. Patients who were well enough spent time in the atrium every day; if they could not walk there themselves, they were wheeled in or escorted by their nurses' aides. Patients in physical therapy were encouraged to walk the length of the atrium with their walkers, guided by their therapists, in full view of a captive audience. Naturally, one would tend to do one's best. The ice-cream parlor opened in the late afternoon during the heaviest period of visiting. People were drawn to the atrium. It allowed the patients to measure their progress vis-à-vis their fellow patients; it served the same function for their visitors, allowing them to view the spectrum of handicaps and infirmities. The atrium also offered residents and visitors freshly popped fat-free popcorn every afternoon—frivolous, perhaps, but surprisingly pleasant.

The consistent level of professionalism in the medical wings also impressed me. Victoria Park's 140 residents were separated into four divisions, each offering different types of care. Hampton housed long-term residents with Alzheimer's disease and other types of dementia; Windsor, on the floor above, was an adult congregate, or assisted-living, unit for people who required minimal help; and Essex and Savoy were for people who needed skilled nursing care, the former for private patients and the latter for Medicare patients. Savoy not only had beds for patients whose short-term stays bridged the gap between the hospital and home, but it was also in the process of installing an acute-care unit.

I liked the atmosphere in the skilled-nursing-care wings. Victoria Park was making a real effort to provide excellent care. I found courteous and helpful registered nurses at the nurses' stations. The wide hallways were carpeted and decorated tastefully. Victoria Park never smelled bad; patients did not have to shout for help. My impression was that most of the patients in the skilled-nursing-care wings were there for short-term stays and knew it. They were separated from the long-term patients, who required qualitatively different types of care. Grouping together the patients who required skilled nursing made it possible to serve them effectively, and the patients were more optimistic about their chances when they were placed with others in similar circumstances.

What set Victoria Park apart from facilities such as The Palms and LovingCare was the matter of ownership. Most nursing homes in South Florida are owned by corporate entities that are loosely known as the "nursing-home industry." Victoria Park, by contrast, was owned by Andy Moller, whose father, Edward Moller, opened the first Victoria Park in Chicago in the mid-1950s, when nursing homes were not particularly fashionable. Edward Moller went on to operate two more Victoria Parks in the Chicago area and was joined by his son in the early 1970s. In 1982, Andy Moller started the Victoria Park in Boca Raton. His daily presence and hands-on style seem to have enabled the facility to achieve exceptional levels of care.

Mother was settled comfortably on top of the bed during the long admissions procedure. The contrast with LovingCare was palpable. We were in a beautifully appointed private room, not unlike a luxurious hotel suite. I sank gratefully into a divinely soft sofa near a window framed by palm fronds while Mother's nurse took her medical history. A host of questions, another examination of Mother's body to detect physical vestiges of old medical procedures—the process was tedious but tempered by the nurse's good-natured approach. She photographed Mother with a Polaroid camera and took her vital signs. Finally we were finished. "Is there anything you need immediately?" the nurse asked.

"No," Mother said.

"Yes," I interjected. "My mother needs a respiratory therapist. She's still breathless and paler than normal."

"I'll send one up immediately. Dinner will be ready shortly." The nurse turned to me and continued. "Why don't you keep your mother company and stay for dinner?"

"No, but thank you. I'll keep my mother company, but I'll skip the dinner," I answered, recalling the many institutional meals I had endured for Mother's sake.

"Please, be our guest. We would like you to stay for dinner. I'll bring you the menu."

So I stayed and was pleasantly surprised by the tasty meal. Mother's food arrived at the proper consistency, and she was able to eat on her own. We were alone at last. A chest X-ray had been taken, and the respiratory therapist had installed a portable oxygen tank by Mother's bedside. Her respiration was beginning to normalize. For now, no more medical procedures. It was the Labor Day weekend, and there was a lull in the normal rhythm of activities. We dined together, chatted quietly, and shared a sense of peace.

On Tuesday, Mother called me early.

"Are you all right, Mom? Why are you calling so early?" I asked warily.

"I'm fine, darling. Happy Birthday!"

"I can't believe you remembered," I said. "I almost forgot about it myself, to be honest. I'll be there soon."

When I arrived, I could not find Mother. She had already been moved to a Medicare room below her private one. Fortunately, she still had a large room to herself, but this floor bustled in a way that the private wing had not. As I bent over to kiss Mother, she said, "I'm so sorry I couldn't give you a card. Go home and pick out the card from my drawer. I bought it several months ago."

"Don't be silly, Mother. I don't need a card. You've already given me the best present by calling me this morning."

"You know what my present is: I'm still alive and hanging in."

"Mother, I know you would never leave me on my birthday. Next year, I expect you to take me out for lunch at an Italian restaurant."

Mother smiled at the thought. Today, however, she had appointments with the dietitian and the therapist and would be visited by the attentive Karen, all in the same morning. The dietitian worked out a high-protein, high-carbohydrate diet, supplemented by several cans of Ensure, to help Mother gain weight without increasing her fat intake. The therapist devised a plan intended to have Mother walking again within the month, and Karen served as a general emissary to advise Mother of her resident rights and coordinate her needs vis-à-vis the available services. She had done her job well. A beautiful bouquet of flowers was waiting for Mother when she arrived in her Medicare room.

Later, Karen intercepted me as I walked through the lobby toward the atrium. "Luisa," she called, "I've finally had the chance to chat with your Mother. Now I understand what you told me about her. She's absolutely delightful. But I realize that your mother is a very sick woman. She's so fragile, she reminds me of a little bird."

I felt the same way. Mother reminded me of an injured wren that was trying as hard as it could to fly again. "I know what you mean, Karen. Mother's so petite and delicate, I thought of that analogy myself."

"I told your Mother that she must eat," Karen continued, "that it's very important for her to eat so she can recover soon. Your Mother was in the middle of lunch when I entered her room, and she seemed determined to finish, even though she was eating so slowly. 'Yes,' she responded, 'my daughter said I must eat to live. I don't have much of an appetite, but I'm going to force myself to eat to get well.'"

"I'm afraid I've badgered my mother about the meals," I said, "but I'm trying to push her to eat on her own. I know she doesn't enjoy eating, but she knows she must eat to stay alive."

"Well, Luisa, I want you to know we'll do everything possible to help your mother get well. We're going to try as hard as your mother is trying."

The grown son of another Medicare patient walked by and turned to greet us. "That guy is really something," Karen said. "He's been here with his father constantly. I see so many men around here like him. Tell me, does your mother have an adoring son, as well?"

I did not know quite how to answer. "Well, let's put it this way," I said. "In our family, I'm the adoring child. My mother has an adoring daughter. The only adoring sons I know are the Latin American ones back in Venezuela."

Now the silence was a bit awkward, but Karen continued. "Your mother must have been older when she had you. You're too young to be dealing with something like this." Then she told me the story of losing her mother suddenly. Karen was in her mid-twenties when her mother died, and twenty years later she still had not gotten over it.

"I'm just young-looking for my age," I told her. "It's hard to appreciate my mother's beauty because she's so ill. She was a natural beauty."

"I understand," Karen said. "I feel for you and your mother. Please remember that you can come to me at any time with any problem. I'm not just saying that to be polite. I really mean it."

"Thank you, Karen. I know you do."

Although Victoria Park handled most bureaucratic matters efficiently, there were problems that seemed inherent in any nursing-home environment. The main one concerned the aides, who sometimes seemed insensitive to their patients' distress. Most of the nurse's aides had come from Haiti, and their English was passable, at best. An enormous cultural rift separated them from their white, middle-class patients. Most patients were too ill to try to bridge this cultural gap, so ultimately it was up to the aides to change. Instead of going over their heads to the administration, Marisa and I decided to take up the matter directly with Mother's assigned aides. We explained that her body ached and she had to be handled gently. Mother had been moved so roughly during her transfer from the bed to her wheelchair that she developed decubitus ulcers on her ankles. Did they feel up to the task? I asked. If not, we would request a change of aides, a step I knew would reflect badly on them. I was always watchful. I observed every interaction between Mother and her aides. I also asked Mother to be as pleasant as possible, no matter how bad she felt, because the quality of the aides' hands-on care would improve dramatically. Mother's new roommate had another approach. She was a robust woman in fairly good health who was recovering from a hip fracture, and she barked at her aides, thoroughly intimidating them.

"Nobody will tell me what to do here," the roommate said. "They're here to help us recover, not to order us around."

Delicate Mother, of course, could not behave that way. We had to appeal directly to the aides' sense of humanity.

• • •

Now that Mother was settled in, we had to deal with Dad, who was still at The Palms. I begged Marisa to return so Dad could go home to a person we all trusted. I would not bring another stranger into the house, and I could not stay indefinitely. Graz had been discharged from the hospital in Caracas and probably would need a few weeks of bed rest. But Marisa, who was living with her boyfriend, refused. Mother encouraged Marisa to stay with the fellow and even offered her a cocktail dress and a zircon "diamond" ring so she would be prepared for a marriage ceremony at any time. Actually, Mother and Marisa worked out their own solution. Marisa drove to Boca Raton every day and helped Mother and Dad, returning in the evening to her boyfriend's house in Pompano Beach. When I left, Marisa began using the family car.

I moved Dad into the assisted-living wing of Victoria Park two days after Mother moved to the Medicare floor. I had checked Dad out of The Palms in less than five minutes and stopped by the nurses' station to pick up his discharge form and the remaining supply of the month's medications. Dad's practical nurse came to say goodbye and wished him luck. "Where are you going, Albert?" Beth asked. "We're going to miss you here."

"I'm going to be with my wife."

"Well, say hello to June for us. We hope she gets better real soon."

I thanked Beth for her attention to my parents. As much as I disliked The Palms, I could not dislike her. "We're not all bad here," she said. "I try to do my work as well as I can, and I was genuinely concerned about your parents."

I drove Dad directly to Victoria Park. I left him with Mother and went through the routine of settling him in. At home I had put a week's change of shirts and slacks on plastic hangers and stored his personal belongings in plastic containers. I wanted everything neatly arranged so it could be packed or unpacked in a few minutes. I put Dad's trusty clock radio and a photograph of him and Mother on their fiftieth anniversary by the bed. I placed his glasses in the top drawer alongside various issues of the large-print edition of Reader's Digest, writing tablets, and several well-sharpened pencils. Then I stored his favorite snacks: one container of raisins and walnuts, another with chocolate kisses, and a large canister of cookies I had baked using one of Mother's recipes. I put five sets of underwear in the dresser, and, moving his roommate's things off Dad's side, placed a box of tissues and a basket of fruit on top. I also cleared a space for Dad in the bathroom and set out his lotions, combs, cup, and tooth gear in a neat row. The room looked very cozy. I was also satisfied that, while Dad had everything he needed to be comfortable, I could pack him up and take him home instantly if I had to.

Dad had problems with assisted living, however. The staff was as kind and considerate as could be, having been informed of Mother's presence downstairs and the reason Dad had come to Victoria Park. But Dad did not get along with his roommate. He treated him as part of the room's furnishings. At the same time, the roommate felt that his territory had been violated. Like the fastidious Felix in the movie *The Odd Couple,* he griped about Dad's behavior. After Dad's first night at Victoria Park, his roommate complained, "You know, your father kept me up all night."

"I'm so sorry to hear that," I said. "What happened?"

"He kept getting up to go to the bathroom and kept flushing the toilet. Then he forgot to turn off the bathroom light."

"I can see where that can become a problem. My father is not used to having a roommate. The only person he's ever lived with is my mother, and now she's in the acute nursing division downstairs."

I knew there was no point in discussing the situation with Dad. He was oblivious of his roommate, even though they ate meals together in the small dining room down the hall. Dad's roommate had lost a leg to diabetes and was confined to a wheelchair, but he appeared to be in fairly stable health otherwise. The room had a pungent odor of stale urine, and papers and clothing were scattered carelessly around. This did not bother Dad, but it bothered me. I asked Karen what could be done about the smell, and she immediately sent someone to clean the rug. At the same time, she must have received news of Dad's roommate's unhappiness, because after a few days Dad was quietly moved to a private room.

"We had the space," Karen said, "and I thought this would be the best solution, as they were not working out together. And, of course, we will not be charging you extra for the private room." She continued, "By the way, your father has been wandering into other people's rooms."

"I guess he's having difficulty finding his way back to his own room. All the doors look alike. Maybe I should put his photograph on his door."

"I think your father should move downstairs to the Alzheimer's wing, Luisa. He'll get more attention there. He's really lost upstairs and seems to be disoriented without your mother."

"No, I don't want that. My Dad is depressed and upset by my mother's condition. If you move him downstairs, his behavior will decline to the level there. He doesn't have Alzheimer's disease."

"True, but we don't want him to wander around aimlessly. Why don't we take your father downstairs during the day for activities, and we'll escort him back and forth to your mother's room, as well."

"I suppose that's O.K.," I said. Karen was a problem solver, and the matter was resolved.

We settled into a routine of sorts. Marisa and I spent the day at Victoria Park, dividing our time between Mother and Dad. I picked Marisa up in the morning, and we drove to Boca Raton together. She went straight to Dad's room to make sure he was properly bathed, dressed, and shaved, and I headed to Mother's. I usually helped her with lunch, then went upstairs to retrieve Dad, taking him to Mother's room for part of the afternoon. Then we switched positions: Marisa helped Mother while I took Dad for a walk on the grounds. Then I escorted him to the main dining room, where we shared an early dinner, then accompanied him upstairs, where I stayed until his bedtime. The staff served tasty evening snacks, and Dad enjoyed a banana, yogurt, and tea before stopping at the desk to kibitz with the night staff, who, as at The Palms, took an instant liking to him.

I often wondered why Dad was so talkative with the staff when he had almost nothing to say to his fellow residents. Silence reigned around the dining-room table in the assisted-living wing. Each diner stared at his plate, immersed in his own world, and no one initiated conversation. When I tried to strike up conversations with Dad's tablemates, they did respond but immediately lapsed into awkward silence. Timothy Diamond, the sociologist who worked as a nurse's aide to write *Making Gray Gold: Narratives of Nursing Home Care* (1992), says that the strange silence during meals is due to the enormous importance of eating, the big event of the day. But I am inclined to believe that the silence is caused by a sense of abandonment among many of the residents. In Dad's wing, there were just as many men as women, if not more, an unusual circumstance in a nursing-home setting, where women who have outlived their husbands predominate. The men I spoke with said they had no one to take care of them or no one who cared enough to care for them. When I explained that Dad was there to accompany his wife, their faces lit up with sympathy, but after briefly commiserating they fell back into silence. Dad also rejected associations with the Alzheimer's patients downstairs. "That woman is crazy; get me away from her," he said when I asked him about a youthful-looking Alzheimer's patient. Yet Dad was animated, almost jovial, with the nurses he liked and hung around the nurses' station to chat. After I tucked Dad in, I returned to Mother, who, thanks to Marisa's ministrations, was freshly creamed and powdered and resting comfortably in bed. We chatted at length—Mother was not an early-to-bedder—and I left reluctantly. I hated to leave Mother, but it was late. I dropped Marisa off at her boyfriend's house and usually stopped at the supermarket or drugstore on my way home.

One evening, as I quickly cruised the market's aisles, I ran into Dr. Klein, the rheumatologist at Coral Bay who had administered the massive dose of prednisone that saved Mother's life.

"How is your Mother coming along?" he asked, genuinely interested.

Dr. Klein was accompanied by his wife, and I replied to both of them, "Well, you won't believe it, but Mother is coming along fairly well. I'm hoping for the best."

"Don't forget to keep me posted," he said. "Your mother is a seriously ill person, and I hope everything works out."

I thanked him. He was a courageous doctor who had spoken frankly without being offensive.

Despite my determination not to overload Mother with impulsive purchases, I found myself buying compulsively at the drugstore while Mother was at Victoria Park. I could not contain myself when it came to pharmaceuticals. Mother needed medicated lip ointment, baby wipes with aloe, witch hazel pads with aloe, tissues with aloe, and mint-flavored waxed dental floss. I bought moisturizing soap bars and gentle cleanser for her skin so she would have a choice. Mother's parched skin soaked up creams, so I bought another moisturizing hand and body lotion.

I completed my selection with a pack of M&Ms and a large bag of Sunkist Fruit Gems to whet her appetite. To keep all the items neatly stored, I bought a bright blue vinyl organizer with zippered pockets that could sit sturdily on her night table. After making my final selection, I was ready to drive home.

• • •

Dr. Dawson, Mother's attending physician at Victoria Park, evaluated her situation and considered her potential for rehabilitation to be good. "Patient has a leg discrepancy with L greater than R by approximately 3/4 inch," he noted in her medical chart. "Estimate 3–4 weeks of progressively active remobilization treatment program for cooperative, alert and motivated, but now extremely weakened 79-year-old woman. Today, Mrs. Margolies is extremely frail and weak; she is utilizing continuous O_2 and is coughing frequently, producing large quantities of phlegm."

I had spoken with Dr. Dawson about Mother's cough. Although she had entered Victoria Park without a cough, within a day of her first shower Mother developed a dry hack. I was concerned about a recurrence of the bronchitis, but Dr. Dawson assured me he would prescribe antibiotics, if necessary.

On September 7, my birthday, Mother's chest X-ray revealed "congestive heart failure, with left pleural effusion." Mother was probably having a flare of her underlying condition, but each new physician interpreted the pleural effusions as congestive heart failure. She was relying more and more on the oxygen tube at Victoria Park, although she claimed she really did not need it. I wish I had seen the report while Mother was at Victoria Park. I learned about it much later and was unaware that she was again suffering from pleural effusions.

Another urgent medical matter intervened that relegated the cough to the background. One morning I found Mother uncharacteristically agitated. "I'm very upset," she said. "I want you to know they're prescribing digitalis again. They said it would help my heart work more efficiently."

"What's wrong with that, Mother?"

"That's the medication that gave me all the trouble at Sacred Heart. I'm afraid I'm going to have a problem again."

Now I was upset. "Don't take any more, Mother. I'll call Dr. Dawson immediately. I don't understand why he's prescribing this medication. You don't have a heart problem. He's obviously unaware of your medical history."

I phoned Dr. Dawson's office and left an urgent message for him to call me at Victoria Park, although I doubted he would be able to find me as I shuttled between upstairs and downstairs. In the evening I called Noel, thinking that his medical clout would help resolve the problem. I wanted him to speak with Dr. Dawson, who might be inclined to take a colleague more seriously. Noel was not sympathetic, though. "Who are you to question the doctors?" he said. "You think that all you have to do is read *The Merck Manual* and you know more about their specialties than they do."

That was not fair. I learned a lot, actually, by reading *The Merck Manual,* a concise compendium (now in its seventeenth edition) of what's what in medicine. It was my own personal medical bible, but Noel was always annoyed when I quoted from it. He admitted that he did not understand much of the cardiological terminology. I was convinced he could have learned the pertinent jargon from *The Merck Manual.*

"That's not true, Noel," I said. "I have a right to question Mother's physicians, a responsibility to question them. It's my obligation to follow Mother's case, because she's in no condition to do it herself. I can ask as many questions as I have to, as long as I do it in a nonthreatening way. After all, doctors are not infallible; they're not gods. And I have to remind you—you're a son, too, not only a doctor."

Noel backed down. "I'll try to call him in the morning."

"It's urgent, Noel. Have you forgotten that Mother had a violent reaction to digitalis and nearly died? You were there. You know all this."

"I'm not so sure that's the way it happened. The whole business about the heart block doesn't ring true."

"It doesn't matter. Mother doesn't have a heart condition and doesn't need that medication. You're her son. It's your obligation, as well, to speak with her physician."

"All right! I'll call him in the morning."

And he did. But just to follow up and assuage my own doubts, I also called Dr. Dawson, getting through late the next afternoon. He had already spoken to Noel and had immediately ordered a blood test. Good thing, too, because the digitalis had begun to build to dangerous levels in Mother's blood. Dr. Dawson discontinued the digitalis at once, taking the matter in good spirits.

But I was appalled. Somewhere in the paper trail of Mother's medical records a clear warning, such as "The patient is highly sensitive to digitalis preparations. Prescribe with great caution," should have appeared. Dr. Dawson did not know about Mother's toxic reaction to digitalis and near-death experience at Sacred Heart. Was it his fault that he prescribed a potentially lethal medication? Probably not. However, he could have asked Mother if she was sensitive to any medications. He did not do so. If Mother had not been alert enough to catch the oversight, she probably would have died a second time around.

I was also disconcerted about why Mother's medical history was lost in the shuffle. True, Mother's medical records and discharge sheet from Coral Bay followed her to Victoria Park. But before that, her medical records were sent to each institution's own records department. Victoria Park had a limited view of Mother's medical history over the past five months and was unaware that she had suffered a clinical death and been resuscitated.

Clearly, the medical records were fragmented. Each institution generated its own set, which could be released only by the written request of the patient. A family member could have access to these records by demonstrating that he or she held a legal power of attorney. I did not think of requesting Mother's records until after she left Sacred Heart, where the ICU nurses had acted as though they were unaware of her hip fractures. I prepared the letters, and Mother signed them. Because of my perseverance, I succeeded in obtaining a complete written history and familiarizing myself with Mother's medical treatment. But the cumulative results of hundreds of lab tests, X-rays, and other procedures were too complex for any one person to grasp. No doctor would have the time or patience to wade through hundreds of pages of medical records; nor were they readily available. How could a doctor tailor the right treatment without knowing exactly what had occurred? Mother's experience with digitalis underscored the need for a mechanism whereby physicians could have a succinct, computerized summary of a patient's treatment and what is permissible or not for that individual.

• • •

It was time for me to go home. Mother looked perfectly poised to succeed, and Dad had adjusted to the new routine. I was frantic to see Graz, but I could not share these feelings with my parents. I went to Marisa.

"Do you think you can handle things for a few days? Can I leave Mother and Dad in your hands? Can you manage the car and run back and forth between Pompano and Boca Raton without feeling overwhelmed?"

"Don't worry, Señora Luisa," she said. "You go home for a few days. I can handle it."

"O.K. You know why I have to leave. I don't know how Graz is coming along—whether he can enroll in his new school or whether he'll have to stay home for a few more weeks."

"I mean it, Señora Luisa, I won't let you down. I'll be at Victoria Park every day, all day. You take care of Graz and come back in a few days."

Fortunately, Marisa had the complete support of the Victoria Park staff. Rather than viewing her as an interloper and hampering her actions, as had happened at The Palms, Victoria Park welcomed her presence and understood the crucial role she played in my parents' care. She not only loved them and displayed great sensitivity to their needs, but she was their link to the outside world, keeping them abreast of matters at home. She was also a reliable source of information. I knew I could call Marisa each evening and she would give me an accurate, up-to-date assessment of my parents' progress.

The day of my departure, September 12, came too quickly. Mother had been at Victoria Park for a full week. She had participated in several therapy sessions and was considered a good candidate for rehab. Her spirits appeared to be lifting. I planned to get an early start and spend a large part of the day there. I expected to have a quiet, pleasant afternoon with my parents. I planned to drive up to Boca Raton without rushing and stop off at the mall to buy Graz jeans. I would return home by 4:00 P.M., when Kathy was scheduled to drive me to the airport. Unfortunately, this idyllic vision was shattered by another unexpected exchange of words with my brother, who called to catch up on the events of the past few days and let me know he would arrive later in the week to visit Mother.

For days I had been observing Mother's new roommate and her relationship with her adult children. She was an elderly woman who had suffered a stroke and was admitted to Victoria Park for therapy. Her grown son and daughter were together at her bedside and were clearly in anguish about their mother's condition. I had to admit that I felt a twinge of envy when I saw grown siblings compatibly sharing their mother's care. My brother and I always managed to miss each other, and we certainly thought along very different lines.

The conversation with Noel was winding down. Against my better judgment, I asked, "Noel, are you going to help me with Mother and Dad? I'm worried about all the expenses."

"I've already expressed my opinion about this. I've already told you what I think."

"Noel, I really don't feel comfortable about bringing this up, but I'm spending hundreds of dollars a day. I'm spending much more than is coming in from both them and me. The nursing-home fees alone are a killer, and now Dad may move to a private room."

"We've been through this before. You already know how I feel. Our parents were saving for their old age. Now they're in it. You should spend that money for their expenses."

"What kind of son are you? It seems to me that your parents are getting the short end here. You have an obligation." Then my tone turned vituperative. "We can go way back, Noel, if you care to. If it weren't for your parents, you would never have finished medical school. If nothing else, you definitely owe them one." I thought of the many roast-beef dinners Mother had lovingly prepared for Noel; the laundry bags of dirty clothing he brought home from the dorm every weekend for her to wash; the term papers she corrected after endless discussions, typing up the final version because Noel had never learned how to type. Mother had catered to his every need and excused her "subservience" by claiming that geniuses needed special care. I could go on and on. I felt like dredging up the entire history of my parents' treating their only son like royalty, but I wisely kept quiet.

"I'm going to make myself clear again, Barbara. You should spend their money for their medical care, and when you run through their savings, then you should go to the government for help."

I did not know what he was talking about. Was he talking about Medicaid and spending down? Was he talking about exhausting their resources and making them impoverished in the space of several months?

"And when you're finished with the government," Noel continued, "then you can come back to me, and maybe then we'll talk. That's my final word on this subject. I'm not going to change my mind."

"Fuck you, Noel," I said bluntly. "Why don't you grow up and start acting like a son? When you start doing that, then maybe you and I will have something to discuss. I have nothing more to say to you right now. Good-bye."

I had lost it again, but he deserved it. I found the entire conversation demeaning. "Go to the government; go to the government." His words reverberated in my head. If I could not depend on my only sibling—the big brother I had so looked up to as a child—on whom could I depend? He did have a valid point; I understood the logic behind the idea of using one's own resources to cover the costs of medical care. But I found Noel's position coldhearted, at best. No doubt, this was one of the lowest moments of the past few months, one that I was unlikely ever to forget.

I could not face my mother until I calmed down. I was still unsteady as I neared Victoria Park, so I turned off at the mall and went on a minor spree. I bought Dad a watch to replace the one that had disappeared at The Palms, cosmetics for myself, and Levi's for Graz. Within forty-five minutes, I was on my way to Victoria Park.

Mother was in the middle of lunch when I walked in. I was pleased to see her eating on her own and beginning to find the food appetizing. "What happened, dear?" Mother asked. "I was starting to worry about you. You said you were going to come early."

"I know, Mother. I'm fine. I'll tell you about it in a few minutes. But let's just sit quietly while you finish your lunch." I was not about to tell all. For a few days I had wanted to tell her about Graz, but I decided to wait until I saw for myself how he was coming along.

"Mother, you know I have to go home because of Graz. He's not even officially enrolled in school yet and I have to get him settled." (This was quite true.) "I'll be back the week after next."

"I feel that something's bothering you. What is it? Do you want to tell me about it?"

"No. It's nothing, really. Noel called me this morning, and I have to admit, we did not have a pleasant conversation."

"Why? What happened, exactly?"

"Well, first of all, he'll be in next weekend. I know you want to see him, and it's just as well we're not coinciding. This way, we'll both keep you busy with our respective visits. But I don't want you to count on him. Don't count on him, because we'll have to manage on our own. You know what I mean."

"I don't need anything from Noel. I would never accept anything from Noel. Dad and I can take care of ourselves." With that, Mother began to cry.

"Oh, please don't, Mummy. Please! I don't want to upset you on my last day here."

"Well, I can see he's upset you. He's very busy. He's always busy. He's too busy to take care of sick parents. I don't want him to feel guilty. It's pointless. There's nothing to be gained from making a grown child feel guilty."

"I agree, Mother, but it hurts. You didn't have to leave anything for your children. You should have spent every last bit of it, enjoyed your money—on dinners, cruises, flowers, anything that gave you and Dad pleasure. But not on this."

"I just hope there's something left when it's all over. You're right. We were too preoccupied about it lasting, particularly your father."

"Mom, that's the way people of your generation behaved. They never got over the Depression."

At that point, Dad walked into Mother's room, accompanied by Marisa, looking very chipper in a striped cotton shirt.

"Dad," Mother said, "you remember that Barbara's going home today. She has to get back to her family."

"You're leaving today?" Dad asked.

"Yes, Dad, I have to take care of Graz for a few days. Then I'll be back to see you."

"Where are you going?"

"To Caracas, Dad."

"You don't have to go to Caracas. You can live here and stay with us."

"Let's go for a walk while we talk about it Dad."

I walked Dad to the hall, and we sat down on the sofa near Mother's room. I could see Dad was getting angry and upset. He refused to look at me. I took his hand and said, "Dad, please don't make this more difficult for me. It's hard enough for me to leave you and Mother, but it's only for a few days, and in the meantime Marisa will be here every day. Graz has been sick, and I have to take care of him, too. Remember, I also have Graziano, my husband. I have a family in Caracas."

"This is not a good time to leave us. This is not the way to do things."

"I know, Dad. It's never a good time, but try to understand. I'll be back soon, and I'll try to bring Graz with me."

"Well, that would be nice."

But Dad was displeased. He turned away and refused to give me a kiss. We returned to Mother's room, and she chided him. "Dad, Barbara has to go home. She has a family there, too, you know."

The matter was settled. Mother made it easier. I was cutting it close. It was time to leave, but I wanted no dreary farewells. I kissed and hugged both of my parents and turned around at the door. "I'll see you both in a few days. And Dad, don't let the bedbugs bite."

Dad smiled, and I made my escape. It broke my heart to walk out that door. Dad had never harbored a grudge against me, and now I was causing him pain. I wondered, as I moved down the corridor, whether I would see my mother alive again. Kathy was already waiting downstairs when I got to the house.

"Give me a call when you're ready to come back and I'll pick you up at the airport," she said. "How long are you going to be away this time?"

"About a week, Kathy. I've learned my lesson. The minute I turn my back, Mother's condition starts to go downhill. I can't leave her alone very long. I won't leave her alone. I'm going to see her through this. As soon as I check on Graz, I'll be back, and then I'm not going to leave Mother until she comes home."

"She'll be fine for a few days. I'll call her every day, and Marisa will be with them all the time. But you seem awfully down."

"I'm feeling down—about as down as you can get." With that comment, I burst into tears and told her the entire story. Kathy, my confidante throughout Mother's tribulations, consoled me the best she could. We talked about the social baggage and unresolved rivalries that siblings often bring to their adult relationship. By the time we reached the airport, I had managed to pull myself together.

Noel flew in from Chicago on Friday and spent the afternoon and the following day with Mother. When I called him on Saturday evening (despite our memorable conversation the time before), he observed, "Mom's having a hard time focusing on things. The television's on, but she's not really watching. The magazines and *Miami Herald* are by her bedside, but they look like they've never been read."

I knew what he meant. I took stacks of magazines to Victoria Park—not her favorites, such as the *New Yorker*, which required long spurts of concentration, but *People* and *Life*, which had a lot of photos. The next day, Mother would insist I take them home, claiming she had already finished them. In truth, Mother was not particularly engaged. She had transcended such mundane matters and now focused solely on her fight to survive. Mother needed all her energy to worry about eating, sitting up in bed, and transferring to a wheelchair or walker. Keeping in tune with the outside world was scarcely relevant.

"I wouldn't worry about it, Noel. Mother has more important priorities right now. So, how has your visit gone? What have you two talked about?"

"We just talked. Nothing special."

But their conversation was special enough that Marisa, as she later confided, felt like an intruder and quietly left the room. Mother reproached Noel about our disagreements, which she knew went well beyond what I had chosen to tell her. We must be friends, she insisted, not enemies. She understood that he was busy, but he must understand that I was carrying the full burden. "Don't worry about us," he had responded. "We're fine. You have to worry about yourself right now." They talked at length; they were alone together. It was a summing up, at least for Mother.

According to the nurse's report, Mother was alert and oriented on the day of her conversation with Noel. She chatted with friends and family. "No acute distress noted," the nurse wrote.

But on Sunday, the day of Noel's departure, Mother's condition changed. She was tired and did not feel well, Noel noted when he said good-bye. Mother was out of sorts in the morning and refused to eat breakfast. Perhaps her condition was related to Noel's departure, for she began to perk up at lunchtime. Marisa helped Mother into her wheelchair, and she ate a little bit. She was still tired, and her body ached. Marisa brought Dad over to keep Mother company. I spoke with Mother in the afternoon, and she said she had had a good visit with Noel—that he was well-meaning but not always able to act on his intentions. The nurse noted that Mother had been feeling very tired in the morning and refused all her usual medications except the prednisone. She apparently had difficulty swallowing during lunch.

Mother and Dad's neighbors Kay and Maury visited briefly in the afternoon and found her agitated and depressed. Kay and Maury were good friends as well as neighbors. Kay called Mother almost every day and dropped by frequently, always bringing a box of candy or another thoughtful gift to cheer her up. They had checked on my parents for years, so it was fitting that they came by to visit on this Sunday afternoon.

Mother was short of breath, yet she insisted on pulling out the oxygen tube. "Now, June," Kay said. "Put it back in so you can talk."

"No. I've had it," Mother replied. "I'm giving up. I don't want to go on. I'm tired of all this."

"Please, June, put the oxygen back so you can breathe more comfortably."

But Kay herself was not so sure. While she admonished Mother, she thought back to a few months earlier when she had taken a good look at Mother at the pool. Mother's arms were like sticks and "she had on that poor brace." She had gone "down to nothing."

"No," Mother answered. "I'm tired of being ill, of living like this." Mother refused to reinsert the oxygen tube.

Marisa had an upset stomach and wanted to leave early. Mother told her not to wait around for dinner to arrive. "I'm not going to eat supper anyway, so you don't have to help me."

"Please, Señora June, drink some Pulmocare."

Mother drank the nutritious liquid, and Marisa left. Perhaps the drink would soothe her throat. Mother's cough had worsened, and she was bringing up yellow sputum.

In the evening, Mother called for the nurse and told her she was breathless and needed respiratory therapy. The therapist came, took one look at Mother, and called Dr. Dawson, asking for an order to send her to the hospital at once. The nurse returned. Mother was wearing her reading glasses, and despite her shortness of breath, she was trying to glance through the Sunday *Miami Herald*.

"Mrs. Margolies," she said, "you're very short of breath, and the respiratory therapy isn't helping you right now. We think you need to be in the hospital. We would like to send you to the hospital right now. Do you agree?"

Mother nodded, and the nurse called 911. Mother was taken to Boca Raton Medical Center, a few blocks east of Victoria Park.

In Caracas, things were quiet for a change. Graz was settled in for a few weeks of rest, and his new school said it would send his work so he would not fall behind. I was leisurely getting ready for bed when the phone rang. Mother's Victoria Park nurse was on the line.

"Is this Mrs. Gasparini?"

"Yes," I said warily.

"Mrs. Gasparini, we've been trying to contact your brother all evening about your mother."

"What's wrong with my mother? My brother was at Victoria Park with my mother all weekend. He's flying home to Chicago right now."

"I'm sorry to have to tell you this, but your mother was taken to the hospital this evening. She had difficulty breathing and was in a great deal of distress. We thought she needed to be hospitalized, where she'll get the attention she needs right now."

"I can't believe this," I said. "I spoke to my mother this afternoon, and she seemed fine, just a little weary. Can I call the hospital to get some news about her condition?"

"I'm afraid you can't do that. They won't take calls at this hour. Call them first thing in the morning."

"Where has my mother been taken?"

"To the emergency room at Boca Raton Medical Center."

"Well, thank you for calling me. It was thoughtful of you to call me long distance."

"Please, we wouldn't think of not calling you. It's our responsibility."

"Well, thank you anyway."

I knew I would not call the hospital in the morning. Everything was ready—my passport, a few hundred dollars and plenty of *bolivares*, my Florida house keys, my parents' paperwork. I threw together my usual outfits in a large handbag. I planned to catch the first flight out of Caracas the next morning and had no intention of waiting around for luggage in Miami. The call was ominous. Now I had the disagreeable task of calling Noel and catching him a few minutes after he walked in the door. There was no way he would be able to comprehend that his mother, with whom he had conversed at length the day before and had been with only a few hours earlier, was now in the emergency room of a Boca Raton hospital.

Nobody at Victoria Park thought about telling Dad. Perhaps it was best that Dad slept peacefully through the night. Marisa told him on Monday afternoon. Marisa was shocked to find Mother missing from her room on Monday morning. She rushed over to Boca Raton Medical Center and persuaded the ICU staff that she was a close friend of Mother's. She was allowed in for a few moments. Mother was heavily sedated, and Marisa caressed her brow, gave her a long look, and left.

Later, Marisa told me she had had a dream that week, a sort of premonition that she did not fully understand at the time. Marisa dreamed that Mother was holding a bag shaped like a human organ and filled with dirty water. In Marisa's native land, this signified that something bad was about to happen. Marisa told Dad that Mother had had to return to the hospital for oxygen therapy. He did not question this explanation, and they spent the remainder of the afternoon together at Victoria Park.

I'd Rather Age in Place
Residential Design for Elder Living

TODAY'S ELDERS should have an inviolable right to remain at home and "age in place." Nursing homes need not be the final destination in the face of deteriorating health. Some 30 percent of American seniors now live alone, valuing their ability to cope with the assorted maladies of aging and rejecting any possible benefits that could be derived from residing in a nursing facility. Most old people cherish their autonomy so highly that they will avoid institutional living at any cost. And according to a recent poll, a significant portion would rather die than live their remaining years in a nursing home.

Old people do not have to remain in the home in which they raised their families. They can relocate to residential housing that is comfortable, functional, and accessible to health-care services. Such surroundings will allow them to coexist with their infirmities without compromising their autonomy. The care will come directly to the home and keep pace with their changing needs. The object is to provide a supportive environment rather than the structured, regimented one in the nursing-home model.

The architect Victor Regnier, who visited 100 assisted-living communities in northern Europe and the United States, notes that the design and service philosophies of the European communities are so radical that they would be considered "illegal" in the United States. They are designed as residential homes, not institutions. "Residents with major mental and physical infirmities were able to grow older in housing that was spacious, complete, and tethered to a range of emergency care and supportive health care services," he writes. "It was a vision I saw only a glimpse of in the United States" (1994:xiii). Regnier uses "illegal" metaphorically to express the difficulties of implementing comparable facilities in the United States. Rules and regulations, state laws, building codes, regulatory agencies, and more, combine with lethargy and cultural conservatism to prevent the residential model of housing the elderly from flourishing.

In the five northern European countries Regnier visited, homelike dwellings served thousands of elderly people by providing necessary support services. Even the severely disabled were able to stay in place because the services adjusted to them. The work of designing innovative housing is highly valued, and architectural competitions are held throughout Europe to encourage professionals to propose new prototypes. I observed a similar approach in Spain's Canary Islands, where architects vied for experimental projects to bring attractive residential housing to growing numbers of old people. By relying on vernacular and cultural traditions, they were able to create workable communities that respond to the needs of aging residents.

"Assisted living"—one popular way to age in place—is a long-term-care solution that allows people to receive the required supports in a homelike setting. The philosophical underpinnings of this type of housing are diametrically opposed to those of the nursing home. The challenge is to provide a continuum of care for people in various conditions of physical and mental health. For assisted living to succeed as a viable housing alternative, it must be perceived as *residential* instead of medical. The elderly recipient must be treated as an independent person who needs some assistance rather than as an infirm patient incapable of caring for himself or herself.

Instead of existing as separate entities, as they do in Europe, assisted-living units in the United States often occupy part of total- or continuing-care communities that offer a spectrum of services. Today, the nursing-home industry faces stiff competition from the growing number of continuing-care retirement communities that include assisted-living divisions. Although the concept of planned communities for the elderly goes back to the nineteenth century, the present-day version generally offers three levels of care: independent residential living, which includes amenities like dining facilities, van transportation, and linen and cleaning services; assisted-living units for people who require some help with their personal needs; and the medical environment of a skilled nursing facility for patients with multiple infirmities. Continuing-care communities move their residents from one area to another, depending on the level of care required. Today, the continuing-care retirement community is being replaced by free-standing assisted-living facilities that are committed to maintaining aging seniors in place, no matter what their medical needs.

The concept of a care community in which seniors are supported in their efforts to live independently is an important one. The anthropologist Otto von Mering notes that the continuing-care community model is a positive one because it offers elders the opportunity to age productively despite their declining health. Further, this type of living arrangement is an expression of the American social movements that drew together like-minded individuals to create special, utopian-like communities to "rediscover their own worth, survivability, and maybe even their souls" (1996:259). Care communities provide ample opportunities to forge new friendships based on common generational interests. They are designed with regard for people's privacy as well as for their desire to form part of a cohesive group. Continuing-care retirement communities have been around for at least a century, but they were considered a minor housing option until well into the 1960s (Regnier 1994:6). The majority of the assisted-living facilities in the United States, estimated at 10,000 by the American Seniors Housing Association, were constructed during the 1990s in response to the nursing-home abuses that were being increasingly reported in the media (Goldstein 2001).

Care communities offer the same basic amenities: studio to two-bedroom deluxe apartments, housekeeping and linen services, and a meal plan consisting of one to three meals in a community dining room. The apartments also have safety features, such as nonslip floors, grab bars in the bathrooms, and panic or call buttons. The common areas generally include a lounge with receptionist, library, auditorium, arts-and-crafts shop, beauty parlor, country store, and snack bar. Some may even offer banking and postal services, making it unnecessary to leave the complex. Recreational facilities usually include a whirlpool, swimming pool, exercise room, shuffleboard, and billiards. Transportation is available to the doctor, the supermarket, and nearby shopping malls. The entire package is rounded out by a monthly schedule peppered with daily events and numerous outings.

The Palms at Palm-Aire, one of the first continuing-care facilities to be built in Florida (where my mother spent a disastrous five weeks), was unique when it opened in the late 1970s because it offered a lifetime care plan to the residents of its comfortable tower apartments. The monthly rental fee not only covered an apartment with all the amenities; it also encompassed skilled nursing care in the adjacent sixty-bed "Health Care Center" free of charge, should the need arise. According to some of the original promotional material, "Lifecare provides you with physical and financial assurances. You maintain your status as an active, independent person. Should anything affect your health during your retirement living at The Palms requiring long-term healthcare, The Palms guarantees that care for only the normal monthly service fee, for as long as you need it." Attractive, yes, but the catch is that the monthly service fee is several times higher than the monthly maintenance charges for a spacious condominium apartment at neighboring Palm-Aire Country Club. Each additional occupant, as well as each visitor, at The Palms (one's adult children or grandchildren, for instance) was charged additional fees. In 1996, a small two-bedroom unit rented for $3,625 monthly for one person, plus $595 for an extra person. Alternatively, by paying a 90 percent–refundable entrance fee of $179,000, plus $12,000 for an extra person, one could lower the monthly charge to $2,445. In contrast, my parents paid a quarterly maintenance charge of $800 for a three-bedroom, two-bath garden apartment and were building equity at the same time. The guaranteed feature of "total" lifetime care may be attractive in theory, but the contrast between the lovely residential apartments of The Palms and the dismal institutional atmosphere of its skilled nursing facility is incongruous. One long-time resident of The Palms who unexpectedly found himself in the skilled nursing center for the first time commented: "This place is a living hell. God forbid the poor soul who is unfortunate enough to end up here." By the time the man needed the skilled nursing facility's services, after living independently in The Palms for more than twenty years, the retirement community had undergone several changes in ownership and management and numerous transitions in personnel. It was coasting on a reputation for excellence that had been forged years earlier.

The Forum Group, an Indiana company, runs thirty-three total-care communities nationwide, among them The Forum in Deerfield Beach and the Park Summit in Coral Springs. Both are full-service rental retirement communities associated with adjoining nursing facilities. The Forum is an exceptionally graceful cluster of buildings that offers independent living without an entrance fee. For $3,000 monthly in 1996, a married couple received a one-bedroom apartment with utilities, weekly housekeeping and linen services, personal laundry service, three meals daily in the dining room, some assistance with daily living activities (bathing, dressing, bedmaking, medication monitoring), transportation within a five-mile radius, and a twenty-four-hour emergency-call service.

The hotel industry has also expanded into the field and is cashing in on the rush to build assisted-living housing. Chains such as the Hyatt and Marriott advertise the resort lifestyle available to seniors who are healthy and wealthy enough to enjoy it. Who is better qualified or better suited than the hospitality industry to offer such amenities? As the Marriott says about its Horizon Club, "More than 65 years of excellence in gracious hospitality shows in every detail." (Rumor also has that residents dress for dinner each evening as if they were on a luxury cruise.) The hotel industry tends to be pragmatic. Marriott's Horizon Club and the Hyatt's Seasons (a "Classic Residence") stress the quality of services available for different levels of care; the four S's—security, safety, social activities, and services—are the hallmark of a "carefree style of life" that will allow one "to cultivate fun and friendships." Seasons is particularly proud of its oceanside site in the heart of Florida's Gold Coast and promotes its resort-like setting as the ideal place for an active, well-rounded retirement. According to a spokesman for Marriott Senior Living Services, "Assisted living is going to be our main focus for the next 5 to 10 years because demand for this product far exceeds supply." The corporation sees the rapid expansion in the assisted-living market as a "natural extension of its hospitality core and plans to pump hundreds of millions of dollars into it" (as quoted in Nordheimer 1996:C3).

As a result of the demographic explosion in the senior population, total-care communities are now a billion-dollar industry and are frequently run by large public corporations such as Alterra Healthcare, the nation's largest assisted-living provider. During the bull market of the 1990s, investors in this thriving industry reaped bountiful returns of nearly 20 percent, and Alterra Healthcare opened two new facilities per week. In 1990, 800 care communities existed in the United States, and after a decade of unsurpassed growth, their numbers doubled. Assisted-living units will continue to grow, spurred by a "surging" market caused by the tremendous dread of nursing homes (Nordheimer 1996).

One must ask whether is it possible for this young industry to grow with integrity. Will it retain its commitment to its philosophy, or will it be subjected to the same abuses that accompanied the expansion of the nursing-home industry? *Consumer Reports* notes that, whereas a maze of regulations protect residents' rights in nursing homes, the assisted-living sector is barely regulated. Strangely, the mom-and-pop operations of the past have reared their ugly heads again in the form of assisted-living arrangements whose contracts and provisions are so vaguely conceived that the situation is tailor-made for abuse (When a Parent Needs Care, Part 3, 1995). The federal government sets no standards, and state regulators are ill equipped to do an effective job. Recent exposés of the quality of care in *Time* and *Money* magazines make it clear that informed consumers must proceed with caution (Geary 2001; Goldstein 2001). The exposés charge assisted-living communities with understaffing, substandard training, neglect, and misleading advertising, and have led consumers to be wary of the assisted-living industry's capacity to provide consistent services.

Total-care communities take advantage of older people's concerns about their ability to continue caring for themselves. "Let us take care of your future" is their subliminal message. "Come to our rental retirement community and enjoy freedom and an independent lifestyle, because we offer security and peace of mind, just in case you become too infirm to live on your own." Take, for example, publicity put out by Adult Communities Total Services (ACTS), the developer of fifteen large communities along the eastern seaboard: "The most important reason for our success might be that people experience real security in knowing that if there is a health problem, a full spectrum of health care is available [at no increase to your monthly fee] including home healthcare, assisted living and 24-hour skilled nursing care in a private on-campus medical center." ACTS invites South Floridians to complimentary luncheon tours to meet like-minded people "who have declared their independence by choosing lifecare retirement living."

Healthy individuals who have spent the past twenty to thirty years living at a distance from their adult children worry about what will happen to them as they grow old and frail. The children often complicate the situation by encouraging their able parents to have a "contingency plan." The children do not want to have to worry about their aging parents and believe that retirement communities will provide a safe environment; the parents are seduced by the notion of not having to impose on their offspring. Structure and security versus freedom and autonomy—it is a tough decision with multiple implications. The Palms, for example, nurtures the fear of future frailty by warning prospective occupants that some 40 percent of seniors will require nursing care. Never mind that this statistic is taken out of context and is misleading. The truth is that less than 5 percent of the senior population lives in nursing homes on any particular day, and relatively few people will require *extensive* long-term care (Difficult Dialogues Program 2002:9).

The catch inherent in retirement communities is simple: You have to be well enough to enjoy the amenities, balancing the risks by calculating your present state of health against the possibility that you will need assistance later on. People confined to wheelchairs or with obvious dementia are ineligible for independent living and for many forms of assisted living. If you wait too long to make the move because you feel you want to stay in your own home, the chances of making it into the independent living quarters of these retirement-care communities decline rapidly. The communities accentuate their attractive amenities rather than focus on care, which they downplay when advertising. Try to see the skilled nursing division when you visit a retirement community as a prospective resident and you will probably be rebuffed, as my parents and I were when we visited a total-care community in Fort Lauderdale a few years ago. Why frighten potential clients by showing them what may await them if they live to a feeble old age?

The truth is that there is little chance of taking care of one's future health needs by buying into a total life-care community when one is still in reasonably good health. Only hospitals are technically equipped to handle medical emergencies, and most nursing-home emergencies are still managed by transferring the resident to a hospital. Why anyone would want to buy into a system that can offer only custodial care down the road is a question that should be answered only after considerable introspection by the elderly and their families.

To round out the picture of eldercare, we must not neglect the burgeoning health-service industry that provides home care by licensed, bonded, and insured health workers. Medicare certifies some 8,000 agencies, but at least 9,000 more that are not certified by Medicare offer some form of home care (When a Parent Needs Care, Part 3, 1995:660). In Florida alone, the number of agencies has grown sixfold in the past decade, to more than 1,300. The full range of services includes companions and homemakers on an hourly or twenty-four hour basis, home-health aides certified to assist with personal hygiene, licensed practical nurses qualified to administer medication, therapists, social workers, nutritionists, and registered nurses. The agencies emphasize not only the medical aspects of home care but also the "art" of caring and their special role in providing compassionate caregivers. The home-health-care sector could take on many of the functions now dominated by nursing facilities if the reimbursement system were reoriented to provide for chronic care rather than short-term acute care.

Medicare reimbursements pay for more than half of all home-health-care expenditures and have grown by more than 500 percent since 1989, from $2.4 billion to $17.7 billion in 1996. This figure constitutes only about 30 percent of long-term-care expenditures in the home. The real obstacle to the growth of home-health-care services originated in the way the Medicare and Medicaid Acts were planned in the 1960s. Medicaid designated the nursing-home institution as the only provider of long-term care, thus eliminating the development of more appropriate community-based alternatives in response to the longevity boom. Medicare reimbursements, by contrast, are pegged primarily to short-term post-hospital care in a skilled nursing facility or at home through the services of an authorized agency. Unfortunately, the "actual use of services is shaped more by economic possibility, historical tradition, political climate, and the culture's welfare philosophy than by objective needs and individual choice" (Topinková 1994:18). Precisely as more and more elderly require continuing coverage for chronic conditions, the political climate encourages the cutting of such services. The only systematic program proposed to provide home-based care to the elderly died along with the Clinton bill in 1992. Since then, the Balanced Budget Act of 1997 slashed by more than $16 billion the Medicare funding that would allow home health care to keep pace with the rising demand of aging baby boomers. As matters now stand, 7.3 million of the 12.8 million long-term-care population are older than sixty-five and manage for the most part at home. The entire field of long-term care is in considerable upheaval because it will eventually have to respond to the new reality of an aging population. The vertiginous growth of home-health-care agencies in the Sunbelt states with large elderly populations demonstrates that today's consumers are demanding to remain at home and be cared for in place.

Home care is probably the wave of the future because the average senior will not be able to afford assisted-living housing. In contrast to northern Europe, where national health insurance plans cover the complete cost of assisted-living arrangements, this type of housing in the United States receives no federal entitlements and must be paid for by the consumer. Most communities have steep entrance fees, which can range from $100,000 to $300,000, depending on the type of unit, and add monthly carrying charges to cover rent, services, and the amenities. These fees are subject to change without notice. Communities that have waived the entrance fee may charge monthly fees of up to $10,000 for basic coverage, effectively prohibiting a huge segment of the elder population from considering this option.

Interest groups are beginning to spring up in states that are heavily populated by seniors to push for effective home care. One such group has appeared at Palm-Aire, the retirement community that once actively sought affluent members in their prime to enjoy the good life centered on the golf course and famous spa. Now its residents are aging and have more serious concerns. In a letter sent to community dwellers by the Broward Homebound Program, Charles Singer, a Palm-Aire resident, wrote,

> I have become painfully aware of the growing number of frail and disabled neighbors in our midst, who face the possibility of requiring admission into a health care facility. You should know, however, that today there are home health services available that bring the caretaker right into your home to provide 'hands on' help. This can prolong and in most cases avoid the need for placement in an institution. It assures the patient the dignity, which comes with remaining in one's own home, in familiar surroundings with loving family and friends. Broward Homebound is a nonprofit, tax-exempt organization that can make this vital service available based on the patient's ability to pay. We here in Palm-Aire can establish a neighborhood support program to make home care available to every resident in our community who may need it.

The program solicited donations of any amount to help the community's graying population age in place. Too often, Palm-Aire's long-time residents simply moved over to The Palms or to The Preserve, a newer, more attractive continuing-care community, without realizing that they had other choices.

The most horrific example of how our present public policy discourages aging in place by denying in-home care was written up in the *Miami Herald*'s *Tropic* magazine a few years ago. Pat Kirkenberg was approaching eighty and lived independently in her own mobile home in South Broward County on a $900 monthly income. She received some housekeeping help from the county's elderly-services agency. One day, Pat disappeared from her house, apparently because an agency caseworker reported that she was incapable of taking care of herself at home. She was whisked away by Broward County officials to a Medicaid-funded adult congregate living facility, a 1950s-style motel on the intercoastal waterway. Her neighbors tried to contact her, but a court-appointed guardian refused to divulge her new location. As one friend and neighbor who checked on Pat several times a day put it, "Even people on Death Row are allowed visitors." Pat was forced to share her room with three other elderly women. Every day she packed the few belongings that had followed her into the facility and announced she was going home. Every day, a staff member said, "Sure, after lunch" or "Sure, after dinner." Meanwhile, in a five-minute bureaucratic hearing attended by a group of local experts, including a prominent gerontologist, Pat was declared incompetent and made a ward of the state. She was not allowed to attend the hearing. Ironically, Pat could afford to live in her own home but could not afford the cost of a nursing home, so she was put in a facility for the indigent against her will.

What did Pat do to deserve this? She lost her property, her possessions, and her civil rights. In a perfunctory test to determine her mental status, administered by the same prominent Fort Lauderdale gerontologist who attended her hearing, Pat was declared mildly demented. "In a five-minute hearing that she did not attend, Pat Kirkenberg lost her right to marry, travel, drive, vote, work, sue, consent or deny medical treatment, choose her place of residence, and decide what happens to her possessions and property. But she gained the protection of the government, which is supposed to keep her clean, well-fed and safe" (Laughlin 1993:13). Pat went willingly because she was told she was being taken to a nice place to paint. Pat's public guardian defended the decision to remove her from her home, insisting it was a "dirty, disgusting and dangerous" place and that Pat was mentally ill. At the same time, the guardian admitted that appropriate community services to help Pat remain in her own home were lacking.

What did Pat's only daughter have to say about all this? From Virginia, she told the reporter over the phone, "Now that she's in a safe place, I don't have to worry about her." Pat had taken in her own mother, then her mother-in-law, and finally her sister-in-law, nursing them until the end. But her daughter, who claimed to love her, insisted it would be too emotionally draining to become any more involved in her mother's life than she already was. No doubt, Pat was an "eccentric old woman" who needed help. No doubt, her home needed a guiding hand to make it more livable according to a social worker's standards. But there was no excuse for turning her into a helpless child, called "cute" and "little" by the owner of the facility, and for destroying a lifestyle that was well suited to her once vivacious personality. I still get chills when I think about how Pat was put away paternalistically with the full backing of public sanctions. Pat not only fell through the system's cracks; she descended directly to hell. And it occurred only because she happened to find herself old and alone toward the end of a long, fulfilling life.

Not all stories have to end like this. I can think of one fine example of aging in place in my own family. My Aunt Gussie and Uncle Sidney, like my parents, had worked out an amiable arrangement for taking care of each other in their old age. They found themselves, at eighty-nine, living in their own apartment in North Miami and managing very well on their own. My aunt was arthritic, had a pacemaker, and was rapidly losing her eyesight, and my uncle, although growing frailer every year, was still in good health. He drove everywhere and escorted my aunt from one errand to the next, so her fading eyesight never had a chance to become an impediment. But when Uncle Sidney died suddenly from a massive stroke in late 1994, Aunt Gussie had to ask herself, "Now what do I do?" Alone and nearly blind, how would she manage to stay in her own home? Her two sons lived up north, and her nephew Mark was preparing to leave Miami after accepting an out-of-state job. My aunt was on her own for the first time in her long life. Marisa went to Miami for a few days to be by her side during my uncle's passing, and it was then that Aunt Gussie prepared to tell her children she had no intention of ever leaving her home. They urged her to move north, but she firmly told them she was staying right where she was. One visit to The Palms to see Mother had been enough to convince my aunt that nursing homes, even under the best circumstances, were not for her. She would have to find a trusted companion like Marisa who could be relied on to carry out caregiving duties. One of Aunt Gussie's sons reminded her that, if this magical being did not turn up, she might have to think about a nursing home. "Don't even bring it up," I advised him. "Your mother will never leave her own home."

Eventually, Marisa herself became Aunt Gussie's trusted companion, providing hands-on help and serving as my aunt's surrogate eyes. Aunt Gussie asserted herself as head of her own household right from the start: no moving things out of their original place, no coming home late at night, no salt in the diet, no mumbling, and no Spanish in the conversation. At the same time, though, she and Marisa did plenty of traveling, eating out, shopping, attending services, visiting doctors, and other kinds of engaging with the outside world. Aunt Gussie achieved a measure of tranquility by taking charge of her own life, thinking ahead to her great-grandchildren, and living among familiar things.

I am sad to say that in the first year of the new century, my Aunt Gussie succumbed to her multiple conditions at age ninety-five. I like to think that staying put in her own comfortable home was her secret tonic for attaining a good old age.

CHAPTER SEVEN

Boca Raton Medical Center

"Your mother's condition is critical."

SEPTEMBER 19–SEPTEMBER 21, 1993: 2 DAYS • Mother had been intubated in the emergency room of Boca Raton Medical Center on Sunday night. I flew from Caracas on Monday afternoon—earlier flights were booked—and saw her during the last visiting period of the day. On Tuesday morning I called Dr. Dawson, Mother's attending physician at Victoria Park.

"Your Mother is in critical condition," he said. "She has an infection in her lungs we have not yet identified, and her lungs have stiffened and filled with fluid. She has a temperature of 102 degrees, and I suspect she has pneumonia as well as congestive heart failure. The ventilator is set at the maximum to increase the pressure in her lungs. Her breathing is very shallow, and she is receiving 75 percent oxygen. Her kidneys are weak and not functioning properly. I don't have the greatest hopes for her recovery and want to know what measures you wish to take. I've already spoken with your brother, and he does not want any extraordinary measures."

"My mother went through a similar crisis four months ago and came out of it," I said. "I'm her health-care surrogate, and I want you to do as much as possible without taking further invasive measures. She has always responded well to higher doses of steroids, and I want her to receive antibiotics and liquid nutrition."

"Do you want your mother to be resuscitated if the situation should arise?"

I hesitated. "No. I don't think my mother would have the stamina to go through that procedure again. And I don't think she was asked whether she wanted to be put on a respirator. She would not have approved. My mother was very clear about that in her living will. I'd like you to try to wean her off the respirator."

"We'll do our best, and I'm sorry, very sorry, to have to give you this prognosis."

On Tuesday, I visited Mother four times: at 11:00 A.M., 1:00 P.M., 5:00 P.M., and 7:30 P.M. I stretched the fifteen- to twenty-minute visiting periods to twice their length before I was asked politely to leave. Mother was fully awake and alert. I still could not reconcile the dreary prognosis with her appearance. I was not as shocked by the ventilator and tubes as I had been the first time and even managed to kid Mother, who responded by squeezing my hand.

"Mother, did you go through all this just to get me up here a few days earlier? I've become a regular customer on American's two o'clock flight to Miami."

Mother studied my face and continued to press my hand as I explained that her doctor would treat her lung infection with heavy infusions of antibiotics. She would also receive elevated doses of prednisone—80 milligrams every six hours. I implored her to fight, and she motioned that she would try. She had gained thirteen pounds in the past two weeks at Victoria Park and seemed to have enough reserve to hold her own. In the late afternoon, she responded to Dad's caresses with tender glances and appeared unchanged. But when I returned at 7:30 P.M., she was thrashing around and restlessly moving her legs in what appeared to be an attempt to find a comfortable position. The nurse assured me that Mother's condition was stable and that she was semi-somnolent because of a recent injection of morphine.

Why was my mother in isolation? I wondered. Was there something about her condition I should know? A sign by her door said, "Do Not Enter," and the nursing staff entered her cubicle wearing masks and gloves. Unfortunately, one of the nurses advised me, this was necessary when patients were admitted from nursing homes. *Staphylococcus aureus,* a common bacterium in nursing homes, was resistant to methicillin, the only backup for the antibiotics that had lost their efficacy. Until the results of the culture were known, the precautions were required.

Mother now fit the picture of a typical dying elderly patient: She was intubated, hypotensive, and suffering from both respiratory and renal failure. Her organs were seriously compromised, and the infection was rapidly overtaking her weakened lungs. I spoke to Mother's nurse from home at 10:45 P.M. Mother's kidneys still were not functioning properly, despite massive doses of diuretics. Her nurse promised to call the doctor and told me to call back before her shift ended at 11:00 P.M. The attending physician (who had never seen Mother) felt that Mother probably was not eliminating the intravenous fluids because she was so dehydrated. He would re-evaluate the situation in the morning; other medications could be tried. Still, Mother's nurse had switched to a different diuretic shortly before I called, but it also was not working.

Noel called me at 11:00 P.M. I told him that Mother's condition seemed stable. Her blood pressure was almost normal; her blood-oxygen level was higher than 90 percent; her pulse was a steady 88; and her heart rhythm was regular. I had felt comfortable about leaving Mother at 9:30 that evening and believed her condition was not as desperate as Dr. Dawson had painted it. After all, he had not seen Mother at Sacred Heart, when she had been much worse.

The local operator interrupted our conversation. "Please get off the phone," she said urgently. "You have an emergency call. The hospital has been trying to get through for the past few minutes."

"Noel, I have to go. I'll call you back later."

The night nurse, who had been on duty for only five minutes, was on the line. "Your mother's pulse is slowing down, and I advise you to come up here immediately."

"I can't believe it," I said. I had spoken to the day nurse not more than twenty minutes earlier, and she had assured me that Mother was stable.

"Well, I'm sorry to have to tell you, but a person's condition in a situation like this can change abruptly. Do you have someone who can drive up with you? I don't think you should drive right now."

"No. I'll come myself. I'll be there in about fifteen minutes."

"I want you to drive carefully. Don't race up here."

Normally, the drive from Pompano Beach to Boca Raton takes a half-hour. I tried not to race, but it was inevitable, and I sped up I-95 at more than ninety miles an hour. I did not want to crack myself up, but I also knew a dwindling pulse was a critical matter. The exits seemed endless. At 11:15, I made a sharp right and drove through the maze of darkened side streets. I had taken Mother to this hospital a year earlier for her bone scan and had been back and forth all day, but I was not sure how to get there at night. Finally, I found the emergency entrance, where the nurse had instructed me to go. A policeman was waiting to escort me upstairs.

I rushed into Mother's cubicle. She was dulled by morphine, yet still alert. She was comfortable and not in pain. Her eyes fluttered open, then closed. The nurse held her wrist: pulse down to 58, down to 30, down, down, down. Just a few seconds later, at 11:25 P.M., Mother slipped away.

I did not know how this could have happened in less than fifteen minutes. Had the day nurse actually checked on Mother when she told me her condition was stable? Did I have the right to doubt her? The heart monitor showed a flat colored line. The respirator was silent.

I wanted to be alone with my mother but without the tubes. "Please, please take out the tubes. Take them all out," I said to the nurse. I waited outside while she and another nurse detached Mother from the machine. They drew the curtains and removed the respirator tube from her trachea, the food tube from her nostril, the IV lines, and the monitor. Then they cleaned the tape marks from her face. It was 11:45. Mother was in a natural state, and that settled the issue of the official time of death. Mother's nurse was kind and brought me a cup of coffee. The ICU was silent. I closed myself in with my mother.

We were alone. This was the last time I would ever see her lovely face. She was warm, in repose, and I sat by her side. The tubes that had impeded my access earlier in the day were gone, and I could finally reach her. Her slim hands were entwined, relaxed across her stomach. She seemed to be alive. Her essence was still palpable in her facial expression, and I could not believe she was actually gone. The moment I had dreaded for months was now upon me. Just a few hours earlier, I had reminded Dad not to lean on the tubes. He tried so hard to get close to Mother, but the tubes were in the way. Earlier, I had wanted to sit on the bed to be closer to her, too, but it was impossible because of the mechanical obstacles. This was not how I had envisioned my mother's death, but who was I to presume how she would die?

I had never expected Mother to be fully awake and lucid at the moment of her departure. I refused to believe she was dying. No one told me, or even encouraged me, to stay by her bedside. She fooled me. Now I felt ashamed. I had pushed her to fight, right to the end. I was wrong to have badgered her. I had refused to accept the inevitable. She never failed in my presence; that was why I was so shocked. I had left her in stable condition, but when I walked out of her room, she began to decline.

The swelling of Mother's hands and arms gave her a childlike grace. I could not bear to leave. I maintained a posthumous vigil, sitting by her side for several hours and reflecting. "Mother, I don't know what you actually died of," I thought. "Exhaustion, wear and tear, a body at war with itself until the end? Why did it have to end like this? Why did God insist on this horrible test?" Perhaps if Mother had been confused or unconscious I would have accepted her death more easily, but this rational departure of which she had been entirely aware was shattering.

I ripped the page from the wall calendar. Tuesday, September 21, in appropriately bold black graphics. Her mother had also died on the twenty-first of the month. What a haunting coincidence. There was nothing to take home, only the skin cream I had purchased the day before. Had I been foolish enough to buy yet another cream, thinking it would keep bad things from happening? Mother had arrived from Victoria Park wearing a hospital gown. Her precious gold locket was missing from her neck, but I was too confused to find out what had happened to it.

The night nurse asked me to sign a form for the death certificate, then asked me for the name of the funeral home. My mind suddenly went blank. I could not remember and promised to call the business office in the morning. Despite her kindness, the nurse was impersonal. Practiced—I suppose one must be that way to survive as an ICU nurse. Earlier, the day nurse had noted that most patients left the ICU alive, despite their advanced ages. It is not every day that a patient dies, even in intensive care. The same policeman returned to escort me downstairs. He did not say a word—he offered not a single condolence, although he knew very well what had just happened.

The ride home at 2:15 in the morning lacked drama. After so many months of excruciating tension, my sense of urgency was instantly deflated. There was no need to rush. Mother was gone, and so was my frenetic sense of purpose. I wanted to speak to

Graziano but called Noel first out of filial loyalty. He was not surprised, and we chatted calmly for a few minutes. We felt the bond of our mutual loss, but he spoiled it by asking, "What have you decided to do about Mother's prepaid funeral?"

"Noel, I know exactly what I have to do. Let's leave it at that. I'll call you tomorrow when I've made all the arrangements."

"Will you have it on Thursday?"

"I have too much to do, too many arrangements to make. It's already Wednesday, and I'll tell you later."

Was it only three hours earlier that we had discussed the possibility of Mother's coming home and walking with a walker? Now I would wake up Graziano. There was nothing he could do, and I would rob him of sleep, but I needed to share this with him. He loved Mother and should know right away.

For months, I had been compulsively driven, so busy devoting my energy to keeping Mother alive that I never envisioned the moment of her death. When she had been on life support at Sacred Heart Hospital four months earlier, I had gone as far as to remove the envelope with the burial arrangements from the desk drawer. I had also ripped out an obituary page from the *Miami Herald*. But that is as far as I went. I refused to contemplate her death. Once the crisis was over, I put the envelope away without opening it and discarded the ripped newspaper clipping. Later, I refused to look over the burial papers, even though Mother had asked me to do that when she was at Coral Bay the second time.

Now I turned my attention to the three huge plastic bags filled with Mother's belongings. I was upset when I discovered that the Victoria Park staff had hastily rolled up Mother's carefully arranged clothes and tossed them into the bags, which they then deposited in the storage room. They had been in a big rush to remove her things from her room, as if they knew she would not return. When I retrieved the bags, the night nurse had remarked, "Oh, your poor Mother. It's for the best. This is not the way to live, to be living on oxygen." I decided to take the bags home when I heard that remark.

One by one, I cut the bags open. Mother's belongings seemed to have accumulated considerably, even though I had prepared only a few days' change of clothing. Several items were missing, including the beautiful rolled pillow I had purchased for her knees. I hung Mother's outfits neatly in the closet and then went about eliminating the most obvious signs of her numerous confinements.

I wanted everything connected with the hip fractures and everything soiled or used to be gone—the extra hospital gowns, the diapers, the plastic washbasins and mouthwash bins, the insulated pitcher, gauze pads, nonstick tape, the ointment for bedsores (expensive, I knew)—I shoved the items into the broken nursing-home bags and dragged them to the garbage bin outside. A large, dirty pillow—not Mother's—which had ended up among her things, the stained booties I had purchased at the Coral Bay gift shop, and the unmatched socks followed. Might as well eliminate the accumulated supplies from prior hospital stays too, I decided. I took the nebulizer's masks, mouthpieces, and boxes of ampoules from the dresser and threw them out. I rolled up two egg-crate mattress covers—those bulky blue foam pads shaped like egg boxes—and forced them down the chute. And one more item—the foam abduction splint, used to separate the legs of the hip fracture patient and prevent a dislocation—I threw out as well.

From the bathroom drawer, I removed the barrier cream for incontinent patients and the institutional mouthwashes and body lotions routinely given to new patients and stuck them in a garbage bag. I opened the small dresser by Mother's side of the bed and reached for the blue waterproof pads that had irritated her skin and the plastic spirometer for exercising her lungs. I tossed them in the bag. I was in a frenzy to erase the physical evidence of her prolonged convalescence. No matter how hard I tried, though, I could not force the portable commode or the special rolling walker with padded arm rests down the garbage chute. So I stuck them into the space between Dad's bureau and the window, where they would be out of my sight when I entered the bedroom. (Later, when I came to my senses, I gave the commode and walker, along with other salvageable items, to a hospice.) Finally, I discarded the last item of the evening: the stained floral sheets I had used on Mother's hospital bed at home, the ones that reminded me of the worst month of my life.

Even though the trips back and forth to the garbage chute were tiring, I did not sleep. I was restless. I pulled out the contract from Levitt-Weinstein, the funeral home, and sat down to read it. My parents had paid for their burial arrangements after Dad's near-fatal heart attack five years earlier. At first, this had seemed somewhat macabre, but now the prearrangements eliminated the need to make hasty decisions under dire conditions. It had been a tough choice for them—to be buried in South Florida, far from their beloved New York.

After a wakeful night, I called Levitt-Weinstein and set up an appointment at the funeral home's Boca Raton chapel. Then I called Marisa, who had stayed by Mother's side until I arrived from Venezuela. She was inconsolable. "Come with me today, Marisa. I really need you," I said.

"Of course. I'll come over right away."

"We have to stop at the hospital first to sign some papers and then at Victoria Park to tell Dad. I don't want to leave Dad alone while I'm at the memorial chapel."

Marisa taxied over, and we drove up to Boca Raton in silence. I had the receipt for Mother's personal effects. The receptionist in the business office was pleasant and brought me a sealed envelope. But her boss was brusque when he told me he had already received a call from Levitt-Weinstein. He did not invite me to sit down; he left me standing in the reception area while he went to check the confirmation sheet I had signed after Mother's death. Was this a harbinger of things to come? Confrontations with people who were too uncomfortable to offer condolences? Over the next few weeks I would come into contact with some people who graciously offered sympathy and others who pretended not to know. Mother's missing reading glasses resurfaced, as did her gold locket, which the emergency-room staff had removed when Mother was intubated. She had never taken it off, not even when bathing, and it had not been removed during any of her previous hospital stays. Mother had tried to give me the heart-shaped locket several years earlier, but I insisted that she keep it. I had had a sense of foreboding when I realized that the locket was missing from Mother's neck. Now I slipped the chain over my head, and we quickly left the hospital.

Dad looked sweet and unsuspecting when I found him at Victoria Park. I had sent Marisa downstairs to take him out of an activity, and she brought him to his room, then discreetly disappeared. We sat down together on the couch, and I took his hands gently in mine. "Dad, I don't know quite how to tell you this. Remember, when we visited Mother yesterday afternoon, and she was resting comfortably. After I brought you back to Victoria Park, I returned to the hospital to say goodnight to Mother. She was still all right, but later I had to return again because her heart was slowing down. Dad, her heart kept slowing, and then it stopped beating. Mother died late last night."

Dad was silent, and a shocked expression washed momentarily over his face. I told him that Mother had left us very gently.

"It's done. It's finished," he said. "How could it come to this? She was holding her own."

"Do you remember when we went to visit her yesterday, she was on a ventilator for the second time? She could not breathe on her own. She was very ill."

"I don't remember. This has completely ruined our lives."

"It's ruined my life, too, Dad. It's something we've had no control over. Mother hasn't had a life to live for the past few months. You haven't; I haven't; Graziano hasn't. Mother didn't want to go on this way."

"She never told me that."

" She didn't want to burden you, because you're not well yourself, but she told me so every day. She told Noel, and she told Aunt Gussie. Sometimes she thought she would make it home. Particularly at Victoria Park, she felt she would go home. She wanted to spare you, Dad. I know that no matter how painful her loss is going to be for me, it will be far worse for you. I'll be with you, Dad. I'll try to help you."

"It's going to be very lonely. And even though this is a beautiful place, it must be very lonely to spend the rest of your life in a nursing home."

"I know what you mean. But there's no reason for you to stay here, Dad. You were only here to be near Mother. I'm taking you home. You belong at home. Marisa has agreed to come back to the house, and I'll go back and forth."

Marisa reappeared, and we accompanied Dad to the dining room. He ate a tuna-fish salad like a zombie while Marisa and I picked at our lunches. I left Dad and Marisa sitting on the terrace while I drove to Levitt-Weinstein. I was nervous. As a lapsed

Jew who had married a lapsed Catholic and lived in a Catholic country for the past twenty years, I knew nothing about Jewish burial rites. Even with the preplanned arrangements, I was there for more than three hours. It was quiet, out of season, as the elderly snowbirds had not yet arrived. Mother's interment was the only one scheduled for Friday. I steeled myself to speak calmly with Jacob Weiss, the funeral director and counselor. His approach was just right—personable without pressure and consistently solemn. I wanted to respect Mother's arrangements for a graveside service at Beth David Memorial Gardens but ordered a casket bouquet of pink and white carnations with baby's breath. Flowers denote happiness in Jewish tradition and are never displayed at funeral services, but Mother loved fresh-cut flowers. Jewish custom also calls for an immediate burial, but I needed the extra day to finish up and give my brother, husband, and maternal aunt enought time to fly in. Graz was still housebound, and I did not intend to bring him to Florida.

"The official mourning period will be very short, only a day," Weiss said. "Saturday is Rosh Hashanah. You will sit *shiva* for one day only."

"Why is that?" I asked.

"Ordinarily, the period of *shiva* lasts for seven days. [Not unlike the Catholic novena of nine days.] But Jewish law dictates that when a religious festival intervenes, this is a joyous occasion and must take precedence over mourning."

How odd, I thought, for one's private sorrow to be superseded in such a way. Of course, only the "official" mourning would be cut short. In contemporary society, only the most religious families maintain this tradition. It struck me that an official mourning period has the same purpose among different religions—to segregate the grieving family from the rest of society for a specified time and acknowledge their loss by ceremoniously paying last respects.

I did not return to Victoria Park until nearly Dad's dinnertime. He was still conversing quietly with Marisa after having spent the afternoon on the terrace.

"Dad, I'm not going to take you home tonight. I don't have any food in the house, and I'll have to spend a few hours calling everybody. I feel terrible about this, but I think it's best for both of us. I'll come back early in the morning to take you home. Do you think you'll be all right?"

"Yes," he said. "I'll be fine. Don't worry."

We escorted Dad to the second-floor dining room and settled him in at the table. I sat with him while Marisa went to his room to start packing his things. I did not tell his tablemates that Mother had just died. I asked the man on Dad's left, who had a head of beautiful white hair, why he was in the assisted-living division of Victoria Park. It was a long story, and he didn't want to go into it. But to sum up, he said, "Nobody wants to be bothered with old people. My children have no time for me." I could imagine the story behind those words and resolved to come back in the future to interview the residents. A woman at the adjoining table was sobbing bitterly and refused to eat dinner.

"What's the matter?" her private aide asked, taking her charge's hands.

"Nothing, nothing, I just feel so alone."

"You're not alone. You have me."

I listened to this interchange with sorrow. Then I led Dad back to his room and helped him prepare for bed, promising to pick him up early the next morning.

I went home to an empty house—poignantly empty, because now I knew my mother would never return. I called her dearest friends and felt the closeness of her presence. Then I went to her bedroom and meticulously arranged her burial clothing on the empty bed. She had already told me what she wanted to be buried in. I set the rosy chiffon suit alongside the accessories, my movements guided by her silent wishes and filled with infinite sadness.

Who Decides?

Resuscitation and an Equitable Decision

MY CONVERSATION with Dr. Dawson was not an easy one and could have come about only after many months of watching Mother's decline and being involved in her fruitless efforts to recover from a double hip fracture. Dr. Dawson was the first of Mother's physicians to broach the matter of continuing her treatment. "How aggressive do you want your Mother's treatment to be?" he asked. Because of her recent intubation, she obviously was no longer in a position to voice her opinion. Whether she wanted to be intubated or had given her approval I never satisfactorily determined. If she had given her consent, it must have been because she was gasping for breath, and the intubation would relieve her discomfort. She probably would have died right then if she had not been put on a mechanical ventilator. But the treatment was initiated against the wishes that were clearly set forth in her advance directives.

Now it was too late to ask the patient about the treatment plan, which is why her attending physician turned to her children. "Pretending that a half-conscious patient fighting hard for breath is able to think, evaluate, and rationally choose and consent is ridiculous," notes Lofty Basta (1996:231). Although Mother had spelled out the dos and don'ts of the treatment she wanted, her written directives once again failed to follow her to the hospital. I felt extremely uncomfortable about discontinuing a treatment that was already in progress because I did not know whether the invasive therapy would save her life or would prolong her death.

Recently I came across an excellent analysis of the problems involved with treating the critically ill elderly by the neurosurgeon Bryan Jennett. He breaks the decision-making process regarding treatment down into three therapeutic categories: life saving, such as cardiopulmonary resuscitation; life sustaining, such as dialysis and tube feeding; and life enhancing, such as coronary bypass. Deciding which therapies to employ should be done in the context of the patient's health status. "There are those who, being previously well, have a sudden unexpected crisis—a heart attack, stroke, or head injury," Jennett writes. "In such instances an initial trial of treatment will almost always be justified before any decision is made about whether to continue treatment. Quite different are patients with progressive disorders in whom a predictable crisis or relapse occurs and about whom some prior discussion about limiting future treatment may have been held with the patient and family. These will include patients with progressive organ failure . . . and those with advanced cancer or dementia. A third category are those already disabled by progressive disease who fall victim to an unpredictable accident or acute illness unrelated to their existing disease" (1994:21). Mother, of course, fell into that third category. Bearing in mind the three broad objectives of treatment outlined by Jennett— saving, sustaining, or enhancing life—can make the decision to treat, continue treatment, or discontinue treatment more a pragmatic matter than an emotional one.

Weighing the expected benefits of treatment against the possible harm enhances the probability of arriving at an appropriate decision. The decision should be seen from the perspective of the patient, who might judge even limited gains quite differently from the family or the medical team. The doctor's task is to set forth the options, discuss them with the patient and his or her caregivers, and achieve a degree of consensus that will enable him to act in the patient's best interest.

But how many of us will ever be exposed to ideal conditions in which the patient, family, and doctor act in unison to reach the "right" decision? With the exception of Dr. Klein, who spoke frankly at Coral Bay, Dr. Dawson was the only physician to give me a clear idea of Mother's prognosis. Perhaps none of her other physicians considered her ill enough to warrant such a discussion. Near the end, Mother's chances were slim and her condition was rapidly deteriorating. Dr. Dawson could offer little encouragement. I had to decide for Mother. And I had to make the right decision. It was a weighty responsibility and far more difficult than making my own decisions. Mother must be permitted to react favorably to the massive infusion of antibiotics, but must be subjected to no more *invasive* lifesaving interventions, I finally decided. And I knew instinctively that she would have been in accord.

Many adult children in my position have to make this type of decision, and the shadow of doubt lingers. Here lies the ultimate mortality lesson—one that we must all accept: There comes a moment when we have to let go and say, "It is time."

CHAPTER EIGHT

Heartbroken

"I have only my memories."

SEPTEMBER 22, 1993–JULY 25, 1994: 10 MONTHS • Dad
was now at grave risk. I wondered how his bereavement would
affect his health. He had always reacted to Mother's medical
crises with tremendous anxiety. They had been inseparable partners for fifty-nine years, and living without his wife was inconceivable. Mother had provided the structure in Dad's life; she had
nurtured him and arranged his day. Could Dad cope without her?
I thought about Richard Nixon, who had succumbed to a heart
ailment eleven months after the death of his beloved Pat. And
Will and Ariel Durant, lifelong partners and working collabo-
rators, died within thirteen days of each other. Less-well-known
couples have suffered similar ends. One of my colleagues lost his
father five months after his mother's death. The father simply lost
his will to live.

Losing an elderly spouse is particularly traumatic for partners
who have rarely been separated. The death of a lifelong partner
accelerates the aging process and frequently portends one's own
demise. This is not merely anecdotal. Studies show that widow-
ers older than seventy are the most vulnerable, experiencing a
48 percent mortality increase during the first three months of
bereavement (Bronte 1993:33). The increased risk encompasses
not only the normal sense of grief but also the loss of a supportive companion who has helped maintain the aging couple's delicate balance. The loss actually begins before the spouse's death,
because the ill person can no longer provide mutual support, sap-
ping the strength of the "well" partner and exacerbating the level
of stress. When elderly spouses compensate for each other's deficiencies, the death of one can have devastating effects on the functional capacities of the other, particularly if the remaining partner is also in poor health. The bereft spouse may lack the social
and psychological support to weather the crisis because he or she

lives far from the adult children or has already outlived many contemporaries. Alone and ailing, he or she may quickly follow the deceased spouse to the grave.

Spousal grief also complicates the grieving children's mourning process—and more so when the surviving parent is chronically ill. Rather than passing through the stages of bereavement, the children are immediately thrust into the role of caring for the remaining, ailing parent. They must sublimate their feelings to function as effective caregivers and may have little time to mourn properly.

Once Mother was gone, Dad complained that I neglected him. He was getting forgetful, he reminded me, and was having difficulty with his balance. Why wasn't I doing something about it? Dad's condition had changed dramatically, but I did not take a good look at him until after Mother's death. His neck had collapsed, and his head was thrust prominently forward, giving him a curved profile. He took rapid, mincing steps to maintain his balance and could barely rise from a chair without falling forward. His elbows were permanently bent into an unnatural position, and he held his arms pressed forward against his torso, with his hands dangling lifelessly. His entire stance was rigid. Even when he slept, he curled up tightly into a fetal position and seemed unable to straighten out.

"Dad," I said one evening while tucking him in, "why don't you try to relax? I'm sure you'll sleep better."

"I am relaxed," he insisted as he coiled in one corner of the queen-size bed, apparently incapable of extending his legs or resting his head comfortably on the pillow.

I was especially alarmed because Dad's physical deterioration seemed to accompany symptoms of apathy and increasing forgetfulness. I decided to take him for a neurological workup. Dr. Hafner recommended David Adler, a neurologist affiliated with Coral Bay whose practice included a large number of elderly patients.

I spoke briefly with Dr. Adler by phone, as did Dr. Hafner, and I took Dad for his exam exactly a week after Mother's death. When Dad was called, I got up to follow him into the examining room. The nurse asked me to wait outside.

"I always accompany my father during his medical appointments," I said.

"The doctor would like to see your father alone," she responded. "When he's finished with the exam, he'll call you in."

I reluctantly returned to my seat. For fifteen years, I had followed both of my parents into the examining room and served as a neutral pair of eyes and ears. This allowed me to stay abreast of their medical histories and remind them of what had been said.

Dad had been inside for a few minutes when the nurse motioned for me to join him. Dr. Adler appeared unhurried and reminded me, as I observed his unruly beard, of an aging Haight-Ashbury straggler.

"I asked your father a few questions, and I'm afraid he was unable to respond very well. Do you want to know how he responded?"

Not really, I thought, suspecting that Dad had failed this "test" miserably. But I replied, "What did you ask him?"

"Your father did not know who the president of the United States is. He said Nixon. He also said that we're in the state of Connecticut, and when I asked him the year, he claimed it was 1910."

"He merely confused today's date with his birthdate. Did you ask him anything else?"

"Yes. He was unable to do some simple calculations."

I did not feel that the results of this cognitive test were especially conclusive. Dad had known the date earlier in the day and probably could have come up with Bill Clinton's name if he had been given a few more seconds to think about it. I was more worried about the sudden onset of his balance and gait problems than his rapid memory decline. I told Dr. Adler about my mother's death and explained that her illness had taken a heavy toll on my father's health. Perhaps he had suffered a series of small strokes, but my gut feeling was that he was in the midst of a severe depression.

Dr. Adler was not impressed with my interpretation and did not take an extensive medical history. He quickly concluded that Dad had moderate dementia, a syndrome characterized by the loss of cognitive abilities, complicated by a Parkinson's-like "syndrome." The causes were probably multi-factorial, he said, and caused in large part by Dad's degenerative vascular disease.

Now I had a new disease to worry about: Dad's descent into dementia with Parkinson's-like overtones. Although I was certain that depression had caused the swift decline in Dad's mental condition, I was not sure what had caused the Parkinson's-like rigidity, imbalance, and shuffling gait to emerge so suddenly. I did not know that more elderly people suffer from the symptoms of Parkinson's than generally suspected.

I wanted Dad to undergo some diagnostic tests, but Dr. Adler felt this was unnecessary. Even if he had suffered several mini-strokes, they might not be apparent in a scan. "What difference does it make what the causes are?" he asked. "One has to deal with the resulting manifestations." I am not a neurologist, but I knew my father better than Dr. Adler did. Six months earlier, Dad had not worried about losing his balance and falling down. I suspected that his fear of falling had an emotional component that was powerfully related to Mother's fall and that this association was an important factor in his present condition.

"Surely, there is some medication that can help my father's memory," I said. "What about tacrine?" Tacrine, marketed as Cognex, had just been approved by the FDA to treat Alzheimer's disease and was being hyped in the press as the new miracle drug for memory problems. A British expert on the effects of aging on the brain had touted it as "the first medication to be shown, unequivocally, to be of any benefit to people with Alzheimer's" (as quoted in Hirschler 1993:6). Others were more cautious, claiming that the drug's effects were modest, at best.

"Don't get your hopes up regarding that one," Dr. Adler said. "The only reason that drug is being promoted is for political reasons. After so many years, this is the answer for all those people clamoring for an Alzheimer's drug, but it's not especially effective." He went on to say that the drug benefited only a small number of patients (about 20 percent) and was most effective in the beginning stages of the disease, when it might have a slight impact on recall. Furthermore, one's liver enzymes had to be closely monitored, and the drug could not slow the degenerative, progressive nature of the disease. He dismissed the idea that such a drug could counteract the memory impairment normally associated with aging.

"What about flumazenil for memory disorders, or melatonin for sleep disturbances?" I persisted.

"No, those are very experimental," Dr. Adler answered. "Maybe sometime in the future we'll have such drugs, but right now we have to content ourselves with what's available. I suggest we try to deal with the Parkinson's-like syndrome. I would like to prescribe Sinemet. It is the least innocuous of the Parkinson's drugs and may help your father's gait. Anything else will just increase his confusion. We'll begin with a half-tab twice daily, increasing to three times a day after two weeks. Come back in a few weeks, and we'll re-evaluate his situation."

I decided to give it one more try. "Well, what about physical-therapy sessions to improve my dad's muscle tone and help his balance?"

"I could prescribe physical therapy for your father, but I don't really see the point. It may help somewhat, but I doubt he'll be able to remember and put the things he's learned into practice."

I thanked Dr. Adler. He was pleasant and straightforward, but I was not happy with the visit. I felt he had written Dad off too quickly. All he had done was glance at Dad—a frail old man with a shuffling walk—to make a quick assessment of his condition. But he could have done all sorts of simple standardized diagnostic tests right in his own office to provide a more rounded picture of Dad's mental status. I knew Dad felt deeply humiliated by his failure to answer three simple questions.

Despite Dr. Adler's opinon, I was sure that some of Dad's symptoms were reversible. But was my gut feeling correct? I could not articulate my concerns to the neurologist. Only several months later, after attending several geriatrics conferences on mental health and dementia, was I able to pinpoint the key to my dissatisfaction: Dementia has a complicated etiology, and a meticulous diagnosis is necessary to determine whether one is dealing with a progressive or a reversible condition. A diagnosis of true dementia certainly cannot be made cursorily.

Sometimes depression can be so severe that it masquerades as dementia. Pseudo-dementia is certainly reversible. Dad did show some signs of depression: The onset of his symptoms was both acute and rapid, he lost weight, and he could not sleep. Perhaps Dad could return to normal by overcoming his depression, though I doubted any pill could help him deal with his loss. I kept Dr. Hafner's warning in mind: Sleeping pills and antidepressants were troublemakers. They might help momentarily, but they would also increase Dad's confusion and interact negatively with his heart medications.

I explained all of this to Dad. I was optimistic that Sinemet, a medication that has been around since the late 1960s, would help his balance, and I cautioned him to be patient for a few weeks. His memory would probably improve, I assured him, as he over-came the immediate shock of Mother's death. I reminded him that the CT scan done just a few months earlier, when he had changed cardiologists, was normal. Dad agreed to cooperate because he was despondent over losing his memory. The anthropologist Melvin Konner put it succinctly when he wrote, "Few things are feared more by older people today than having a wise old age turned into a mewling, doddering, tantrum-filled second infancy; than being robbed of memory itself, one of the things that most makes life—especially later life—worth living" (1987:105).

• • •

Dad's mental condition had started to deteriorate when Mother's physical condition worsened. He became increasingly forgetful, and his short-term memory disappeared at a frightful pace. When he went to the kitchen for a glass of water, he forgot what he wanted once he got there. His ability to concentrate and his atten-tion span were limited—he read the headlines but not the text, and he read small sections of a book on organic healing over and over. He started Gay Talese's *Unto the Sons*, a marvelous book about growing up in New Jersey as the son of an Italian emigrant, and got stuck on page 159, which he kept rereading. Dad refused to give up on the Talese book, insisting he had only a few hundred pages to go. He lost all interest in answering the phone, opening his mail, and following the plot of a weekly situation comedy. His night wandering grew more frequent, and he had trouble find-ing his way to the bathroom and back. When I was around, I often had to rescue him from the bathtub at the crack of dawn, when, in a semi-somnambulant state, he assured me it was time to awake and shower. I was particularly upset to learn that he did not remember how to adjust the showerhead after turning on the bathtub taps. I found out about this by accident when he insisted I call a plumber to fix the broken shower. Outside his cozy home environment, his spatial disorientation was obvious. He could not leave Mother's hospital room without getting lost.

Dad tried to compensate for his forgetfulness by using any substitute that occurred to him while he fished for the right words. I constantly had to reassure him that nobody would take his home away, and we went over his bank and stock statements every day. He had no doubt that their illnesses would leave them not only homeless but also penniless. One day he left me a note: "June needs a permanent person to take care of her. I also need a permanent home to take care of me. So it goes. The only way to beat it is to die early." I tried hard to assuage his fears and knew that he believed me when I spoke to him. Dad also had moments of complete mental acuity, and we discussed Mother's condition and chances for recovery in a straightforward, logical way.

By the time Mother died, Dad had visited her several times daily in four different hospitals, and he had bounced back and forth between home and two nursing homes to be with her. The ponderous toll on Dad's health over these months was obvious. Scientists have noted that the increasing poor health of one spouse is the strongest predictor of the other spouse's failing health. When Mother fell, Dad was perfectly capable of meeting his own personal needs. Five months later, he required total care. Dad accepted some of the care because it was convenient. Why should he shave himself when Marisa did such a splendid job? Why bother setting the table or shucking the corn when I was there to do it? Generally, though, Dad was not faking. He could no longer dress himself. I laid out his clothes in the morning and helped him into them after a shower, assisted by Marisa. In the evening I helped him into his pajamas. He could not unbutton his shirt and tore the buttons apart in frustration. Yet in the early morning, no matter how wakeful Marisa or I had been, he would get up in a jacket or shirt and pants, having changed by himself during the night. Sometimes the pajamas were missing; sometimes he placed his clothing over his pajamas. At other times, he scattered miscellaneous pieces of clothing around the bedroom. He had no recollection of doing any of this. When I asked him why he got dressed in the middle of the night, he replied that he had to get ready for work. Dad's dexterity was gone, and we had to brush his teeth, trim his nails, and rub his dry skin with lotion—in short, do whatever was necessary to present Dad to the world as a well-groomed and neatly dressed gentleman.

In the midst of all this, Dad said that he wanted to start driving again. He could probably function on automatic pilot, but it was clearly out of the question. "No, Dad," I said. "I don't think this is a good time to think about driving when you're having problems with your balance."

"Well, maybe you're right," he said.

I knew that the issue was not the driving but his growing sense that he was losing his independence. I shuddered to think what might happen if Dad did take off in the car. I instructed Marisa to put away the extra keys and keep her own set in her bag. Then Dad found another issue: "I'd like to buy a new car. I've been thinking about it for a while now."

"I know, Dad, you mentioned it before Mother fell," I answered, "but you were still driving then. Do you think it's a good idea to buy a new car for Marisa to drive? When I took the Toyota in for an oil change, your old friends at the shop said it was still a great car. As a matter of fact, they told me to congratulate you for taking such good care of it."

I could see that Dad was not moved. "Well, maybe I'll wait a while until my eyesight improves, but I'd still like to get a new car."

Dad had more trouble finding the right words for objects and frequently left his sentences dangling. His conversations with me were disjointed. When I asked him a question, he responded with an entirely unrelated matter. Dad dealt with his memory loss by inventing elaborate stories that impressed me with their clever juxtaposition of vivid details. Sadly, none of them was vaguely true. Dad fooled a lot of people at first, but he could not fool himself. He knew he had a big problem but thought he might be able to salvage some remnant of his past by reconstructing a new reality. This ruse, called *confabulation*, is deployed to compensate, however inadequately, for the extensive memory loss that so profoundly demoralizes and humiliates the dementia patient.

Dad also had moments of excessive restlessness. He wandered from room to room, talking animatedly to himself or an invisible party. He frequently moved his hands up and down in the air, creating strange kinetic patterns with his darting fingers. When I was not looking, he tied the sheets or pieces of clothing into knots so tight that I needed a screwdriver to pry them loose. He compulsively moved papers from one place to another in no particular order, then rolled them into balls. Then he lost interest and discarded them. He tore apart magazines for no reason and bunched up his clothing with rubberbands. He folded, unfolded, and refolded the kitchen towels and aprons in tiny, neat squares. He stuck pins in the kitchen bulletin board, making thousands of tiny slivers on the notes.

Dad was having increasing problems with his balance and looked as if he would fall over when he arose from a chair. I bought him a three-prong aluminum cane to lean on and tried to teach him to use Mother's walker when he got up, but he could not remember no matter how many times we went over it. I lived in constant terror that he would fall and, God forbid, fracture a hip. The pressure of watching Dad around-the-clock—not only to protect him from himself but also to determine whether he was showing new signs of physical or mental diminishment—was exhausting.

I do not doubt that Dad missed Mother profoundly, even though he rarely verbalized his feelings. When I finally returned to Caracas in late October, I wondered whether he remembered her death. When I called, he told me that Mother was shopping or in the kitchen cooking. The conversation faltered, because Dad did not have much to say.

"Shall I call Mother? Would you like to talk to Mother?"

"No, Dad. You know that Mother is gone. You do remember that, don't you? Mother died in September, and we went to her funeral together."

"Yes. I forgot, but just for the moment. I'll never forget. It was so big. That's one thing I'll never forget."

I vacillated between humoring Dad and pulling him back to reality. After all, to mourn properly you must have an ongoing memory of your loss. Dad reminded me of the story the novelist Isabel Allende tells in *Paula* (1994) about her father-in-law. He had retreated into oblivion shortly after attending his wife's funeral, and a curtain of senility descended on him from which he was never able to recover. Was this also Dad's way to protect himself from the pain of losing his dearest companion?

When I returned to Florida three weeks later, I realized that Dad had not forgotten. He wrote notes to himself—almost doodles—that he left scattered on his desk, in the kitchen, and slipped into newspapers, magazines, and books. "June," "June Margolies," "Yukie, Yukie"—Dad wrote Mother's name and childhood nickname over and over, filling the page and its margins with her name and address. More notes surfaced as I did the paperwork—"Albert and June," "June and Albert," "June and Nemie [Dad's nickname]," "Yukie and Nemie." Mother had been named after her mother's baby brother, Yankel, and was called Yukie by her mother. I could not remember how Dad's nickname originated. Wherever I placed a pad and pencil for Dad to jot with, he left this written memorial to his departed wife.

"I know Mother is really gone," he told me. "I know Mother has left us. How could this happen? My whole life is turned upside down. How could this happen to me?"

I had heard this lament before. Several times, Dad had reiterated his list of ailments, expressing surprise that so many could befall one person. Now he had to continue alone. How could I comfort him except to say that we shared the loss, however unequally, and that I would always take care of him? Dad rarely complained, and I knew this was his way to express grief.

"I have nothing to look forward to," he said. "I see the future. I know it. The grim reaper is coming for me, too."

I wished I could have the old Dad back—the one who chatted with me late into the night and relished storytelling; the one who called me long-distance on the spur of the moment, when everyone else was sleeping, just to say hello; the authentic father who said how he truly felt. Now I had to guess his feelings and make do with fleeting moments of clarity. I had to accept Dad's mental and physical deterioration and acknowledge my own limitations in relieving his suffering. I also had to be honest with myself: Dad probably would get worse. He had become one of the frail, vulnerable elderly, and his condition could change in an instant.

• • •

Mother came to me one evening as I napped on the couch. Her head floated just above my own and seemed to be encased in a brilliant globe. She was shouting, warning me, calling for help, yet no sound escaped from her lips. Her face was contorted in pain. She was suffering, I knew, and wanted to warn me about something, something to do with Dad. I could not understand. I awoke with a start. "Mother, Mother," I cried, "tell me what you want. Is it about Dad? Don't leave me, Mother, please!" Mother continued to cry for help as her face faded away.

I had just flown to New York after visiting Dad two months after Mother's death and had fallen asleep on the sofa. Was this just a dream, or was Mother really trying to reach me? I knew that her soul was not at peace, that she had not yet found her final resting place. I shivered. She was waiting for Dad. I was devastated. I had wanted a sign, but all I saw was her suffering face.

Dad had not improved after completing the eight-week course of Sinemet. His short-term memory was gone. He seemed to be emotionally anesthetized and not especially interested in what went on around him. Bits of history occasionally filtered through, but in many ways Dad had already undergone a social death. Nearly his entire life story was now out of his grasp.

Dad snapped out of his trancelike state once. It was three months after Mother's death, and New Year's Eve was approaching. Graziano had accepted an invitation to be a scholar-in-residence at the Getty Center in Los Angeles. Before we left Caracas, I had mentioned to Graziano that I wanted to ignore the holidays and spend a few quiet days with Dad before flying to California. He agreed. But a week later, at Dad's home in Florida, Graziano suggested opening a bottle of champagne to bring in the new year. "No," I said. "No champagne. I don't want to celebrate."

"Don't be silly," he answered. "We're not celebrating, just making a small toast."

"Graziano, please understand, I don't want to open a bottle of champagne. I don't even want to stay up, and I'm certainly not in the mood to celebrate."

"You're being ridiculous."

"Maybe, so, but I'd like you to respect my feelings."

The argument escalated—in front of our son, in front of my father, right in the middle of dinner. It was clearly my fault. I had no patience with my husband or the holidays or any other intrusion on my private grief.

Dad listened to all this and suddenly perked up, becoming his old self. "I think you're being unreasonable, Luisa," he said. "I don't think Graziano has been out of place or done anything to justify your anger. Why are you acting this way? Now let's sit quietly and finish our dinner."

I simmered down, surprised and silenced by the unexpected clarity of Dad's words. I was thrilled to hear Dad sound like his old self. But I had spoiled my family's New Year toast and behaved badly in front of my ailing father.

"You're right, Dad. I guess I'm in a bad mood and haven't learned to cope with holidays in Mother's absence," I said. Dad looked at me, then went back to his usual phlegmatic state. New Year's Eve was ruined. The next day, however, Dad did not remember a single aspect of this unpleasant exchange.

• • •

We were comfortably installed in an apartment in Santa Monica, and I expected to bring Dad and Marisa to the West Coast for a few weeks. Dad's condition was stable, and Dr. Hafner said it would be safe for him to fly. Then, on January 17, a big earthquake hit Los Angeles, trashing our first-floor apartment. We moved to a hotel in Marina del Rey as aftershocks continued to open jagged cracks in our apartment's walls. Dad certainly could not come to Los Angeles under these circumstances. I would have to go to Dad.

Dad always sounded wonderful on the phone. His voice never lost its youthful timbre, and even though his conversation was halting, we still chatted away. But Marisa's reports were disconcerting. I did not doubt that the repetitious patterns of bizarre behavior that she described—the "getting stuck" syndrome discussed in *The 36-Hour Day* (Mace and Rabins 1981)—had claimed another victim in my poor dad.

Two weeks before I was scheduled to visit South Florida, Marisa called with disturbing news. Dad was feeling unwell and lethargic. He had fallen out of bed at dawn and called for her. She found him sitting on the carpet with a small cut on his forehead. I asked her to pass the phone to Dad. Although he reassured me that he felt fine and would ring for Marisa when he wanted to get up during the night, he could not remember to call for help.

Dad had fallen a few times during the past year, and I was petrified that he would fracture a bone. I had tried to accident-proof the house. I padded the living-room coffee table with heavy blankets and placed pillows near the sliding glass doors. I moved the rocking chair away from the bed. I installed a raised toilet seat with handles and additional grab bars in Dad's bathroom. I stuck a broom handle in the shower-door track to prevent Dad from showering unsupervised. I told Marisa I would call Associated Nursing to hire a nighttime aide.

"No," she said. "I can manage. I'm a light sleeper, and I'll hear Mr. Albert if he gets up. I'm going to sleep on the couch for the next few nights. I don't like the way the aides talk to your dad. They're impatient, and they don't know how to be gentle. They'll only bother him. Then I'll have to check on the aide and make sure she's not sleeping herself."

"We'll talk about it when I arrive, but please be sure to shower when Dad's sleeping so you don't leave him alone."

By the time I reached Florida, the only evidence of Dad's fall was a small scab on his forehead. Marisa had been doing a splendid job of caregiving. Dad was calm and impeccably groomed. The patches of dry skin that had plagued him were gone; his mustache was neatly trimmed; his bushy black eyebrows were carefully combed; and his cotton shirts were ironed. Marisa kept a close eye on Dad's keys, wallet, and glasses—possessions he had to have with him at all times. I made sure he always had $100 in his wallet so he could take us out to lunch and pay for the gas. Marisa also had taken my admonishments to keep Dad physically active seriously, and she cajoled him into a daily routine he clearly relished. Twice a day, Marisa walked up and down the catwalk with Dad, and she had him doing relaxed calisthenics. When the weather permitted, they walked in the shallow end of the pool.

I felt that as long as Dad could stand on his own feet and walk, he would survive. Physical mobility was the key. As Walter Bortz has shown, mobility and the life force itself are inextricably bound. The risk of death among the elderly increases in direct proportion to their difficulties in moving around. If Dad could just maintain his current level of wellness, I would be satisfied. But what if Dad had a stroke or another heart attack? I did not think he would survive these catastrophes, and even if he did, the consequences were too terrifying to imagine.

After Mother's death, away from the stress of the hospital setting, I had plenty of time to think through the ethical and moral issues and had made some fundamental decisions on my own about Dad's care. Several months earlier, Dad had signed a living-will declaration, a health-care-surrogate form, and a durable power of attorney form, all sanctioned under Florida law. These documents reiterated Dad's long-standing objection to prolonging his life by using heroic measures, and they legally allowed me to make all health-care decisions on his behalf. Dad also signed a general power of attorney designating me to act on his behalf in all matters. I was in no mood for fruitless discussions with my brother about nursing homes. But Noel surprised me by saying how impressed he was with Marisa's devotion to Dad and how pleased he was with my decision to care for Dad at home. Dad's experience at Victoria Park had been good, thanks to the kind, concerned staff. But the miserable memories of The Palms were indelible.

I was equally determined that Dad would never return to the hospital, where he might become the unwilling subject of overzealous attempts to prolong his life. Perhaps if Dad had his wits about him he would be able to survive another hospital stay intact, but he could not do so in his present condition. What Dad needed was care at home. Mother and I had discussed this many times. She felt that, if she predeceased Dad, he should go directly to a facility because he would not be able to function on his own.

But these discussions were clearly theoretical, and I was sure that if Mother had had the chance to rethink the matter after her own experience at The Palms, she would surely agree I was doing the right thing.

I personally gave copies of Dad's living will and health-care-surrogate forms to his physicians. I also left phone and fax numbers at which I could be reached at any time. I put two sets of the documents in brightly colored binders on Dad's desk. Marisa had witnessed and signed the forms, and we went over the contents several times. She understood Dad's feelings and mine. We reviewed the emergency procedures again and again. I told her she must react to changes in Dad's condition calmly. If he complained about chest pains, she should put a nitroglycerin tablet under his tongue, make him a cup of heavily sugared tea, and call me immediately. This would keep her busy for a few minutes so we could assess the situation, by which time a crisis might be averted.

This approach was anti-medical but sanely humane. I did not want to think beyond that point. I knew if Dad went back to a hospital, he would become confused and agitated and probably would be sedated and restrained. He might end up in an ICU, where he would be attached to monitoring and lifesaving equipment. His heart was so damaged that he would not live through it, and the process of saving his life would in fact be a futile prolonging of his death. Dad was right where he wanted to be and was adamant about never returning to the hospital. When it was his time to go, he wanted to be home. I prayed Dad would not have an incident that would require me to violate his wishes, because if he went to a hospital, I would not be able to buck the system.

Leaving Dad to return to California was almost unbearably difficult. I felt a tremendous responsibility toward Dad and knew I could not let him down. He had been sweet and trusting, imploring me to stay longer. I did, but it was now time to return to Santa Monica for the conclusion of Graziano's fellowship.

"Do you have to leave?" Dad kept asking.

"I wish I could take you with me, Dad, but we're packing up to go home."

"Stay a few more days," he urged.

"I already have. I wish I could stay even longer, Dad. I'm going to miss you terribly, but I can't leave Graziano and Graz alone any longer. I'll be back next month, and then we'll spend the rest of the summer together."

Things were quiet for a few weeks, but on July 6, Marisa called me in Los Angeles with bad news. Dad lost his balance rising from his chair and had fallen, hitting his arm on the glass door. Graziano, who was en route to Caracas, stopped in Florida to check on Dad. He said that Dad had a badly bruised arm, was unresponsive, and did not seem to know him. Marisa, however, claimed that Dad was fine and had suffered no ill effects from the fall.

"Marisa," I said, "please keep an eye on Dad, and try to avoid any more falls. If you think he's not feeling well or has one of those episodes you've been telling me about, call me immediately. Don't tell me about it later."

Another call came on July 15. "Mr. Albert had another fall," Marisa said, "this time when he went to the bathroom. He hit his head on the tile floor."

I was upset that Marisa had been showering when this incident occurred. I had asked her to shower while Dad was sleeping, but I tried not to place blame. The damage had been done. "What happened, Marisa? Is Dad O.K.?" I asked.

"He's having an episode again, but he seems to be coming out of it."

"Marisa, put my father on the phone."

"Dad, can you hear me? Tell me what happened?"

"I felpudit en barrrrrseeemmmmme, ugugugugugugu."

I could not understand a word he said. He was talking gibberish. "Dad, speak more slowly," I implored, "and repeat what you just said."

"Ohh, dorshinsleee barrseemmmeee, ugugugug."

"Dad, put Marisa back on the phone *now!*"

But Dad did not put Marisa back on the line. He held on to the phone, and she finally took it from him.

"Marisa, you never told me that Dad's speech sounded like that. You must realize he's had some sort of neurological episode, maybe even a stroke. I'm going to call the neurologist right now, and I'll get back to you in a few minutes. Meanwhile, call Dr. Hafner and set up an emergency appointment today."

Dad's speech was aphasic. Perhaps he had had small strokes during his earlier falls. "Abrupt, little worsenings" is how Sherwin Nuland describes the barely perceptible, irregular series of strokes that lead to multi-infarct dementia (1994:67). I called the neurologist and insisted that Dad be given an imaging scan that afternoon. Something was brewing, but I did not know what. Dad was sleeping excessively during the day. As soon as he sat down in his favorite chair, he fell asleep, yet the minute he retired for the night, he was up, wandering back and forth between his bed and the bathroom. A pattern emerged in which Dad slept profoundly for an hour or two in the late evening, followed by several hours of wakefulness. We tried herbal teas with honey, warm milk and soda crackers, snacks, reading aloud, chatting—nothing seem to help Dad achieve a normal sleep pattern. I refused to use sedatives. They might help correct Dad's sleep disturbances but would add to his confusion.

Later that day Marisa told me that Dad could not have a MRI because the scan would interfere with his pacemaker's electrical impulses. I wondered why the neurologist, who was well aware of Dad's chronic heart condition, had not anticipated this problem. A CT scan was scheduled for Monday, when Dad also had an appointment with Dr. Hafner. His speech had returned to normal, and aside from the bruise on the right side of his face, he did not seem to be experiencing other ill effects from the fall.

The weekend passed miserably. I vacillated between flying to Florida at once and waiting until I received the CT scan results. Graz and I planned to leave Los Angeles the following week, anyway. I had already shipped most of our books and papers to Caracas. Better to pack up the remnants and be ready to leave immediately, I thought. It was impossible to concentrate on work, but the packing was necessary and would keep me busy. Graz could always follow after he finished summer school. It was time for me to face an unpleasant truth. Dad could not be left alone. He needed twenty-four-hour surveillance to prevent these constant falls.

On Monday morning, a call from Dr. Hafner woke me up. "I have your father in my office right this minute," he said. "I don't like what I see. Your father is very confused, and I think he's dehydrated. He could expire anytime. I want to put him in the hospital right now to hydrate him."

"Dr. Hafner, I don't want my dad to go to the hospital," I said. "It will only confuse him more. I'm afraid he'll get worse in the hospital. Can't you hydrate him in your office?"

"No, I can't do that. I don't have the equipment here. Furthermore, he may have a subdural hematoma, and we'll have to do a scan immediately."

The doctor's warning that Dad "could expire anytime" was terrifying. It also created an obvious dilemma: Although I did not want Dad placed where he could be subjected to futile procedures to save his life if something went wrong, I also did not want my actions to be responsible for his untimely death.

"I'll tell you what," Dr. Hafner continued, "I'll put him in for twenty-four hours as an outpatient, but we won't check him in. We'll observe him, and if he's better after the hydration, he'll go home."

"Dr. Hafner," I reasoned, "my father cannot stay alone in the hospital. I want Marisa with him every minute. It's better all around. He'll cooperate with the treatment, and I'll feel easier."

"Well, I'll bend the rules. Don't worry about it. Now, suppose your father gets worse?"

"Could we take it one step at a time? I don't know why, but I just feel he'll get better. It will take me ten to fifteen hours to get there from California, even if I leave right away, so I'd rather wait a few hours. We're leaving for Florida next week, anyway, but if the situation warrants I'll come tomorrow."

Dr. Hafner gave Dad the phone, and I explained the procedure to him. I assured him he would stay in the hospital only overnight. Marisa promised that she would not leave his side, and I agreed to call them at the hospital in a few hours.

"She's a tough one, that daughter of his. Very stubborn," Dr. Hafner commented to Marisa when he got off the phone.

I went to the Getty Center to pack. A fax was waiting for me there from the head nurse on Dad's floor, asking me to call her about an affidavit. Because Dad had a living will (which Dr. Hafner did mention to her) and did not have the capacity to make medical decisions, she wanted me to notarize the affidavit, stating clearly what life-prolonging procedures I might wish to withhold, and return it immediately.

"Is this really necessary?" I asked when I called. "My father is only going to be on the floor twenty-four hours for intravenous feeding."

"Yes," she said. "There should be a Coral Bay form."

"How strange. During all the months my mother was hospitalized, I was never asked to sign an affidavit, even when she was unconscious in the intensive-care unit at Sacred Heart," I pointed out.

"Maybe your mother didn't have a living will," the nurse said.

"Of course she did. But I doubt that her living will ever followed her into the hospital."

I signed the proxy, permitting only continued hydration, the reason for Dad's hospitalization, and requesting that ventilation, dialysis, and artificial resuscitation be withheld. Although I was convinced that preventing these heroic measures was right, marking them negatively, one by one, was difficult. I then went to a bank to have the form notarized and faxed it back to Coral Bay. I was impressed that the hospital was taking the matter seriously, and I felt relieved that Dad would not be subjected to unwanted procedures that might merely prolong his death.

Dr. Hafner's voice boomed over the telephone early the next morning, "Luisa, your father was dehydrated, severely dehydrated," he said, with relief. "He's much better—revived, more alert. I'm sending him home and will take him off the diuretic for a few days. Have Marisa call me if there's the smallest change. There is no subdural hematoma; the CT scans were normal. Now, another matter: What are you going to do about your father? He's going to need more care. Why don't you think about taking him home with you?"

I appreciated Dr. Hafner's call. He knew I was upset about handling this from so far away, and I had to admit that he was genuinely concerned about Dad. He had shown the same qualities with Mother. He had a knack for looking at the whole patient;

he also had a comforting manner and was considerate of the patient's family.

"Believe me," I answered, "I think about that all the time. I know my dad wants to stay at home, and I'll evaluate the situation when I see him. Either I'll shuttle back and forth between Caracas and Pompano Beach or I'll take him home with me."

"Fine, call me as soon as you get in, and by the way, I was very impressed with Marisa. She was level-headed and is obviously very devoted to your father. You're lucky to have her."

I was on the phone constantly over the next few hours. I called the home-health-care agency that had worked so well when Mother came home. Next I spoke with Kathy, who had been notified of the situation by Marisa and promised to coordinate the agency's schedule. I wanted aides with him every second. Marisa would balk, but she was exhausted. Kathy also commented that Dad's color was good; he was very alert, and he insisted on sleeping on the living-room couch when he got home. Actually, from the moment the hydration began to revive him, Dad had wanted to dress and go home. "I have no business being in the hospital," he told Marisa while she persuaded him to wait for Dr. Hafner.

Kathy was at the house when Sandra, the home-health-care nurse, arrived to do an evaluation, and she and Sandra updated me every few hours. "Your father is very gentlemanly," Sandra said over the phone. "We had a nice conversation, and he told me about his childhood and his work. He's very tired right now, but I want to assure you that he's fine. His vital signs are good, and his lungs are clear. I want you to know that I'll be checking on him every day and will monitor the aides. We'll take good care of him in the next few days." Sandra could not have been more compassionate.

Dr. Adler, Dad's neurologist, was not so kind. In fact, he was brutally blunt. "Your father has a cerebral disorder, a type of dementia," he said. "Fortunately, the CT scan showed that a subdural hematoma did not occur when he fell. But he was severely dehydrated and had enormous fluid and electrolyte imbalances that could only be corrected by hydration. I want to emphasize that your father went through his reserve, and that's why he's having increasing problems with balance and gait. The loss of brain cells is affecting his motor functions."

"Surely there's something we can do," I said.

"You're already doing it," he continued. "You're giving your father supportive care. I'm going to be honest with you. This is the end play for him. Just try to make him as comfortable as possible."

What more was there to say? I thanked Dr. Adler for speaking clearly even as I resented the crassness with which he had delivered the prognosis. Neurological forces were assaulting Dad's mind and body that did not make much sense to me. His CT scan had not shown abnormalities. His body was failing him—going haywire. Is this what Adler meant by "end play"?

Or was Dad simply dying of "old age"? Although old age is not a disease, the older we grow, the less resistance we have to a number of diseases. Nuland notes that he "never had the temerity to write 'Old Age' on a death certificate, knowing that the form would be returned . . . with a terse note from some official record-keeper" (1994:43). Many in my parents' generation called the process "nature taking its course"; Nuland calls it "as insoluble as it is inevitable." But it is not politically correct to say someone has died of old age, he notes, to admit that life "simply sputters out."

Dad was giving up without protest. He sat for hours in his favorite chair, lost in inner reverie, and had to be prodded to open his eyes. He still enjoyed meals but appeared to have no interest in the external world. In fact, he seemed to have let go of his own hold on life ten months earlier, when Mother left him. "Now we have a whole new ballgame," he said. "I have only my memories. That's all I have—the past—because I have no future; only death." What was there to live for except continued grief and unwanted solitude? I knew I could no longer motivate him. The time comes when even a devoted daughter cannot will a parent to stay alive.

• • •

For months I put off writing about Dad. There were no traumatic upheavals; no prolonged suffering, as with Mother. Yet Dad's calm departure was infinitely sorrowful. It marked the end not only of his physical existence but also of a devoted relationship that had defined my childhood and the kind of adult I would become. My family of procreation as my brother and I had known it was now gone. Dad scarcely slept the last night of his life. He was up several times to go to the bathroom; he told a few stories and finally settled down for a few hours of rest. He was napping peacefully when his breathing suddenly grew rapid and labored. Dad's aide ran to get Marisa, who had been sleeping in the next room and rushed in to embrace him. Dad glanced at Marisa, gave a deep sigh, and took his last breath.

I knew that my father had experienced a natural death, that it was his time. The paramedics who came to the house early that morning, however, refused to see it that way. In a panic, Marisa had dialed 911, and the paramedics appeared with all their technological paraphernalia. They were going to try to resuscitate Dad, even though it was apparent that he had already died. "No!" Marisa shouted at them. "Mr. Margolies has a living will that says he does not wish to be resuscitated." She retrieved the yellow folder from Dad's desk, ran back to the bedroom, and waved it under their noses.

They finally ceased their preparations to revive Dad, covered him with his blanket, and went to the living room to wait for the police. Marisa called Kathy, then returned to the bedroom to uncover Dad. Kathy arrived and took charge. She hugged Marisa, who had just witnessed death for the first time, and together they waited for the police. When two policemen arrived, Kathy called Dr. Hafner, who confirmed the cause of death over the phone. The paramedics could not leave until the police arrived.

"Why the police?" I asked Marisa on the phone.

"They had to certify that Mr. Albert died of natural causes."

I was sad that Marisa had not been able to spend a few quiet moments alone with Dad, as I had done with Mother. Paramedics, the police, Kathy, the doctor, phone calls back and forth—it was a jarring experience that allowed little time to come to terms with the poignant ending of a human life.

"You know, we all have to die sometime," Dr. Hafner said to comfort me. "I don't want you to feel guilty. You did everything you could to care for your father. We don't always have to look for a cause. I'm not sure I know the cause myself—a stroke, a heart attack, maybe—your Dad just petered out. It was his time to go." Yes, I thought, it is best to think about death in terms of its natural biological course. Dad had had a good death, a natural death, a death without impediments, a gentle death in his own bed, in his own home.

Dr. Risden called right away. "I want you to know how truly sorry I was to hear about your dad," he said, "and, of course, your mom. They were among the nicest people I ever knew. I can't say that about all of my patients, but I was especially fond of your parents. I'm grateful to have had the chance to treat such lovely people."

The year's mourning period for Mother had not yet concluded. Making the arrangements for Dad was eerily familiar and somewhat easier. But it was also far more sorrowful. When Mother died, I still had Dad, and caring for him kept me occupied. Now, the finality of the double loss forced me to acknowledge that my life as a daughter was over.

The rabbi intoned:

> For everything there is a season, yet whenever parting comes, it comes too soon. Death is a destination at which we arrive stage by stage in a sacred pilgrimage from birth to death. Death is not the enemy of life but its friend. Knowing our years are limited makes them ever more precious. Night is coming. It's time to come home; you're tired. Lie down at last in the quiet nursery of nature and go to sleep.
>
> The children who have witnessed the relentless decline of their parents with such sadness and discord finally concur when paying tribute to the memory of their father. We were fortunate to have had a good and kind father who took care of our mother and took care of us. But of more importance, they provided structure for their children by taking care of each other. Their loyal companionship enabled them to confront life's vicissitudes and surprises. They depended on each other and needed to be together. Perhaps it is fitting that their earthly separation was so abbreviated. Now we'll pray, but later we'll remember to tell our own children about the moral legacy their grandparents left us. Amen.

EPILOGUE

En Route

I do feel that life will not be long,
And yet I'm filled with melodies and song,
I go along so smooth and serene,
What is my life, but an incomplete dream?
My days are filled with plans and schemes,
That shine on me with full-ray beams.
I look to heaven—to be informed,
But it will not say—how long, how long.
   —June A. Margolies

"WHAT IS IT, after all, to die?" asked Nanda in Antonia White's *Frost in May*, the moving story of a young girl's experiences at a Catholic boarding school. Mother had marked the passage describing Nanda's impressions upon the death of her favorite nun, Mother Francis:

> It is to say good-bye to everything in this world—to fortune, pleasures, friends—a sad irrevocable good-bye. It is to leave your home forever and to be thrown into a narrow pit with no clothes but a shroud and no society but reptiles and worms. It is to pass in the twinkling of an eye to the unknown region called eternity, where you will hear from the mouth of God Himself in what place you are to make that great retreat that lasts forever.... Think of your friends who have gone before you.... From the grave they cry out to you: "Yesterday for me and today for thee." Ever since the day of your birth you have been dying: every hour of play or study brings you a little nearer the end of your life. (White 1933:100)

Watching my mother die over five months was lonely, terrifying, and seemingly endless. Even when I realized she could not last much longer, I held out hope. When Dad followed ten months later, I was not surprised. It was fitting they were together. We were appalled at what they had been through—Mother's fruitless suffering and my father's rapid decline while he watched his wife and waited helplessly. My uncle swore that none of this would happen to him, and true to his word, he passed away less than twenty-four hours after suffering a major stroke. Other family members, still in their prime, whispered, "Please, don't ever let this happen to me." The specter of fighting so hard to regain one's health and yet not being able to win the battle was something to be avoided at all costs.

I did not do what a lot of newly bereaved people do. I did not read any how-to books about grieving; I did not blame the doctors; and I did not want to settle any accounts. I accepted my parents' deaths. But I was also obsessed with them. I did a lot of sitting and not much talking. I brooded, too exhausted to talk to anyone who was not aware of my situation. I had no desire to participate in professional activities and burst into tears at unexpected, but always private, moments.

Our society is not sensitive to the loss of an elderly parent. When we lose a child, others understand that it is one of the most tragic events that can occur. When we lose a spouse, we are expected to grieve for a long time. When a child loses a parent, it is devastating, but an adult's loss of an elderly parent is considered entirely normal, well within the usual turn of life's events. This does not temper the adult child's emotional response when it actually occurs. Others might be surprised at the depth of sadness that can follow when one loses an elderly parent. The adult child may continue to assess the meaning of the parent–child relationship and the quality of the tie long after the parent's death. Anthropologists at the Plisher Research Center in Philadelphia have concluded that a parent's death represents not only a significant loss but also a life-course transition (Rubinstein 1995). The parent's death may bring about important shifts in emotions and social interactions that have a tremendous impact on the life of the surviving adult child.

Adult children are not supposed to complain, or even grieve for very long. The death is "fitting," and support is missing. There are no comments about "not dying in vain." Instead, the reaction all too frequently is, "Well, she lived her life," or "It was all for the best," or "He's better off this way." Many people feel awkward about mentioning the parent's death to the grief-stricken child. Only other grieving adult children and their parents' contemporaries understand the loss and are willing to talk about it.

Even though the death movement took off more than thirty years ago with the publication of Elisabeth Kübler-Ross's *On Death and Dying* (1969), and gained considerable momentum with the publication of Sherwin Nuland's *How We Die: Reflections on Life's Final Chapter* (1994), the subject of a parent's death is still taboo, because it forces us to focus on aspects of aging that are not pleasant and foists into our consciousness the realization that life's stages are preordained.

When a parent dies after a traumatic illness that caused prolonged pain and suffering, the sadness is redoubled. Who can bear to watch the mother or father we have had by our sides all our lives fall apart, knowing that there is not much we can do except offer comfort and support? When it is over, we engage in emotional postmortems, asking whether we did the right thing. No matter what we did or how we acted, we think, it probably would have been better to have done the opposite.

Instead of fading, my sense of loss grew stronger over time. Things were happening in the world and in my life I could not share with my parents, sentiments I could no longer express. I was the one who paused while the world continued. People went about their usual business, yet nothing seemed normal to me. I felt acutely alone. My mind may have tricked me into thinking that I saw my father sitting in his favorite chair or that my mother came to me in a vision, but I knew that my parents had gone on a voyage of no return. I doubted that I would regain my old exuberance or enjoy my life again.

Then came the reckoning. Every death involves a tremendous amount of paperwork, but a parent's death requires the breaking up of a household and the systematic divestment of cherished belongings. Many children dismantle their parents' homes virtually overnight. They are often sorry afterward. Others savor each speck of writing and take months to review their parents' affairs. From such slow and thorough reviews come the many memoirs on aging parents and their passing written by adult children who are simply not ready to surrender the relationship. They commit to paper the sentiments and memories that remain, an act that helps them come to terms with their loss. I had hundreds of my mother's unpublished poems, diaries, and scattered writings;

I also had my parents' love letters and volumes of their corre-spondence with me.

Only after my mother died did I discover the cache of poems she had written about love and life. To my surprise, she had not given them much importance compared with her children's verses, written later. She never spoke of her early poems nor brought them out to show me, although we talked about the children's poems all the time. When Mother died, a wonderful rabbi named Karen Kedar officiated at her service. She came to my parents' home, conversed with my father, and spent the rest of the afternoon reminiscing with us about Mother and the extraordinary relationship my parents had enjoyed. She was calm and unhurried as we looked at family photographs. "You know," I said, "perhaps I can go through my mother's poetry and read one of her poems at the service tomorrow." Surely I would find something appropriate among the children's verses. Instead, I found a thick folio with hundreds of unfamiliar poems written in Mother's beautiful cursive script. In the days following her service, I read through her love poems and her life poems many times. They helped me through the early months of her absence. They helped me remember the woman my mother was before she fell and broke her hips, and they helped me understand the woman who faced the twilight of her life with such tenacious courage.

In addition, I had Mother's medical records—526 pages of them, to be exact—to document the last 147 days of her life in seven different medical facilities. I felt that they would provide the answers to what had gone wrong. I questioned the medical records as if they were living anthropological informants and carted them back and forth with me, each one neatly stacked in its own col-ored folder. I used my mother's medical records as primary research documents in piecing together the story of why she had died from a broken hip when she had access to the best medical treatment in the world. Only then was I was finally able to appre-ciate many of the nuances that had not been apparent to me while I was caring for her.

If I learned anything from the records, it was that despite the odds, the outcome could have been different. The answer was really rather mundane. Each complication, although it had been brought about by the original hip fractures, was treated as a separate medical episode. No one person oversaw the general picture or coordinated the general treatment plan. No key figure emerged who could assume responsibility for coordinating my mother's treatment and monitoring her progress. The original goal—to regain her mobility and independence—was pushed to the background as one crisis followed another. As it turned out, my mother's chronic condition was of pivotal importance in the final outcome. It compromised her health along the way and transformed what might have been an uneventful recovery into a series of acute medical crises.

Some of the medical personnel involved in Mother's ongoing crises were unaware of either her hip fractures or her underlying condition. No general picture, no holistic vision existed, of who she was and how her treatment should be managed. Most physicians do not follow their patients into nursing facilities; nor do the medical histories. Each time my mother changed facilities, she started all over again with a new attending physician and a fresh medical history. The ethicist Eric Cassell's caveat that the therapeutic value of current hospital medicine is largely untapped is timely: "It is unfortunately common for a patient to become caught up in a parade of tests, treatments, and subspecialists with no physician clearly responsible for the whole problem; on occasion the patient is cared for by a 'team' and cannot figure out the politics of responsibility and leadership—with the result that despite so many caregivers, the patient may be essentially alone at critical junctures" (1991:69).

In the absence of proper management, errors are made and oversights occur. They are not intentional. Many oversights go undetected because the patient is too ill to articulate his or her concerns or a family caregiver-advocate is not present. The best orthopedic surgeon, the best cardiologist, the best internist—all are helpless, despite their best intentions, to treat patients successfully without appropriate management. A comprehensive approach is imperative: The special needs of each patient should be addressed by a medical team that follows him or her through the recuperation period and is watching for emerging problems before they become unsolvable.

If only I had known then what I know now. It took several years of researching hip fractures for me to realize that my concerns about Mother's medical treatment were common—so much so that the American Academy of Orthopaedic Surgeons organized a consensus conference in 2001 on improving the care of hip-fracture patients. The participants concluded that hip-fracture recovery is a slow process that often takes more than a year. Hip-fracture patients are exposed to a variety of health-care providers and are frequently moved from facility to facility. The care is so fragmented that the patient's primary physician may not even know about the hip fracture. "This lack of continuity can result in inadequate or inappropriate care," conclude the experts, "as different providers work in a vacuum, without the benefit of shared expertise" (National Consensus Conference 2002:671). Patients simply cannot be rushed through the system in shortsighted attempts to cut costs. The lack of coordination is a serious problem that compromises the patient's final outcome.

My mother's hip is scarcely unique. The same fate looms for many Americans who reach the end of life's journey as members of the growing population of frail elderly. Future elder boomers will not escape the age-related diseases that are the wave of the twenty-first century. The drama of degenerative diseases, with their seesaw patterns of ups and downs, demands that high technology take a back seat, that physicians practice the "art" of caring, and that family caregivers learn to give generously of their resources. Providing decent care is a worthy goal we must collectively bear in mind if we are to treat the elderly the way we will want to be treated when it is our turn.

Most of us are novices at the complicated task of caring for an ailing parent. We each have to start from scratch as we embark on a difficult voyage—one of navigating through a complicated health-care system whose ethos has not yet caught up with the changing needs of an aging society. If I had known what I later learned through hands-on care, I might have been a more empowered caregiver who could have cushioned her mother from some of the indignities that overtook her as her health failed.

I can offer the following modest note to those initiating private journeys of their own through the medical labyrinth of eldercare:

Do your best. Unfortunately, our health-care system has made few provisions for long-term care, and caregivers will be forced to make countless decisions that are rarely clear-cut. Accept the system's imperfections and shortcomings as you do your best to comfort a failing parent who has you to depend on. Avoid sibling dissension at all costs, because you, the principal caregiver, feel frustrated and angry. When nature finally prevails and takes away the loving parent who held the family together, the nasty residue of conflict will linger precisely when you need a sibling to support you and share the pain.

I did not recognize the nature of my own lessons until I exchanged viewpoints with others who had had similar experiences. There are no easy formulas, and few guidelines exist to help us become competent caregivers. But by valuing our best efforts, we can eventually come to terms with the loss we tried so hard to prevent.

I have laid bare my mother's medical history because there is a story to be told and there are lessons to be learned. For many months, I relived my mother's fall and tried to understand what went on thereafter. My intense involvement is over now. The story is told; the lessons are imparted. That is all that remains. I think about my parents, sustained by my memories, and accept the finality of their passing.

References

Abel, Emily K. 1991. Who Cares for the Elderly? Public Policy and the Experiences of Adult Daughters. Philadelphia: Temple University Press.

Advance Directives Save Medicare Dollars (Briefs). 1994. Ageing International 21(2):9.

Agich, George J. 1993. Autonomy and Long-Term Care. New York: Oxford University Press.

Aharonoff, Gina B., Michael G. Dennis, Ashgan Elshinawy, Joseph D. Zuckerman, and Kenneth J. Koval. 1998. Circumstances of Falls Causing Hip Fractures in the Elderly. Symposium: Update on Fractures of the Hip. Clinical Orthopaedics and Related Research 348:10–14.

Allende, Isabel. 1994. Paula. New York: HarperCollins Publishers.

American Heart Association. 1980. Heartbook: A Guide to Prevention and Treatment of Cardiovascular Diseases. New York: E. P. Dutton.

America's Bone Health: The State of Osteoporosis and Low Bone Mass in Our Nation. 2002. Washington, D.C.: National Osteoporosis Foundation.

Aronovitz, Leslie G. 2002. Nursing Homes: Many Shortcomings Exist in Efforts to Protect Residents from Abuse. Testimony before the Special Committee on Aging, U.S. Senate. Washington, D.C.: United States General Accounting Office (GAO).

Avorn, Jerome L. 1986. The Life and Death of Oliver Shay. In Our Aging Society: Paradox and Promise. Pifer, Alan, and Lydia Bronte, eds. Pp. 283–297. New York: W. W. Norton.

Báez, Gustavo. 1997. Un último encuentro con Darcy Ribeiro. La Brújula, El Universal (Caracas), March 21–April 3, 62:5.

Basta, Lofty L., with Carole Post. 1996. A Graceful Exit: Life and Death on Your Own Terms. New York: Plenum Press.

Battin, Margaret Pabst. 1994. The Least Worst Death: Essays in Bioethics on the End of Life. New York: Oxford University Press.

Beck, Melinda. 1994. A Lesson in Dying Well. Newsweek, May 16:58.

Behar, Ruth. 1991. Death and Memory: From Santa María Monte to Miami Beach. Cultural Anthropology 6(3):346–384.

Blasszauer, Bela. 1994. Institutional Care of the Elderly. Hastings Center Report 24(5):14–17.

Bortz, Walter M., II. 1991. We Live Too Short and Die Too Long. New York: Bantam Books.

———. 1993. The Physics of Frailty. Journal of the American Geriatrics Society 41(9):1004–1008.

Brakman, Sarah-Vaughan. 1994. Adult Daughter Caregivers. Symposium. Caring for an Aging World: Allocating Scarce Resources. Hastings Center Report 24(5):26–28.

Brody, Elaine M. 1981. "Women in the Middle" and Family Help to Older People. Gerontologist 21(5):471–480.

Brody, Elaine M., Christine Hoffman, Morton H. Kleban, and Claire B. Schoonover. 1989. Caregiving Daughters and Their Local Siblings: Perceptions, Strains, and Interactions. Gerontologist 29(4):529–538.

Brody, Jane E. 1999. Falls by Elderly, a Perilous yet Preventable Epidemic. New York Times, June 8:F7.

Bronte, Lydia. 1993. The Longevity Factor: The New Reality of Long Careers and How It Can Lead to Richer Lives. New York: Harper Perennial.

Burgio, Kathryn L., K. Lynette Pearce, and Angelo J. Lucco. 1989. Staying Dry: A Practical Guide to Bladder Control. Baltimore: Johns Hopkins University Press.

Butler, Robert N. 1975. Why Survive? Being Old in America. New York: Harper and Row.

California Nursing Homes. Federal and State Oversight Inadequate to Protect Residents in Homes with Serious Care Violations. 1998. Testimony before the Special Committee on Aging, U.S. Senate. Washington, D.C.: United States General Accounting Office (GAO).

Callahan, Daniel. 1987. Setting Limits: Medical Goals in an Aging Society. Washington, D.C.: Georgetown University Press.

———. 1993. The Troubled Dream of Life: Living with Mortality. New York: Simon and Schuster.

Carlson, Margaret. 1995. Back to the Dark Ages. Time, October 30:63.

Carson, Ronald A. 1994. Clarifying the Issues of Active Euthanasia. Paper presented at the American Gerontological Association, Los Angeles.

Cassell, Eric J. 1991. The Nature of Suffering and the Goals of Medicine. New York: Oxford University Press.

Charmaz, Kathy. 1991. Good Days, Bad Days: The Self in Chronic Illness and Time. New Brunswick, N.J.: Rutgers University Press.

Cousins, Norman. 1979. Anatomy of an Illness as Perceived by the Patient: Reflections on Healing and Regeneration. New York: W. W. Norton.

———. 1983. The Healing Heart: Antidotes to Panic and Helplessness. New York: Avon Books.

Cowley, Geoffrey. 1994. Too Much of a Good Thing. Newsweek, March 28: 50–51.

Cummings, Steven R., D. M. Black, M. C. Nevitt, W. Browner, J. Cauley, K. Ensrud, H. K. Genant, L. Palermo, J. Scott, and T. M. Vogt. 1993. Bone Density at Various Sites for Prediction of Hip Fractures: The Study of Osteoporotic Fractures Research Group. Lancet 341:72–75.

Daniel, John. 1996. Looking After: A Son's Memoir. Washington, D.C.: Counterpoint.

Daniels, Norman. 1988. Am I My Parents' Keeper? An Essay on Justice Between the Young and the Old. New York: Oxford University Press.

Dargent-Molina, P., F. Favier, H. Grandjean, C. Baudoin, A. M. Schott, E. Hausherr, P. J. Meunier, and G. Bréart. 1996. Fall-Related Factors and Risk of Hip Fractures: The EPIDOS Prospective Study. Epidemiologie de l'Osteoporose. Lancet 348(9021):145–149.

De Beauvoir, Simone. 1964. A Very Easy Death. New York: Warner Books.

Diamond, Timothy. 1992. Making Gray Gold: Narratives of Nursing Home Care. Chicago: University of Chicago Press.

Difficult Dialogues Program. 2002. Aging in the 21st Century. Consensus Report. Stanford: Stanford University, Institute for Research on Women and Gender.

Dubler, Nancy, and David Nimmons. 1992. Ethics on Call: Taking Charge of Life-and-Death Choices in Today's Health Care System. New York: Vintage Books.

Emanuel, Ezekiel J. 1991. The Ends of Human Life: Medical Ethics in a Liberal Polity. Cambridge, Mass.: Harvard University Press.

Ervin, Mike. 1994. Muzzled in a Nursing Home, the Spirit Is Extinguished. Los Angeles Times, May 6:B7.

Ettinger, Bruce, and Deborah Grady. 1993. The Waning Effect of Postmenopausal Estrogen Therapy on Osteoporosis. New England Journal of Medicine 329(16):1192–1193.

Family Caregiving in the U.S.: Findings from a National Survey. Final Report. 1997. Washington, D.C.: National Alliance for Caregiving and American Association of Retired Persons (AARP).

Foner, Nancy. 1994. The Caregiving Dilemma: Work in an American Nursing Home. Berkeley: University of California Press.

Frassetto, Lynda A., Karen M. Todd, R. Curtis Morris, Jr., and Anthony Sebastian. 2000. Worldwide Incidence of Hip Fracture in Elderly Women: Relation to Consumption of Animal and Vegetable Foods. Journal of Gerontology: Medical Sciences 55A(10):M585–M592.

Friedan, Betty. 1993. The Fountain of Age. New York: Simon and Schuster.

Geary, Leslie Haggin. 2001. Close to Home. Money, July:98–103.

Gillick, Muriel R. 1994. Choosing Medical Care in Old Age: What Kind, How Much, When to Stop. Cambridge, Mass.: Harvard University Press.

———. 2001. Lifelines: Living Longer, Growing Frail, Taking Heart. New York: W. W. Norton.

Gilpin, Kenneth N. 1994. Vital Signs Improve for the Nursing Home Industry. New York Times, February 7:5.

Goldstein, Andrew. 2001. Better than a Nursing Home? Time, August 13: 48–53.

Grady, Deborah. 2003. Postmenopausal Hormones—Therapy for Symptoms Only. New England Journal of Medicine 348(19):1–3.

Grodstein, Francine, Thomas B. Clarkson, and Joann E. Manson. 2003. Understanding the Divergent Data on Postmenopausal Hormone Therapy. New England Journal of Medicine 348(7):645–650.

Groopman, Jerome. 1997. The Measure of Our Days: New Beginnings at Life's End. New York: Viking.

Guberman, N., P. Maheu, and C. Maille. 1992. Women as Family Caregivers: Why Do They Care? Gerontologist 32(5):607–617.

Gubrium, Jaber F. 1993. Speaking of Life: Horizons of Meaning for Nursing Home Residents. New York: Aldine de Gruyter.

Gunderman, Richard B. 2002. Is Suffering the Enemy? Hastings Center Report 32(2):40–44.

Hardwig, John. 2000. Spiritual Issues at the End of Life: A Call for Discussion. Hastings Center Report 30(2):28–30.

Harper, Cristine. 1997. Overview of Osteoporosis (Shedding New Light on Osteoporosis and Fall Prevention). Paper presented at the 43rd Annual Meeting of the American Society on Aging, Nashville, Tenn.

Harrington, Charlene. 2001. Does Investor Ownership of Nursing Homes Compromise the Quality of Care? American Journal of Public Health 91(9):1452–1455.

Hayflick, Leonard. 1994. How and Why We Age. New York: Ballantine Books.

Heat Wave Spawns Landmark Settlement against Sun. 2001. Long-Term Care Report 3(18):141.

Henry, Jules. 1963. Human Obsolescence. In Culture Against Man. Pp. 391–474. New York: Random House.

Hinton, Richard Y., Dennis W. Lennox, Frank R. Ebert, Steven J. Jacobsen, and Gordon S. Smith. 1995. Relative Rates of Fracture of the Hip in the United States. Journal of Bone and Joint Surgery 77-A(5):695–701.

Hirschler, Ben. 1993. The Start of a New Era. Daily Journal (Caracas), October 3:6.

Hooyman, Nancy R., and Wendy Lustbader. 1986. Taking Care of Your Aging Family Members: A Practical Guide. New York: The Free Press.

Horowitz, Amy. 1985. Family Caregiving to the Frail Elderly. In Annual Review of Gerontology and Geriatrics. Pp. 194–246. New York: Springer Publishing.

Illich, Ivan. 1976. Medical Nemesis: The Expropriation of Health. New York: Pantheon Books.

Jacobsen, Steven J., Jack Goldberg, Toni P. Miles, Jacob A. Brody, William Stiers, and Alfred A. Rimm. 1990. Regional Variation in the Incidence of Hip Fracture: U.S. White Women Aged 65 Years and Older. Journal of the American Medical Association (JAMA) 264(4):500–502.

Jennett, Bryan. 1994. Treatment of Critical Illness in the Elderly. Hastings Center Report 24(5):21–22.

Jorm, A. F., A. S. Henderson, R. Scott, A. E. Korten, H. Cristensen, and A. J. MacKinnon. 1995. Factors Associated with the Wish to Die in Elderly People. Age and Ageing 24:389–392.

Kane, Rosalie A. 1995–1996. Transforming Care Institutions for the Frail Elderly: Out of One Shall Be Many. Generations 19(4):62–68.

Kannus, Pekka, Jari Parkkari, Seppo Niemi, Matti Pasanen, Mika Palvanen, Markku Jarvinen, and Ilkka Vuori. 2000. Prevention of Hip Fractures in

Elderly People with Use of a Hip Protector. New England Journal of Medicine 343(21):1506–1513.

Kaye Abraham, Laurie. 1994. Mama Might Be Better Off Dead: The Failure of Health Care in Urban America. New York: Harper and Row.

Kayser-Jones, Jeanie. 1995. Decision Making in the Treatment of Acute Illness in Nursing Homes: Framing the Decision Problem, Treatment Plan and Outcome. Medical Anthropology Quarterly 9(2):236–256.

Kayser-Jones, Jeanie, and Marshall B. Kapp. 1989. Advocacy for the Mentally Impaired Elderly: A Case Study Analysis. American Journal of Law and Medicine 14(4):353–376.

Kidder, Tracy. 1993. Old Friends. Boston: Houghton Mifflin.

Koch, Tom. 1990. Mirrored Lives: Aging Children and Elderly Parents. Westport, Conn.: Praeger.

———. 1993. A Place in Time: Care Givers for Their Elderly. Westport, Conn.: Praeger.

Koenig, Ronald. 1980. Dying vs. Well-Being. In Caring Relationships: The Dying and the Bereaved. Kalish, Richard A., ed. Pp. 9–22. Farmingdale, N.Y.: Baywood Publishing.

Konner, Melvin. 1987. Becoming a Doctor: A Journey of Initiation in Medical School. New York: Viking.

Kübler-Ross, Elisabeth. 1969. On Death and Dying. New York: Macmillan.

Lane, Diane C. 2001. Money Ills Haunt Nursing Homes. Special Report: Part 2 of 4. Sun-Sentinel, Fort Lauderdale, March 5:1A, 14A.

Laughlin, Meg. 1993. Pat Doesn't Live Here Anymore. Tropic, Miami Herald, September 12:6–21.

Levine, Carol. 2000. The Loneliness of the Long-Term Care Giver. In Always on Call: When Illness Turns Families into Caregivers. Levine, Carol, ed. Pp. 71–80. New York: United Hospital Fund of New York.

Lewin, Tamar. 1996. Ignoring 'Right to Die' Directives, Medical Community Is Being Sued. New York Times, June 2:1, 14.

Lukert, Barbara, and Lawrence G. Raisz. 1990. Glucocorticoid-Induced Osteoporosis: Pathogenesis and Management. Annals of Internal Medicine 112(5):352–364.

Mace, Nancy L., and Peter V. Rabins. 1981. The 36-Hour Day: A Family Guide to Caring for Persons with Alzheimer's Disease, Related Dementing Illnesses, and Memory Loss in Later Life. Baltimore: Johns Hopkins University Press.

Martin, Richard J., and Stephen G. Post. 1992. Human Dignity, Dementia and the Moral Basis of Caregiving. In Dementia and Aging: Ethics, Values and Policy Choices. Binstock, Robert H., Stephen G. Post, and Peter J. Whitehouse, eds. Pp. 55–68. Baltimore: Johns Hopkins University Press.

Mauss, Marcel. 1954. The Gift. London: Cohen and West.

Melton, L. Joseph, III. 1993. Hip Fractures: A Worldwide Problem Today and Tomorrow. Special Issue. Hip Fracture and the Medos Study. Bone 14, Supplement 1(7):S1–S8.

Miller, Charles W. 1978. Survival and Ambulation following Hip Fracture. Journal of Bone and Joint Surgery 60-A(7):930–934.

Mitchell, Peter. 1996. Nursing Homes Get U.S. Action on Complaints. Wall Street Journal, March 13:F1, F4.

Moller, David Wendall. 1990. On Death without Dignity: The Human Impact of Technological Dying. Amityville, N.Y.: Baywood Publishing.

Moody, Harry R. 1992. A Critical View of Ethical Dilemmas in Dementia. In Dementia and Aging: Ethics, Values and Policy Choices. Binstock, Robert H., Stephen G. Post, and Peter J. Whitehouse, eds. Pp. 86–106. Baltimore: Johns Hopkins University Press.

Moody, Raymond A., Jr. 1975. Life after Life: The Investigation of a Phenomenon—Survival of Bodily Death. New York: Bantam Books.

Morse, Melvin, with Paul Perry. 1994. Parting Visions: Uses and Meanings of Pre-Death, Psychic, and Spiritual Experiences. New York: Villard Books.

Murphy, Robert F. 1987. The Body Silent. New York: Henry Holt.

Mutran, Elizabeth J., Donald C. Reitzes, Jana Mossey, and Maria Erlinda Fernández. 1995. Social Support, Depression, and Recovery of Walking Ability following Hip Fracture Surgery. Journal of Gerontology: Social Sciences 50B(6):S354–S361.

Nash, Mary Louise. 1980. Dignity of Persons in the Final Phase of Life: An Exploratory Study. In Caring Relationships: The Dying and the Bereaved. Kalish, Richard A., ed. Pp. 62–70. Farmingdale, N.Y.: Baywood Publishing.

National Consensus Conference on Improving the Continuum of Care for Patients with Hip Fracture. 2002. Journal of Bone and Joint Surgery 84-A(4):670–674.

New Century Dictionary of the English Language. 1946. New York: D. Appleton-Century.

Nordheimer, Jon. 1996. A Mature Housing Market: Growing Business of Not-Quite-Nursing-Home Care. New York Times, April 10:C1, C3.

Nuland, Sherwin B. 1994. How We Die: Reflections on Life's Final Chapter. New York: Alfred A. Knopf.

Olivier, Laurence. 1982. Confessions of an Actor: An Autobiography. New York: Simon and Schuster.

Olson, Laura Katz. 1993. The Political Economy of Productive Aging: Long-Term Care. In Achieving a Productive Aging Society. Bass, Scott A., Francis G. Caro, and Yung-Ping Chen, eds. Pp. 167–185. Westport, Conn.: Auburn House.

Ouslander, Joseph G. 1998. The American Nursing Home. In Brocklehurst's Textbook of Geriatric Medicine and Gerontology. Fifth Edition. Tallis, Raymond, Howard Fillit, and J. C. Brocklehurst, eds. Pp. 1559–1565. London: Churchill Livingstone.

Paradis, Norman. 1994. Making a Living Off the Dying. New York Times, June 12:4HR.

Parker, Martyn J., and Christopher R. Palmer. 1995. Prediction of Rehabilitation after Hip Fracture. Age and Ageing 24:96–98.

Pear, Robert. 2000. U.S. Recommending Strict New Rules at Nursing Homes. New York Times, July 23:1, 15.

Percy, Charles H. 1974. Growing Old in the Country of the Young. New York: McGraw-Hill.

Polich, Cynthia, Marcie Parker, Margaret Hottinger, and Deborah Chase. 1993. Managing Health Care for the Elderly. New York: John Wiley and Sons.

Post, Stephen G. 1991. Justice for Elderly People in Jewish and Christian Thought. In Too Old for Health Care? Controversies in Medicine, Law, Economics and Ethics. Binstock, Robert H., and Stephen G. Post, eds. Pp. 120–137. Baltimore: Johns Hopkins University Press.

Quill, Timothy E. 1993. Death and Dignity: Making Choices and Taking Charge. New York: W. W. Norton.

Regnier, Victor A. 1994. Assisted Living Housing for the Elderly: Design Innovations from the United States and Europe. New York: Van Nostrand Reinhold.

Riley, John W., Jr., and Matilda White Riley. 1994. Beyond Productive Aging: Changing Lives and Social Structure. Ageing International 21(2):15–19.

Rosenfeld, Stephen S. 1977. The Time of Their Dying. New York: W. W. Norton.

Roszak, Theodore. 2001. Longevity Revolution: As Boomers Become Elders. Berkeley: Berkeley Hills Books.

Roth, Philip. 1991. Patrimony: A True Story. New York: Simon and Schuster.

Rowe, John W., and Robert L. Kahn. 1987. Human Aging: Usual and Successful. Science 237(4811):143–149.

Rowles, Graham D. 1994. Evolving Images of Place in Aging and 'Aging in Place.' In Changing Perceptions of Aging and the Aged. Shenk, Dena, and W. Andrew Achenbaum, eds. Pp. 115–125. New York: Springer Publishing.

Rubinstein, Robert L. 1995. Narratives of Elder Parental Death: A Structural and Cultural Analysis. Medical Anthropological Quarterly 9(2):257–276.

Rutman, Deborah. 1996. Caregiving as Women's Work: Women's Experiences of Powerfulness and Powerlessness as Caregivers. Qualitative Health Research 6(1):90–111.

Sankar, Andrea. 1994. Images of Home Death and the Elderly Parent: Romantic versus Real. In Changing Perceptions of Aging and the Aged. Shenk, Dena, and W. Andrew Achenbaum, eds. Pp. 105–114. New York: Springer Publishing.

Sarton, May. 1973. As We Are Now. New York: W. W. Norton.

Seaver, Anna Mae Halgrim. 1994. My World Now: Life in a Nursing Home, from the Inside. Newsweek, June 27:11.

Selzer, Richard. 1993. Raising the Dead. New York: Whittle Books in association with Viking.

Solomon, Caren G., and Robert G. Dluhy. 2003. Rethinking Postmenopausal Hormone Therapy. New England Journal of Medicine 348(7):579–580.

Starkman, Elaine Marcus. 1993. Learning to Sit in Silence: A Journal of Caretaking. Watsonville, Calif.: Papier-Mache Press.

Stini, William. 1995. Osteoporosis in Biocultural Perspective. In Annual Review of Anthropology 24. Pp. 397–421. Palo Alto: Annual Reviews.

Talese, Gay. 1992. Unto the Sons. New York: Alfred A. Knopf.

Tarlow, Barbara. 1996. Caring: A Negotiated Process that Varies. In Caregiving: Readings in Knowledge, Practice, Ethics and Politics. Gordon, Suzanne, Patricia Benner, and Nel Noddings, eds. Pp. 56–82. Philadelphia: University of Pennsylvania Press.

Taylor, Nick. 1994. A Necessary End. New York: Doubleday/Nan A. Talese.

Thomasma, David C. 1991. From Ageism toward Autonomy. In Too Old for Health Care? Controversies in Medicine, Law, Economics and Ethics. Binstock, Robert H., and Stephen G. Post, eds. Pp. 138–163. Baltimore: Johns Hopkins University Press.

Thompson, Mark. 1997. Fatal Neglect. Time, October 27:34–38.

———. 1998. Shining a Light on Abuse. Time, August 3:42–43.

Tinetti, Mary E. 1988. Risk Factors for Falls among Elderly Persons Living in the Community. New England Journal of Medicine 319:1701–1707.

Topinková, Eva. 1994. Care for Elders with Chronic Disease and Disability. Hastings Center Report 24(5):18–20.

Tseng, Brian S., Daniel R. Marsh, Marc T. Hamilton, and Frank W. Booth. 1995. Strength and Aerobic Training Attenuate Muscle Wasting and Improve Resistance to the Development of Disability with Aging. Special Issue. Workshop on Sarcopenia: Muscle Atrophy in Old Age. Journal of Gerontology: Medical Sciences 50A:113–119.

Vesperi, Maria. 1983. The Reluctant Consumer: Nursing Home Residents in the Post-Bergman Era. In Growing Old in Different Societies: Cross-Cultural Perspectives. Sokolovsky, Jay, ed. Pp. 225–237. Belmont, Calif.: Wadsworth Publishing.

Vladeck, Bruce C. 1980. Unloving Care: The Nursing Home Tragedy. New York: Basic Books.

Von Mering, Otto. 1996. American Culture and Long-Term Care. In The Future of Long-Term Care: Social and Policy Issues. Binstock, Robert H., Leighton E. Cluff, and Otto Von Mering, eds. Pp. 252–271. Baltimore: Johns Hopkins University Press.

Weaver, Peter. 2000. Justice Joins Drive on Nursing Homes. AARP Bulletin 41(7):9, 12.

What Do We Owe the Elderly? Allocating Social and Health Care Resources. 1994. Recommendations of a Joint International Research Group of the Institute for Bioethics, Maastricht, The Netherlands and The Hastings Center, Briarcliff Manor, N.Y. Hastings Center Report, Special Supplement 24(2).

When a Parent Needs Care: Ratings of 43 Chains. 1995. In Search of the Right Home. (Part 1) Consumer Reports, August:518–528.

———. 1995. Who Pays for Nursing Homes? (Part 2) Consumer Reports, September:591–597.

———. 1995. Can Your Loved Ones Avoid a Nursing Home? The Promise and the Pitfalls of 'Assisted Living.' (Part 3) Consumer Reports, October: 656–662.

White, Antonia. 1933. Frost in May. New York: Dial Press.

Wicclair, Mark R. 1993. Ethics and the Elderly. New York: Oxford University Press.

Wiener, Joshua M., and Alison Evans Cuellar. 1999. Public and Private Responsibilities: Home- and Community-Based Services in the United Kingdom and Germany. Journal of Aging and Health 11(2):417–444.

Zuckerman, Joseph D. 1989. Health Care Teams Offer Effective Approach to Hip Fracture Treatment. Arthritis Today 3(6):9.

Zuckerman, Joseph D., J. A. McLaughlin, G. B. Aharonoff. and K. Koval. 1993. Hip Fractures in the Elderly: An Interdisciplinary Approach to Management. Facts and Research in Gerontology 7:163–169.

About the Author

LUISA MARGOLIES is Clinical Research Director of the Hip Fracture Research Project of South Florida; she serves as a consultant on aging-in-place as well as on housing, assistive technology, and universal design for the elderly. She also is Director of Ediciones Venezolanas de Antropología in Caracas, Venezuela. For more information, visit www.MyMothersHip.com.